The Maple Tree Behind
The Barbed Wire:
A Story of Survival from the Czestochowa Ghetto

by Jerzy Einhorn

Memoirs

Title in Swedish: Utvald att leva

**Originally Published in Swedish by
Albert Bonniers Förlag, 1996**

Translated by Joan Tate

Published by JewishGen

An Affiliate of the Museum of Jewish Heritage - A Living Memorial to the Holocaust
New York

The Maple Tree Behind The Barbed Wire
A Story of Survival from the Czestochowa Ghetto
by Jerzy Einhorn

Title in Swedish: *Utvald att leva* (Chosen to Live)
Originally Published in Swedish by Albert Bonniers Förlag, 1996

Third Printing: March 2019, Adar II 5779
Second Printing: May 2015, Iyar 5775
First Printing: April 2013, Iyar 5773
Translated by Joan Tate
Editors: Bernard Jacobson and Joel Alpert
Layout: Joel Alpert
Image Editor and Cover Design: Jan R. Fine

Published by JewishGen, Inc.
An Affiliate of the Museum of Jewish Heritage
A Living Memorial to the Holocaust
36 Battery Place, New York, NY 10280

"JewishGen, Inc. is not responsible for inaccuracies or omissions in the original work and makes no representations regarding the accuracy of this translation. Digital images of the original book's contents can be seen online at the New York Public Library Web site."

The mission of the JewishGen organization is to produce a translation of the original work and we cannot verify the accuracy of statements or alter facts cited.

Printed in the United States of America by Lightning Source, Inc.
Library of Congress Control Number (LCCN): 2013938073
ISBN: 978-1-939561-06-0 (hard cover: 346 pages, alk. paper)

... to whoever destroys a life,

it is as if he had had destroyed a whole world;

to whoever saves a life,

it is as if he had saved a whole world.

Mishna, Sanhedrin 4:5

JewishGen and the Yizkor Books in Print Project

This book has been published by the **Yizkor Books in Print Project,** as part of the **Yizkor Book Project** of **JewishGen, Inc**.

JewishGen, Inc. is a non-profit organization founded in 1987 as a resource for Jewish genealogy. Its website [www.jewishgen.org] serves as an international clearinghouse and resource center to assist individuals who are researching the history of their Jewish families and the places where they lived. JewishGen provides databases, facilitates discussion groups, and coordinates projects relating to Jewish genealogy and the history of the Jewish people. In 2003, JewishGen became an affiliate of the **Museum of Jewish Heritage - A Living Memorial to the Holocaust** in New York.

The **JewishGen Yizkor Book Project** was organized to make more widely known the existence of Yizkor (Memorial) Books written by survivors and former residents of various Jewish communities throughout the world. Later, volunteers connected to the different destroyed communities began cooperating to have these books translated from the original language—usually Hebrew or Yiddish—into English, thus enabling a wider audience to have access to the valuable information contained within them. As each chapter of these books was translated, it was posted on the JewishGen website and made available to the general public.

The **Yizkor Books in Print Project** began in 2011 as an initiative to print and publish Yizkor Books that had been fully translated, so that hard copies would be available for purchase by the descendants of these communities and also by scholars, universities, synagogues, libraries, and museums.

These Yizkor books have been produced almost entirely through the volunteer effort of researchers from around the world, assisted by donations from private individuals. The books are printed and sold at near cost, so as to make them as affordable as possible. Our goal is to make this important genre of Jewish literature and history available in English in book form, so that people can have the personal histories of their ancestral towns on their bookshelves for themselves and for their children and grandchildren.

A list of all published translated Yizkor Books can be found at:
http://www.jewishgen.org/Yizkor/ybip.html

Lance Ackerfeld, Yizkor Book Project Manager
Joel Alpert, Yizkor Book in Print Project Coordinator

JewishGen
Yizkor Book Project

This book is presented by the
Yizkor Books in Print Project
Project Coordinator: Joel Alpert

Part of the
Yizkor Books Project of JewishGen, Inc.
Project Manager: Lance Ackerfeld

These books have been produced solely through volunteer effort
of individuals from around the world. The books are printed and
sold at near cost, so as to make them as affordable as possible.

Our goal is to make this history and important genre of Jewish
literature available in English in book form so that people can have
the near-personal histories of their ancestral towns on their bookshelves for themselves and for their children and grandchildren.

Any donations to the Yizkor Books Project are appreciated.

Please send donations to:
Yizkor Book Project
JewishGen
36 Battery Place
New York, NY 10280

JewishGen, Inc. is an affiliate of the
Museum of Jewish Heritage
A Living Memorial to the Holocaust

The Maple Tree Behind the Barbed Wire

Cover of the Original Swedish Book

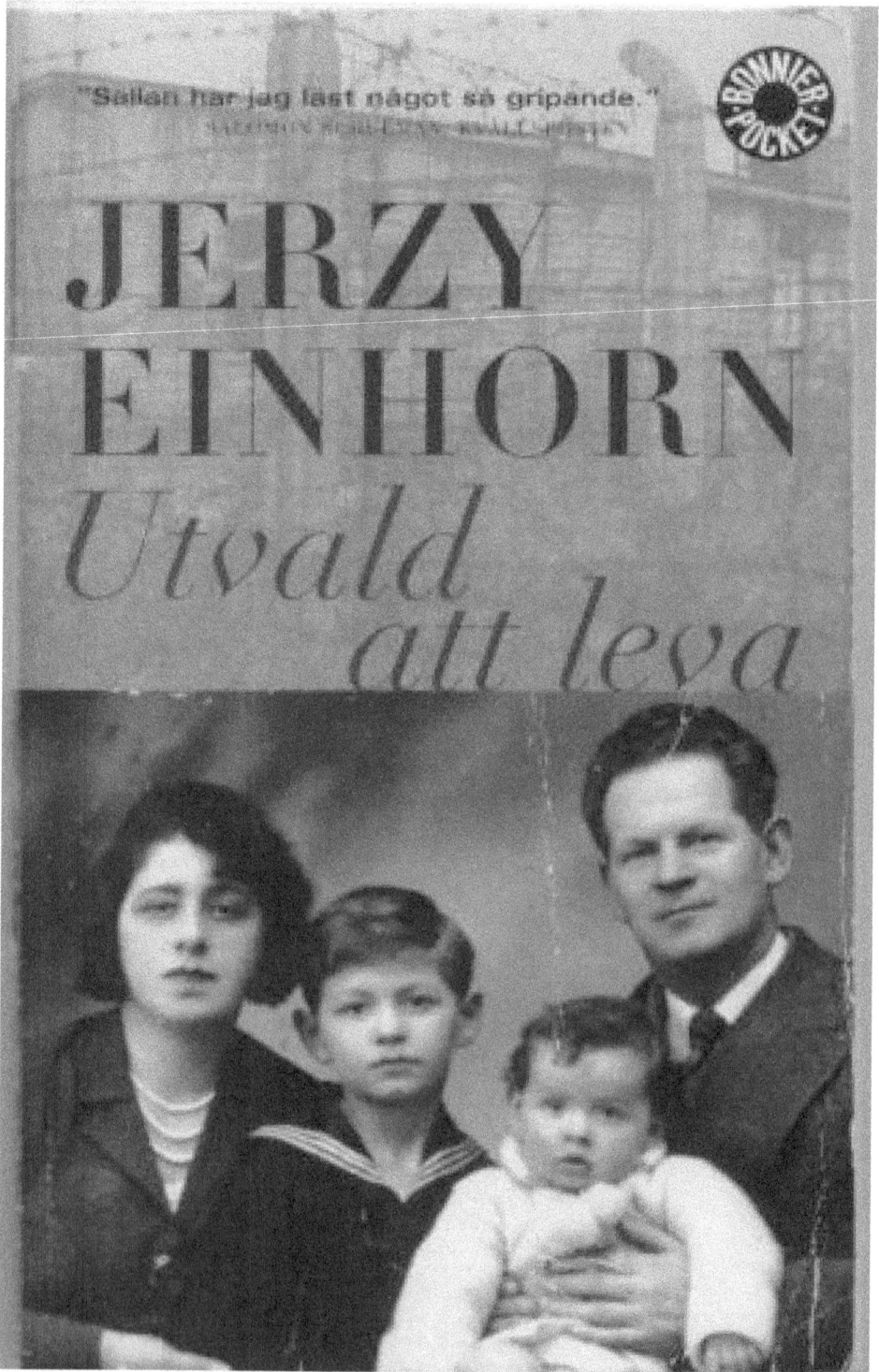

FOREWORD

For the Publication of the English Translation

When we sat down to write the Foreword to this book, to our surprise we found that we shared the same experience: for the longest time each of us had avoided reading The Maple Tree Behind the Barbed Wire, and then, when we finally did, we couldn't put the book down. Is it OK to say that a book written by one's own father is very good? Maybe not – but we will anyway.

Already as small children, we knew that our parents had lived through the Holocaust. Our mother told us in detail about her years in the Warsaw ghetto and the subsequent years of hiding in the Polish capital. In an unsentimental and natural tone of voice she told us about her experiences, but it was still obvious to us that her survival was miraculous (only a few hundred individuals survived the entirety of the Warsaw ghetto). In contrast, our father told his story in such a way that we got the impression that he had been through something resembling a summer camp – "they called it 'Hasag-Spa,'" he'd say, and smile. Not until we read this book did we realize that this was very far from the truth.

So was it only to protect us, his children, that Jerzy told this modified version of events? Probably not. As he writes in his Preface to this book, some of his memories lay deeply hidden, and recalling them required a huge emotional effort. He told us that it was sometimes like watching a film, but a film without sound, a silent movie. There were fragments that we had heard before: the wise father, Pinkus, who saved his son Roman by so brilliantly testing the woman who was to hide him; Pinkus' conversation with the two German officers who asked him about Germany's future; and then the "*maple tree behind the barbed wire.*" This was not to be the title the book had in its Swedish version, but it was the title our father liked the best. That maple tree was the only greenery he saw from within the ghetto.

Since our parents passed away, we have gathered information that was not available when the book was written. About Jerzy's maternal grandparents – who died during the war – we now know that they ended their lives in the Lodz ghetto together with several of their children. The grandparents died at a hospital inside the ghetto. Even the cause of death is provided in the meticulous lists the Nazis wrote, that now are accessible on the website of JewishGen.org. Grandmother Szprynca died on January 6, 1942, 68 years of age, by "marasmus senilis", which translates as "progressive atrophy of the elder". Only twenty days later her husband Szyja died, 74 years old, from the same cause. In all likelihood they starved to death.

The Maple Tree Behind the Barbed Wire

From other lists provided in the JewishGen Holocaust database we have also discovered that Jerzy's uncle, Maurycy Ajnhorn, arrived at "Lager II" in Buchenwald on January 1945, a week after he left Hasag-Pelcery. Where Maurucy eventually died we cannot know for certain.

Also with regard to the difficult process Jerzy had to go through in order to get permanent residency in Sweden we now know more. It was – just as Jerzy suspected – the letters that his parents sent to him (under pseudonym) to the student organization in Uppsala, which prompted a "friend" of Nina's and Jerzy's to contact the police. Distrust of aliens is one of the less appealing characteristics of humans. As Jerzy himself said: "The fundamental problem of the human being is the fact that he distinguishes between 'us' and 'them'."

It was important for our father to write these books – The Maple Tree Behind the Barbed Wire, and the sequel; It is about Human Beings (which depicts his time as a physician in the Swedish health care system). These books, we believe, for him constituted something of a closure. Possibly, he would not with such stoic calm have lived through his terminal illness – which was diagnosed the year after the second book came out – if he had not finished writing them. And when he had finished the second book he was very adamant that there would be no more books. During his last week in life, he once said: "My work is finished. What more is there for me to do?" He also told us that he had lived a good life and that he was content.

And he most certainly lived a full life. Jerzy Einhorn came to Sweden as a poor student and became the head of one of the most acclaimed cancer clinics in Europe. He sat on the Nobel Prize committee for Medicine and Physiology, and became an avid advocate for the improvement of the health care system in Sweden. This commitment also became the impetus for his becoming a Member of Parliament after retiring from the Karolinska Hospital and Institute. Jerzy Einhorn very much was a public figure, known and admired by most Swedes.

One aspect of our father's personality deserves special respect and admiration. In spite of all that he went through, and in spite of all the evil he experienced close-up, he remained strong in his conviction that humans are essentially good. Even in encounters with people that were known to have held Nazi sympathies during the 1930s he refrained from passing judgment. We can perhaps all learn something from this approach.

After the war, Jerzy was separated from his family. He came to Sweden, married Nina and had us. His parents and brother went to Canada. The family remained dispersed, which was a great sorrow to

The Maple Tree Behind the Barbed Wire

Jerzy. He tried to compensate by visiting them as often as he could, and was a very dedicated member of his original family. His mother Sarah, who, when he was in his sixties, chided him for not looking both ways when he crossed the street; his father Pinkus, whom we never met, and who was presented to us as a pillar of wisdom; his brother Roman, who chose the same profession as Jerzy, and towards whom Jerzy always felt like a big brother.

Jerzy and Nina Einhorn received their respective cancer diagnoses one day apart, in August of 1999. Jerzy only lived eight months, Nina an additional two years. This book was published in its Polish translation two weeks after her death. In her place we traveled to our father's hometown Czestochowa and brought the Swedish version of The Maple Tree Behind the Barbed Wire as a sort of guidebook. All the houses that Jerzy lived in are still there. They all are situated along the same street, the long Aleja NMP. What is remarkable, however, is that the memory of what happened barely remains in the population of this city. Admittedly, the elderly couple that opened the door for us in one of the houses knew that there had once been a Jewish ghetto in the neighborhood, but not that they themselves lived within the former ghetto borders. And young people we met did not know that before the war, every third person of their city had been a Jew, and almost all of them had perished. It is remarkable how quickly history fades, although building remains. And this is a reason as good as any that this book should exist and be read.

Now it is also available in the English language. And for this we are most grateful.

Lena and Stefan Einhorn

March 31, 2012

Stockholm, Sweden

DEDICATION

This story is dedicated to:

... The 56,000 Jews in Czestochowa ghetto whom the world allowed to die in silence - with sorrow and eternal loss,

The barely 5,200 survivors of the Hasag prison camp who built up new lives with their souls severely damaged - with respect and admiration,

My parents, Pinkus and Sarah, who gave me a good start in life and prepared me for what was to come,

Nina who gave me a good life - with my great gratitude, warm admiration, deep respect and boundless love.

I have written this story primarily with my grandchildren Dan, Michael and little Kim in mind - I hope they will read it, sometime in the future.

The Maple Tree Behind the Barbed Wire

TABLE OF CONTENTS

PREFACE

This is not an autobiography. I have no intention of drawing a picture of myself, or my life. My story is about people I have met, events I have experienced and what happened to the Jews of Czestochowa - I am one of them.

Nor is this book a historical document. I have not kept a diary, so may have names of people, streets and towns wrong, as well as dates, sequences of events and important details. But all events described here, occurred, all the streets and people did exist.

My story is based on individual events of which I have detailed memories. I remember houses, streets, stairways, rooms, furniture, people, faces, facial expressions, individual words and whole sentences. These events formed my personality. I shall try to reproduce for the reader as best I can these memories and my reflections, not just those I had when the event occurred, but also those I have today.

But memory is imperfect, particularly when concerned with events that happened long ago. In order that my account should be as correct as possible, I have interviewed several of those people who survived the Czestochowa Jewish ghetto with me: my mother's youngest sister Karola, who died recently, my younger brother Roman, who lives in Canada, Heniek Epstein, Sonja Frucht, Jurek Igra and Henry Frydman - all of whom live in Florida - Chaimek Rotenstein and Heniek Ufner, both of whom live in New York, Mietek and Renia Szydlowski who live in Argentina, Ignaz Jacoby who lives in Frankfurt and Abraszka Wilhelm who, as I do, lives in Stockholm. All these people - except Jurek Igra - were in the Hasag-Pelcery prison camp with me, and several of them are named in this book.

Karola, Roman, Heniek Epstein, Sonja Frucht and Chaimek Rotenstein were around when I was a child and Heniek Ufner sat at the same desk at the Czestochowas Hebrew School. Outside the ghetto in the Jewish resistance movement, Jurek Igra was active.

I have also had help from the following people and organizations: Judith Kleiman, head of the reference division, and Dany Uziel at the Yad Vashem's archives in Jerusalem, who have helped me with several of the illustrations in this book, the Red Cross archives in Geneva, Dr Helena Rotsztein who lives in Lòdz, Dr Jan Jagielski of the Jewish Historical Institute's document department in Warsaw, Senior Rabbi Morton Narowe, and Karol Martel, once lecturer in philosophy at Warsaw University. The recently departed Rector of Uppsala University, Professor Martin H:son Holmdahl, has compiled the documentation which provides the background to events that occurred when Nina and I left the medical faculty in Uppsala.

The Maple Tree Behind the Barbed Wire

It took a distance of fifty years for me to be able to confront certain memories from the depths of my memory and analyze why those events could have happened. This caused me very great anguish. When I was working my way through the story, my anguish began to be possible to deal with - the wounds are still there, but I am able to look at them.

Nothing of what I have experienced has shaken the conviction I have inherited from my father - Pinkus Mendel Einhorn - that human beings are basically good, but also more easily influenced than we imagine. At the same time, I have realized that people can be strong, cope with greater stresses and strains than we think, yet maintain their dignity and an undestroyed faith in other people and in humanity.

CALENDAR

Czestochowa is an industrial town in southwest Poland, known for the Jasna Góra monastery and the Black Madonna - a place of pilgrimage for Roman Catholics.

1765. First note of 75 Jewish settlers in Czestochowa.

1827. 1,141 Jews constitute 19% of the population of the town.

1862. The Jews are moved out of the secluded Jewish quarters.

1921. According to the Polish constitution, Jews become citizens, formally with equal rights.

1938. December 31st. 28,486 Jews constitute a third of the population of the town.

1939. September 1st. German troops cross the Polish border and the Second World War begins.

    September 3rd. German troops take Czestochowa.

    September 4th. "Bloody Monday", the first pogrom, several hundred Jews killed in Czestochowa.

    September 16th. Judenrat (Council of Elders) is appointed with Leon Kopinski as chairman.

    December 25th. The second Jewish pogrom, our Great Synagogue is burnt down.

1940. August. 1,000 Jewish men between 18 and 25 sent to Cieszanow forced labour camp. None survives.

1940-41. Autumn and spring. Evacuation to Czestochowa of 20,000 Jews largely from smaller communities in Southwest Poland.

    April 9th. Establishment of the ghetto.

1941. August 23rd. The ghetto is closed. It is calculated that there are 56,000 Jews in the ghetto. Some escape, many are killed.

1942. September 23rd-October 5th. Over 39,000 Jews were sent to Treblinka concentration camp, and over 2,000 were shot on the spot. The remaining 6,500 Jews moved to the small ghetto.

1942. December. The remaining Jewish resistance groups united into ZOB - the Jewish resistance organization.

The Maple Tree Behind the Barbed Wire

1943. January 4th-5th. The first armed resistance, 525
Jews shot or deported.
March 20th. Remaining intellectuals (127 people) in
the small ghetto are granted safe-conduct out of
the country, then executed by firing squad at
the Jewish Cemetery in Czestochowa.
April-June. Several ZOB groups leave the ghetto and
join the Polish left-wing guerillas.
June 26th. Liquidation of the small ghetto. The
remaining ZOB groups in the ghetto offer
resistance. A thousand people killed, the rest
taken to four prison camps associated with the
Hasag factories in Czestochowa.
July 20th. 400 prisoners executed.
August 2nd. Uprising of Jewish prisoners in
Treblinka extermination camp.

1944. Autumn. After the evacuation of Jewish prisoners
from other camps, about 12,000 prisoners are left
at Hasag.

1945. January 15th and 16th. The Germans deport up to
6,000 prisoners from Hasag prison camp - few
survive.

1945. Night of January 17th. Thirteen Soviet tanks
enter the suburbs of Czestochowa and liberate
the remaining 5,200 Jewish prisoners.

1946. June. 2nd, 167 Jews remain living in Czestochowa.
July 4th. Jewish pogrom in Kielce. This is
followed by pogroms in several places in Poland.
The majority of Jews in Poland and nearly all in
Czestochowa leave the country.

CHAPTER I

The World To Be Exterminated

Sarah Marries Pinkus

My father Pinkus Mendel Einhorn was born in 1886, into an orthodox Jewish home in Zawiercie, an industrial town which when Poland was divided between Prussia, Austro-Hungary and Russia, came to be included in the realm of the great Russian Empire. After the division of Poland, the majority of the world's Jews became subjects of the Russian Czar.

My paternal grandfather, Chil Josef Einhorn, whose Hebrew name I was to inherit, was an orthodox butcher. Chil Josef had no children in his long first marriage. When his first wife died, he married again and his second wife, who was to be my grandmother, gave birth to two boys in quick succession, Pinkus and Maurycy. When she was to give birth for a third time, both my grandmother and the child, a girl, died. Grandfather married yet again at seventy-two, a marriage arranged between himself and the bride's parents. His third wife was much younger than he was and she was not kind to the two boys.

Chil Josef and his third wife had met only once before their marriage and even then in the presence of witnesses. According to tradition, they were not to meet again until the marriage ceremony beneath the traditional canopy. Waiting alone under the canopy, Chil Josef heard his bride crying and refusing to come. He broke with all traditions, went into the room where she was being prepared for the marriage ceremony and said: "Don't delay the marriage. I am not getting any younger. I'll just get older if you wait." Then she stopped crying and married Chil Josef. Grandfather, just as my father Pinkus did, found it easy to express himself in words with conviction. Grandfather, just like my father, was very strong both physically and mentally, and he remained vigorous well into old age.

Chil Josef wants Pinkus, his elder son, to be a scholar, to go to the orthodox schools in the Jewish ghetto where the family lives. Pinkus is educated in a cheder, which he starts at when he is five. He has to learn to read, scan the texts of the Bible and do sums. The intention is that he is to continue in a senior religious school, a Yeshiva, perhaps become a rabbi and not a butcher like his father. But Pinkus — that new times are coming and the gates of the Jewish ghetto have been opened. Pinkus wants to go to an ordinary school and not spend the remainder of his schooldays debating different interpretations of the Talmud.

At thirteen he runs away from home in nothing but the shoes on his

The Maple Tree Behind the Barbed Wire

feet and the clothes he is wearing. By chance, he ends up with a tailor — and becomes a tailor. He did not, as he had hoped, succeed in going to an ordinary school, but on the other hand he acquired a profession — and that with a vengeance.

As a lone thirteen year-old, he starts his professional career by working for his keep and board in a basement room with no window, a room, which is both the tailor's workshop and the family's dwelling. He works his way up from sole assistant to a poor tailor hardly able to support his family by patching the worn clothes of other poor Jews, to being employed by increasingly better professionals. He finally ends up in the workshop of the master of master tailors, Kusnir. At this workshop, clothes are made for ministers, ambassadors, the president himself in Warsaw, the new capital of the resurrected Poland, one of the largest countries in Europe, at the time with 36 million inhabitants, of whom 3.5 million were Jews.

When Pinkus considers he has learnt his profession, he wants to open his own tailoring establishment somewhere where he has a chance to be the best. He moves to Czestochowa, an industrial town the size of Malmö close to the German border, and then rapidly becomes the best tailor in town.

Pinkus is an artist. Slim men with sloping shoulders become elegant gentlemen. Fat men become a little slimmer, the stooped more straight-backed, the short a little taller. Every man wants him to make his clothes. He increases his prices and employs more assistants.

Pinkus is mostly happy, always understanding and generous, eager to teach his assistants what he himself, knows. He becomes sad only when someone does not wish to learn. Why are you here if you don't want to learn? Many seek work with him, but he does not want his business to grow too large. "What is important is to maintain the quality," he says to his assistants in the workshop.

The tailoring business goes well, but Pinkus does not attend to his finances. His needs are small. He lives simply and not particularly healthily. He keeps food and money in an icebox, which is daily filled with fresh ice by an ice purveyor, even in summer wearing thick padded clothing. Pinkus likes ice cream very much and his icebox is full of ice cream. He eats irregularly, often simply ice cream. He does not allow himself time, nor has he any interest in buying or cooking any other food, and he does not bother much about what he eats.

Pinkus loves his work and he loves reading. He has never learnt to write, but he can read Yiddish - a mixture of German and Hebrew with elements of Polish and Russian. Pinkus speaks Polish with a strong accent, but manages all the same. He is a skilled professional, and Yiddish is also the main language of many of the people around him. He devours the classic Russian writers - Gorky, Tolstoy. Dostoevsky and Turgenev, weighty literature emerging from a melancholy people in oppressive Czarist Russia. He becomes absorbed in the works of the

The Maple Tree Behind the Barbed Wire

German philosophers - Kant, Schopenhauer and Nietzsche - reads Jewish writers such as Chain Bachman Safari. Maimonides is his favorite. Periodically he reads German writers such as Goethe, Heine and Schiller, and he likes Ibsen and Hamsun best of the Nordic writers, though Strindberg not as much. He has read all of Byron and much else by English, French and Spanish writers, and when he is in a good mood he quotes from Cervantes. Everything is translated into Yiddish, and the two rooms behind the tailor's fitting room looks like a minor public library. That is also where he lives.

When Pinkus is thirty-eight, he knows he is sufficiently secure to be able to support a family. He goes to Zdeunska-Wola near Lódz and starts courting Sarah Blibaum, who is thirteen years younger and who is to become my mother.

Sarah is the middle child of nine siblings, eight girls and a boy, in a Jewish orthodox family that has just left the ghetto. Like Pinkus, Sarah has the courage to break with orthodox traditions, wears modern clothes and acquires a profession. Sarah's parents, my maternal grandfather and grandmother Szprynca, are not at all pleased, but nevertheless are more understanding than Pinkus' father, or else Sarah was stronger and more independent. She is still living at home and shocks her parents, brothers and sisters, relatives and neighbors with her extravagances.

Much later, her youngest sister tells me during a late night conversation in Toronto shortly after Sarah's death in May 1989, about how Sarah's siblings admired her for her self-confidence and her strong will, for her courage in resisting surrounding pressures. Karola tells me how the young Sarah might come home from work one summer's afternoon in a hyper-modern wide-brimmed hat with a shiny black hatband. Sarah took paid employment instead of marrying in her teens, which at the time was customary in Jewish orthodox families. She trains to be a dental technician, but does not practice her profession for many years to come.

Sarah is a beauty with thick dark hair and fair skin, has a lovely walk, straight-backed with head held high, her flashing but gentle smile brightening her face, a birthmark on her left cheek making her handsome face even more expressive. She has good taste, dresses well but not provocatively, an unusually elegant woman at whom men turn round to look, which I don't like. She always knows what she wants and she usually also gets it.

When Pinkus meets Sarah in Zdunska-Wola, in a flash he falls in love. It's her or no one, he says as he proposes.

The Maple Tree Behind the Barbed Wire

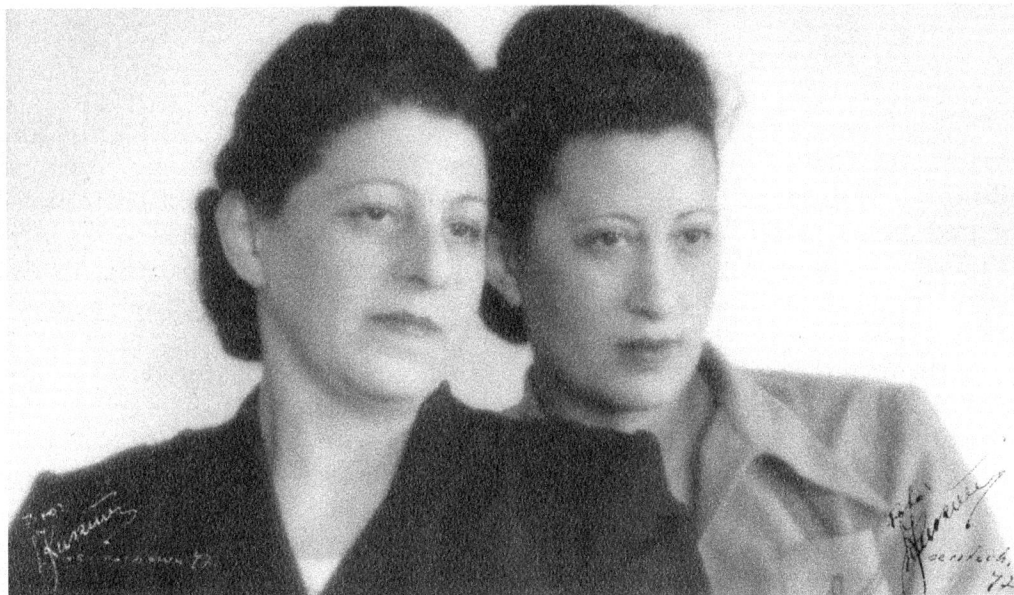

Like Pinkus, Sarah has the courage to break with orthodox traditions, wears modern clothes and has acquired a profession. Much later, her youngest sister, Karola, tells of how the siblings admired Sarah for her courage and strong will, because she dared to resist the pressures around her. Of nine siblings, only these two sisters were to survive the war. (The photograph was taken in Czestochowa in 1947, before Karola leaves for Israel and Sarah for Canada.)

Sarah does not reject him. He is a handsome man — and she is taken with the swiftness of his decision to propose and his firm behavior, but she wants time to think. Pinkus is sick with longing and anxiety. His hopes increase when Sarah writes that she would consider coming to see him in Czestochowa, an unusual suggestion in their circles in the 1920s.

Sarah and Pinkus meet at the most elegant tea-rooms in town - Krysztal - near the railway station, then she inspects his living quarters, the books in great disorder, the ice-box which also serves as his safe, the badly equipped and scarcely usable kitchen — which Pinkus has tried to tidy up for Sarah's visit — and the workshop. They have dinner in the Europa restaurant, one of the finest in Czestochowa - and talk a great deal. Before Pinkus sees Sarah to the railway station, she says she would very much like to marry him. She does this despite seeing his bachelor den, or perhaps just because of that. It is clear to Sarah that there is a lot to do, and that he needs her.

After their wedding, Pinkus has no chance against Sarah when they disagree, which happens. But Sarah respects Pinkus and loves him, and Pinkus loves his Sarah, although he is not very good at showing his feelings. This big muscular handsome man is shy with women. I was born barely eleven months after the wedding.

Family, Friends and Acquaintances

Pinkus occasionally travels to textile factories in England and Poland, to buy or order cloth. Sarah is afraid of being on her own, so Pinkus acquires a dog. He chooses an Alsatian bitch called Lotte, bred at pedigree kennels in Vienna. The young dogs there have to learn to understand their future owners, and the owners have to learn to live with their dogs, so each owner has to partake in the puppy's upbringing.

Lotte was there when I was born, and she is one of my very earliest memories. She is a big, strong, wise and thoughtful dark-brown Alsatian, who has close contact with Pinkus, but if necessary also with Sarah. Lotte not only obeys orders, but it is quite clear she also understands a great deal of what Pinkus says and desires — sometimes I have the impression that they talk to each other.

When I was born, Pinkus stops traveling to purchase cloth, but Lotte stays and makes her mark on the atmosphere of our home. She is security itself, not least for me — no one can harm us while we have Lotte. If anything unusual happens, she knows it before we have noticed anything. She raises her wise head, pricks up her pointed ears, looks all round with her brown eyes, takes a walk round, then lies down again if she reckons the danger has passed. In the middle of the night, she may get up and go to stand over by the door, as if she heard everything, even when she is asleep. It is lovely growing up with Lotte, but she no longer exists once I start school. She dies young from a paralysis, which starts in her hind legs.

Lotte lies down in the soft bedding in her basket, still listening and watching when she thinks danger is threatening, then tries, but is unable to get up. Lotte suffers and we suffer with her. I miss her terribly, but forever in the future I am to keep the security she gave me when I was small and never had to feel defenseless.

My favorite places are my father's workshop and the fitting room with its big mirror, where customers tried on their suits. To have a suit made by Pinkus Einhorn, customers have to come at least four times, to choose the cloth, order and take measurements for the first and second fitting, and then the final fitting, when they may take away the suit — if it fits, otherwise they have to come back several times.

My earliest memory is of the gilt-framed mirror in Pinkus' elegant fitting room falling over on to me and breaking. Luckily the side mirrors fold inwards, so I am lying in a tent, paralysed with terror, in a pile of various sized sharp pieces of mirror-glass. I have sufficient good sense not to move, and I lie still and am scared. For the first time in my life, I realise I am in danger, and after a while I am also frightened Pinkus will be angry. How will he be able to receive his customers without a mirror?

The Maple Tree Behind the Barbed Wire

But Pinkus isn't angry. Carefully, he lifts up the big wooden frame. Strong as he is, he can do that alone. He keeps talking all the time to calm me, telling me to lie still and not move. He carefully picks up all the big pieces of glass, then the smaller ones, wishing to do this all himself, while everyone else in the room stands round in a semi-circle looking on. When I can just glimpse his face, I see that it is rigid and tense, and he goes on talking to me as he removes the last pieces of glass, then slowly and cautiously lifts me up and presses me hard to him. He holds on to me for a long time, saying not a word. It's terrific. It feels safe, and he allows himself to show his feelings. He is pale and I can see tears running down his cheeks. Sarah is frightened and is not allowed to take over for a while, and I have not even a scratch. Pinkus asks Heniek Epstein the bookkeeper to phone the glazier, for the mirror has to be mended quickly, and Heniek is to ask if we may borrow another mirror meanwhile. Pinkus says, apparently calmly, that everyone is to go back to work. I am four and have never before seen and am never again to see my father weep.

I am proud of my father. He seldom raises his voice, is strong, wise and kind — strong, wise and kind, a fine combination. He sees a lot, but says little, understanding that people do not always behave, as they should. I never hear him reprimand anyone, except as a teacher in his workshop, nor do I hear or see him appear superior to anyone, whether child or adult, for that would have been alien to his personality. But nor do I ever see him behaving subserviently — despite everything that happens to us. He has a natural dignity and authority, my father Pinkus has.

Pinkus is not good at small talk. When he says something to me, it is always thought through and important, and I also restrain my empty chatter when with my father. But when I turn to him, he listens and treats what I have said seriously, although I am only five. I cannot remember him ever prattling with me, but I know he loves me — it is better to show your feelings than to talk about them.

There is room for ten employees in my father's workshop, never more. All are robust men who speak a rich Yiddish. You do not always understand what they mean — no subtle ambiguities, no unnecessary circumlocutions or false politeness, but a firmly rooted friendly and warm atmosphere. I am the apple of the workshop's eye and they speak Polish to me. Despite this, I quickly learn to understand and speak the coarse-grained Yiddish of the workshop. Polish is spoken in the fitting room.

Two of the long walls in the fitting room are covered with specially made cupboards running from floor to ceiling and filled with cloth. The best cloth comes from Manchester in England, the next best from Bielsko in Polish Silesia, and no poor quality cloth is found in Father's workshop. I learn the tailoring terms, single or double-breasted jackets, trousers with or without turn-ups, worsted, cheviot or gabardine.

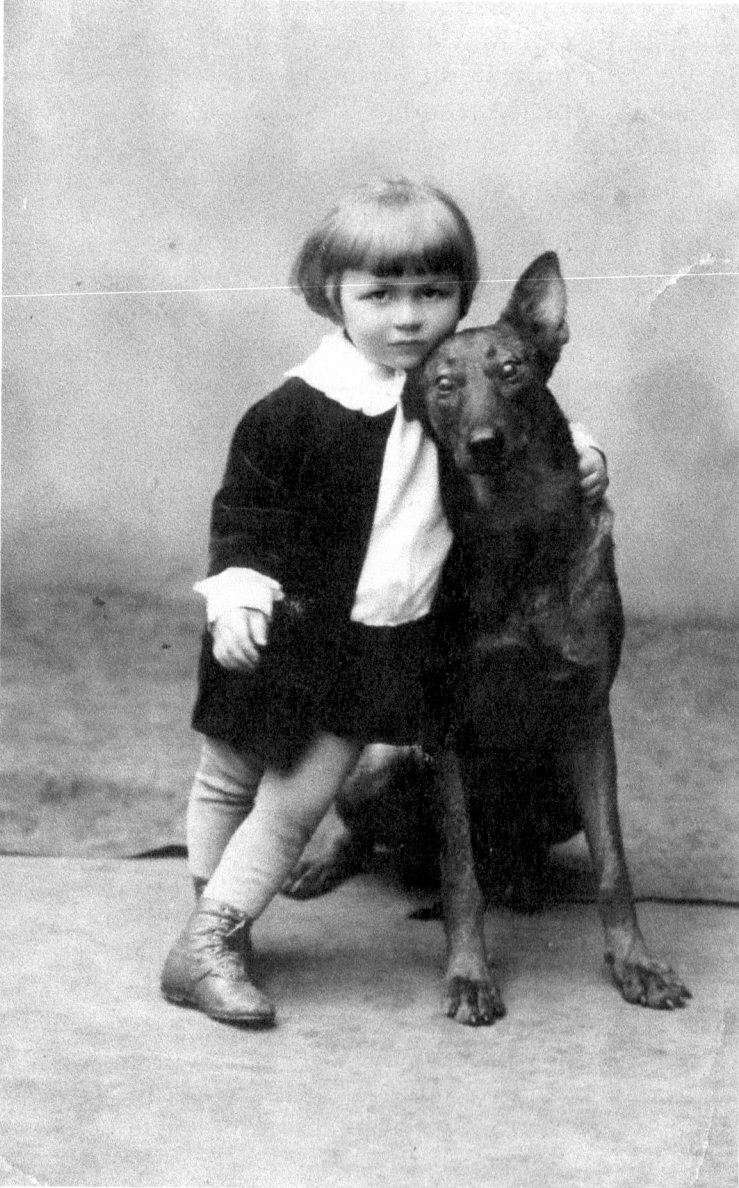

Lotte was with us at home when I was born. She is a big strong, wise and thoughtful dark-brown Alsatian, and she is security itself. It is wonderful to grow up with Lotte. In future I am always to keep something of the security she gave me when I was small.

The Maple Tree Behind the Barbed Wire

The big mirror in its gilt frame dominates the room, the two side-mirrors necessary for the customers to be able to see themselves in the mirror from the front, the side and from behind. The elegant Heniek Epstein, with his slanting smile and pomaded black hair brushed back, is always to be found in the fitting room. He is the favorite with the ladies. Urbanely, he entertains the customers when Pinkus is not there, though when my father comes into a room, with his natural authority, he takes over.

When I am in the fitting room, I sit quietly on my stool below the window behind the left-hand mirror, listening to Pinkus as he receives his customers. Sometimes a customer notices me sitting there and extracts me from of my hiding-place to speak to me, usually amused and friendly, but sometimes — like Dr Goldman the gynecologist — protectively and superior, which I dislike. A constant question is — what are you going to do when you grow up? What a stupid question, a tailor, of course, like my father. But sometimes it is trickier. Which God do you believe in, our Christian God or the Jewish God? There is only one God, I say, the difference being that we pray differently. Pinkus always seems satisfied, sometimes even proud, but he never comments on these conversations, and I am never corrected.

After the mirror fell on to me, I am no longer allowed to sit on my stool behind the mirror. When I dare to do so a few months later, Pinkus pretends not to see me; Heniek Epstein looks surprised but says nothing.

Our living quarters are behind the door at the very back of the fitting room, and in there is my mother Sarah's safe world. Sometimes, Sarah is troubled by having to go through the fitting room to get into our home, but all the same, things are good in our two rooms and kitchen — the living room with its heavy furniture and pictures on the walls, and the bedroom where my father, mother and I sleep. My bed is at the foot of my parents' bedstead.

Sarah is queen of her little realm, but I can see that she is respected outside our home as well, for her personality and bearing, and also as Pinkus' wife. I am often allowed to go with her when she goes shopping, and even more often when she is to meet friends. It is exciting, too, when Sarah comes home after she has been out without me, for she has parcels with her, sometimes for me. I am inquisitive about what is in the parcel, but most of all about what is in her black handbag, which I'm never allowed to open.

I feel I have nothing in common with the children playing in our courtyard, or with the children of our acquaintances. I have no playmates of my own age and like being at home best, in the workshop, in the fitting room, or when I go out with my beautiful self-confident mother.

The Maple Tree Behind the Barbed Wire

One day in the late spring of 1931, when I am almost six, Sarah and Pinkus want to talk to me. They ask me if I want a brother or sister. Pinkus is radiant with happiness, Sarah in high spirits. I want to have a brother. What name do you want for him? Roman, I say. Sarah happens to reading a book about a Roman to me.

A few weeks later I am sent away to stay with my Aunt Bela, one of Sarah's older sisters. Like Sarah, Bela married a man from Czestochowa and they live in an elegant apartment in ulica Katedralna 7, an apartment house, which takes up a whole block and is owned by Bela's husband, Ignas Enzel. He is very rich and they have one of the first cars in town with a chauffeur of their own. Enzel is learning to drive, but it is not going well. Bela and Uncle Enzel like me, but things are not good between them and I hear them constantly quarreling, although they try not to when I am with them.

A few days later, Bela takes me home in the car. I am to meet the little brother Roman the stork has brought. I may go into our bedroom, but only for a short while. Sarah is in bed, clearly weak and tired, Dr Kluczewski is with her as well as a nurse. I don't even think of questioning what Bela has said and Pinkus has not denied that it is the stork, which has brought Roman.

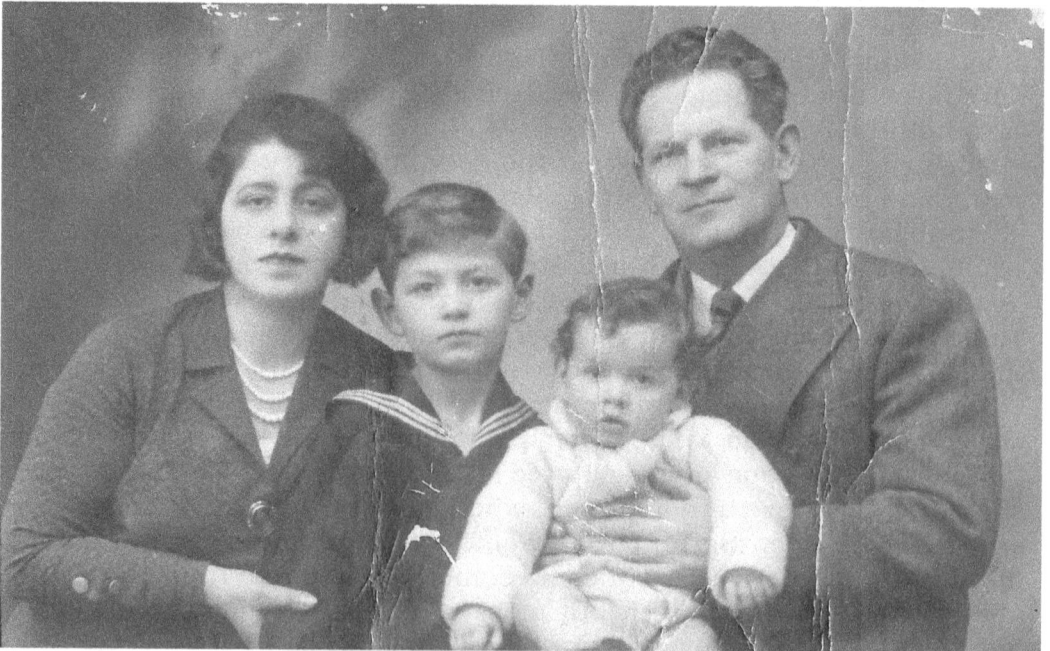

My memories from childhood are bright and warm. Sarah gives me unlimited uncritical love. My father gives me security, treats me seriously, and shares his wisdom with me. We cannot choose our parents and some are lucky, others not. I was lucky. When this photo was taken, I am six, and am to be seven in July.

The Maple Tree Behind the Barbed Wire

But why is Sarah so tired and why does she have to have Dr Kluczewski and a nurse with her? Something is not right, it seems mysterious, and why was I not allowed to be at home when Roman came? Would I have frightened the stork away? I seem to be the only one who is wondering and not understanding. I usually get honest answers to my perpetual questions, but for some reason I don't ask any this time.

Roman does not look like any little children I have seen so far. He is small and wrinkled. I am not allowed to touch him, only look at him for a little while before being shooed out of the bedroom and taken back by Bela. But I have a brother, anyhow. I am no longer alone and it became a boy and he was called Roman, as I had wanted. When I go home another week later, I have to move into the sofa bed in the living room, as Roman has taken over my place in the bedroom.

Sometimes I am allowed a sip of the sweet kosher-le-pesach wine during the Passover Seder meal, the solemn Jewish Easter meal. I look forward every year to exactly the same meal, when we all sit together round a beautifully laid table, although it is boring with hour-long prayers in Hebrew. I also find it hard to understand why the wine, which Sarah puts out in a silver tankard on the table, may not be finished up when the Passover meal is over and the prophet Elia has not come, although the front door has been open all evening. Anyhow, how could he possibly have time to go to all the Passover seder meals in all the Jewish homes in only two evenings?

Pinkus comes home early one afternoon with a large dark-brown wooden box. It is a crackling radio with a crystal receiver. Everyone in the workshop and several neighbors gather in our living room to listen. How can it be possible that we can hear people speaking or music played in another house or in another town? When I ask, Pinkus tries to explain, but I find it hard to grasp and give up.

I am constantly asking questions, not satisfied with evasive or off-putting answers, and I do not give up until someone tries to explain and I realize I am too small to understand. But I rarely give up altogether and usually come back after a while when I have had time to think about the answer, sometimes several hours or days later. I think slowly, but can be stubborn and persistent. Despite this, my parents never tell me to be quiet, not even when we are with strangers and I persist in asking.

We are a large family of relatives, mostly on Sarah's side, and we have a great many acquaintances. But we have only a few friends, all of them Jews. Christians can have business connections with us Jews, but otherwise they live in their own private world into which we seldom have entry. Sarah is the one to see to it that we mix and meet other people. If Pinkus had been the one to decide, we would not have met anyone else apart from customers, the employees in the workshop and a few real friends. To Pinkus, that should be enough.

Sarah tries to widen the family circle of friends and has arranged for Pinkus and her to be invited to dinner with some acquaintances one evening. Pinkus has not said he does not want to go, but when it is time for them to go, he goes to the little sofa in the living room and pleads: "I'm tired, can't you go on your own and make my excuses?" Sarah is upset. I feel sorry for Sarah, but am pleased Pinkus is staying at home with me. Sarah methodically builds up a circle of acquaintances that suits them both, partly the initially unwilling Pinkus, and partly on her own conditions.

Getting Pinkus to go with her to the theatre or cinema if there is a good film on works well. She can even occasionally get Pinkus to go with her to a restaurant, as long as it is alone with Sarah. Even better is to go to Warsaw to Uncle Maurycy's or to the Wajnapel's - Father's friend from his apprentice days in Kusnir's tailoring workshop — just as it is to invite them to us in Czestochowa.

Pinkus likes going to art exhibitions, though Sarah does not. Pinkus likes art and is able to distinguish talent among the young artists. He invites them back home to us and talks to them about their ambitions and problems. But he is not keen to go out to dinner to talk about nothing. Pinkus loathes small talk, wasting time on nothing.

"Life consists of time, time is the most valuable thing we have," Pinkus says to me. You should try not to waste time, but on the other hand you can't always avoid it. A profoundly imprinted way of thinking from studies of the Talmud makes itself felt when Pinkus talks to me about on the one hand and on the other hand. You have to know what you want and be able to choose, but you also have to accept that things will not always be as you want them to be, to live with that and not fret, that's all part of the conditions of life. There is always on the one hand and on the other hand, Pinkus says. "But you may never consciously harm other people" — this Pinkus doctrine is deeply imprinted in me as well. "But on the other hand, you can harm people in other ways apart from just physically" — couldn't Pinkus have not said to Sarah earlier that he did not intend to go out to dinner with her that evening?

My maternal grandparents move to Lódz. In the summer of 1931, just after my sixth birthday in July, I go to stay with them in the country where they have rented a cottage and I am to spend a few weeks with Grandfather Szyja and Grandmother Szprynca.

The Maple Tree Behind the Barbed Wire

My maternal grandfather is an orthodox Chassid, seldom having his hair cut and never shaving. He has a long black beard, always wears full length black Chassid clothes, a little round cap with a small peak in front on his head, which he always wears, indoors and out, and I wonder whether he sleeps in it. Grandfather Szyja drinks hot strong tea like poor Russians - na prekuska. He pours the hot water from the constantly boiling samovar on to a dish he holds in his left hand, then sucks the tea through a sugar lump he holds between his front teeth, and he can be heard all over the room. Every weekday morning he puts on tefilin straps, winds the black leather prayer straps tightly round his left arm and round his head so that the little black box of phylacteries with the texts from the Talmud ends up right in the middle of his forehead, and then he prays. He often goes to his synagogue, but never asks me if I want to go with him. Grandfather seems stern, never looks at women, hardly even at Szprynca, is taciturn and explains nothing. I am used to asking questions and there is a great deal I would like to ask about, but for some reason I do not, and even today I regret that I never even tried.

Grandmother Szprynca is the wife of an orthodox Chassid. In Szyja's presence, she is nearly always silent, but she likes talking to me and fusses rather clumsily over me all day. It is clear they both want me to be happy with them. But nonetheless I am not very, but I don't want to say so to Sarah so as not to hurt her, for they are her parents and my grandparents. But I don't have to go there again. Sarah has perhaps understood, or else my grandfather and grandmother did not want me to come, although Grandmother has not much say in it. Is it like this in all Chassid homes or is it just Grandfather who is so morosely domineering and Szprynca so submissive and silent? Was she like that before she married?

Grandfather and Grandmother did not survive the war. Hardly any of the many Chassidim in Poland did. Of their nine children, only my mother and Karola survived - the youngest — but not the lovely Bela, who managed to dispose of three husbands and live in three different countries, nor kind Rachela who lived in Gdansk, had many daughters but no son, nor Rózia who never married and lived at home with us, nor the only son — the family black sheep — who gambled away money on cards, nor the other three daughters, who were all married and had children. Of all their emancipated sons-in-law and daughters-in-law, of all their many grandchildren scattered all over Poland, only my father, Roman, Ignas Enzel and I were left after the war. All the others are gone.

The Maple Tree Behind the Barbed Wire

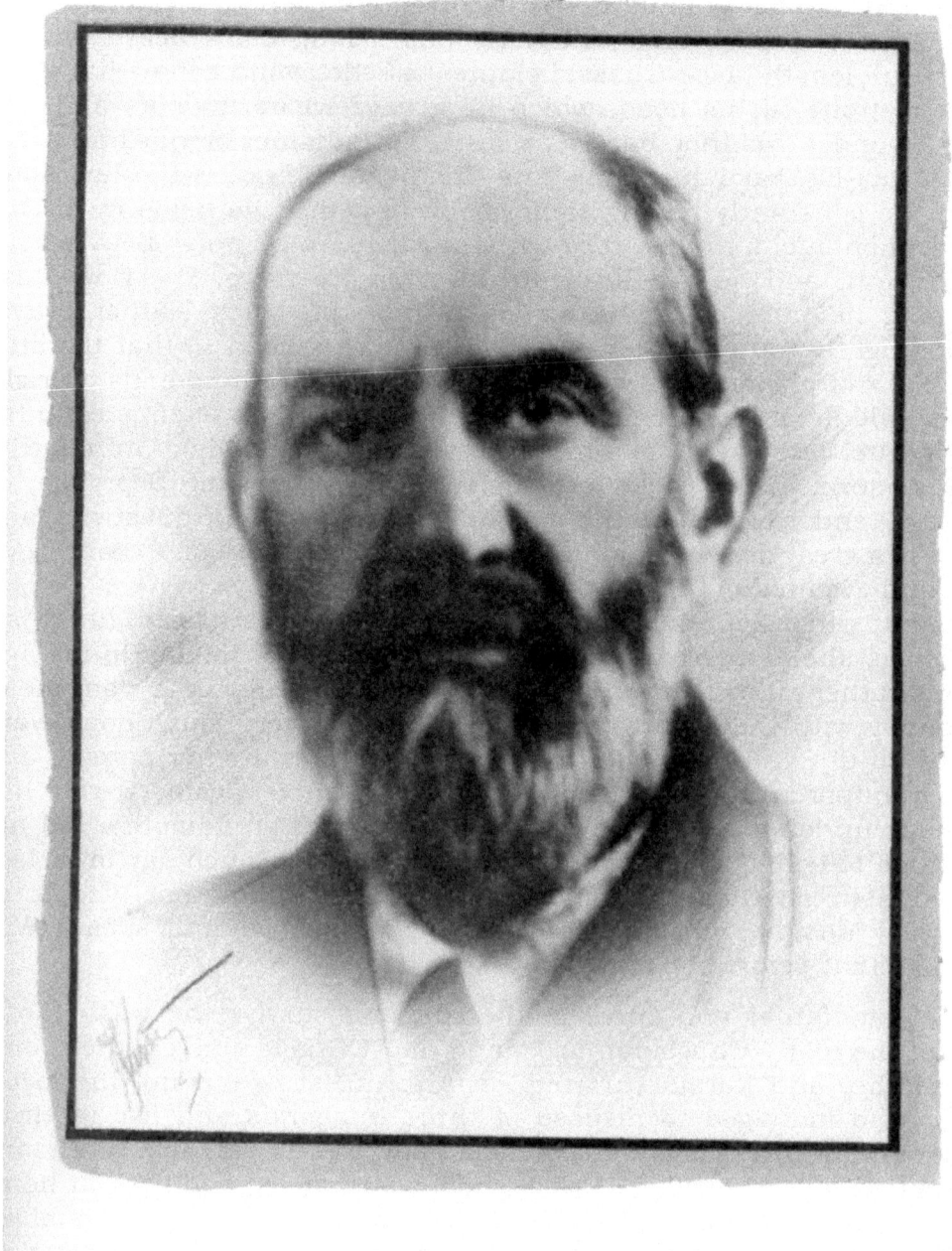

My maternal grandfather is an orthodox Chassid. He has a black beard and wears full-length Chassid clothes. He often goes to his synagogue, but never asks me if I want to go with him. Grandfather seems stern, is taciturn and explains nothing. This last photograph of him was taken in the autumn of 1939. Only a few of Poland's many Chassids are to survive the war - Szyja is not one of them

The Maple Tree Behind the Barbed Wire

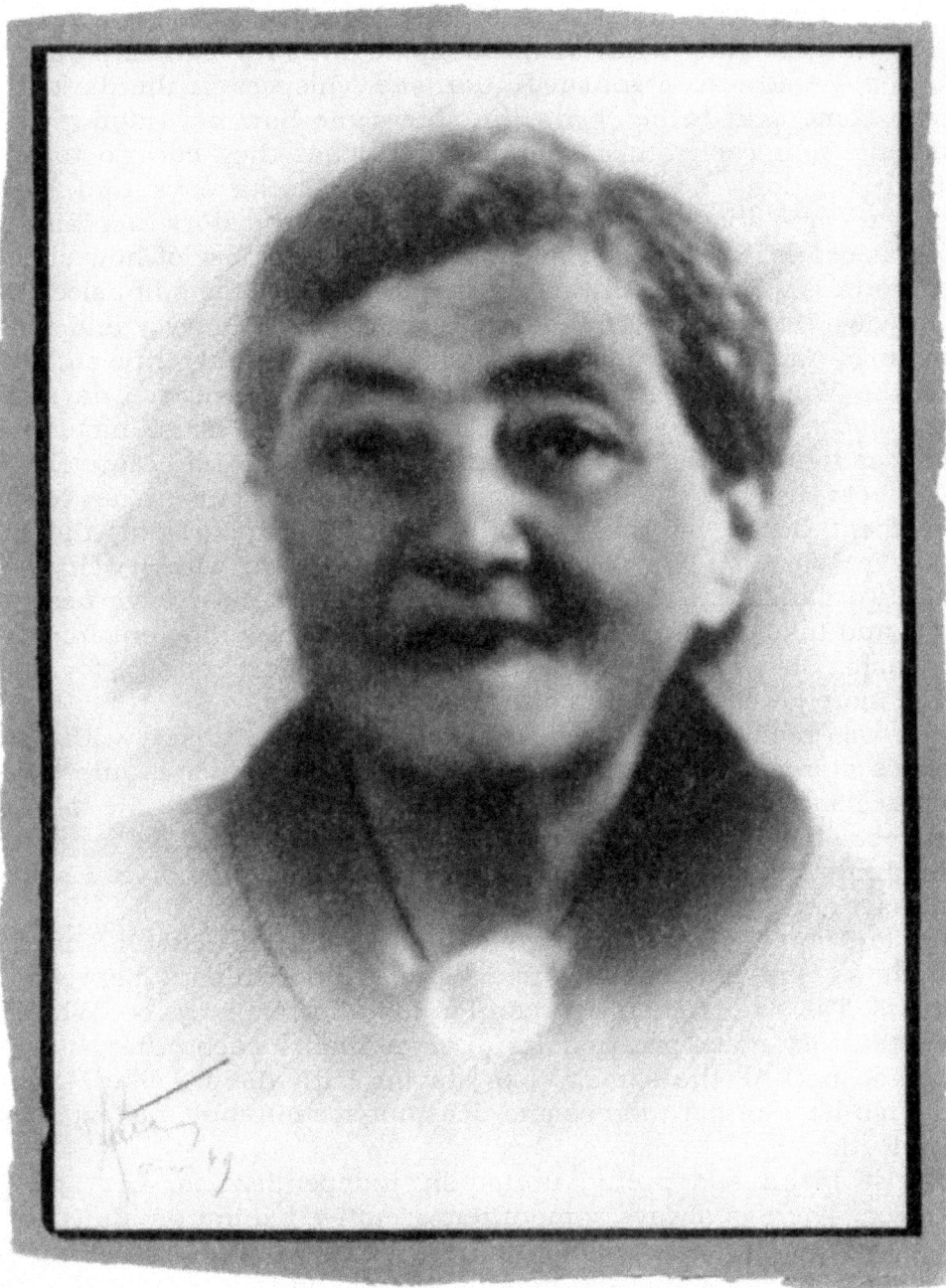

Grandmother Szprynca is the wife of an orthodox Chassid. In Grandfather Szyja's presence, she is usually silent, but she likes talking to me and fusses over me all day. Is it like this in all Chassid homes? Was Grandmother so submissive before she married? Szprynca does not survive the war.

The Maple Tree Behind the Barbed Wire

The best thing I know is when we are on a visit to Warsaw. Sometimes we stay with Pinkus' brother Maurycy, who has a daughter called Rutka. When I am alone at home with my contemporary but much more advanced cousin Rutka, she whispers in the dark that I am to come over to her bed. She shows me how boys and girls are different from each other, and tells me what they can do together, though we don't do it, we are too small. Rutka says that is how children come about, and that the story about the stork is a fairy tale. I fall asleep in Rutka's bed and have a faint memory of how shocked our mothers were when Sarah that night transfers me half-asleep back to my own bed. Before I fall asleep again, I hear Maurycy and Pinkus laughing and saying: what does it matter, they are only little children.

At the Wajnapels', Father's friend from his apprentice days, it is more lively. It is Wajnapel who makes clothes for ministers and ambassadors now, as well as for the president himself, Moscicki. The Wajnapels live in a big many-roomed apartment in an elegant apartment house on the corner of ulica Marszalkowska, the main street in Warsaw. Mrs. Wajnapel is always laden with jewelry. They have two daughters and two sons, of whom the elder is to become a tailor and take over his father's business. Sarah is different from Mrs. Wajnapel. She does not have to make any effort, either, for she is much more jewelry beautiful even without jewelry.

It is also really festive when the Wajnapels come to stay with us, for Sarah's dinners are sumptuous. After a while, dinner is interrupted, the guests can go and lie down to rest for a while before the meal and the festivities continue. Many years later, I was to experience something similar at the aristocratic Japanese home in Osaka of Professor and Mrs. Testsuo Taguchi.

Uncle Maurycy's wife Magda is never satisfied. That is hard for Rutka, as she notices how tense the relationship is between her parents. There is tension between Pinkus and Maurycy too. Whenever we meet, they make great efforts to be cordial to each other, but their wives do not. All the same, I like staying with them. I like Maurycy, although he is rather morose and does not seem happy, but most of all I like Rutka.

She is blond and pretty, unusually independent for her age, but reserved. There is always some ulterior motive behind anything Rutka says. I notice she is not always honest, perhaps because she has had to adapt to circumstances at home and has had to mature earlier than other children. Yet I feel I have more in common with Rutka than with any other contemporary. I like her very much and we were always to feel warmth for each other. Rutka is the only one in my father's family to survive the war, but her soul is damaged and things do not go well for her when she tries to put together her ravaged life after the war.

At the Wajnapels, every day is festive. The youngest daughter Barbara's room is white, Ewa's is pink, and the governess, who prefers

The Maple Tree Behind the Barbed Wire

to speak French when I am not there, has her room next to the girls. The big salons are handsomely furnished and there are always fresh flowers and different kinds of sweets, cakes and nuts in silver and cut glass bowls there. Several of the rooms have windows facing on to the main street and I can see a great deal as I sit there looking out on to ulica Marszalkowska. I like doing that, but seldom have the opportunity.

Wajnapel and Pinkus are good friends and like being together. Just as Pinkus had, Wajnapel has worked himself up from nothing, and with mild superiority he regards what his wife is making of their life, of the home and children. It is clear he thinks much of the extravagance is unnecessary and prefers to talk about cloth, suits and next year's fashions for men, for he and Pinkus have much to learn from each other.

Most of all, I like it when Wajnapel and my father talk about the old days, and then I hear about the young Pinkus, things he has never told me. Wajnapel hopes his elder son will take over the business. But the son is arrogant and a wastrel, as extravagant as his mother. The younger son is like his father, but he wants to be a doctor. That any of Wajnapel's daughters should show an interest in anything as banal as a tailoring business is inconceivable.

One evening Barbara wants me to get into her bed, and she also wants to talk to me about what happens between boys and girls. The door is open to Ewa's room, so she must hear what we are talking about. I would prefer to get into Ewa's bed, but I don't dare - I have always been attracted to older girls and women.

Although I like being at the Wajnapels, I would not like to live their artificial lives, with no contact with their father's work, what makes all this prosperity possible.

In the long run this is not to make any difference. Only the younger son, who is studying medicine in Paris when war breaks out, is to survive. The rest of the family are among the first to perish. They are not equipped to cope with the trials to come. It is sad that this handsome, happy family should have to be wiped out and disappear into oblivion - Barbara and Ewa with their great expectations and who experience very little of life, happy Mrs. Wajnapel and clever professional Mr. Wajnapel. Why? They never harmed anyone, they threatened no one, and making clothes is a fairly harmless occupation.

Although in many respects I develop slowly, or perhaps because of that, at a very early stage Pinkus and Sarah want me to learn to be independent. They give me twenty-five groszy to go on my own to the tearooms, a zloty to go to Abramowicz' restaurant, or fifty-five groszy to go to the cinema. One day I see a beggar on my way to the tearooms, a young woman with a child in her arms. She holds out her hand, is fairly insistent, and somewhat at a loss I give her my twenty-five groszy — no hot chocolate and pastry for me at the tearooms. When I go back home and tell my mother, I am given tea and a cake but am not allowed to go on my own to the patisserie any longer, or to Abramowicz, who has the best hot dogs with mustard in town, but I am still allowed to go to the cinema on my own.

There are three separated sections at the cinema, the tickets to the cheapest seats in the front rows costing fifty-five groszy. With a ticket of that kind, you may go into to the cinema whenever you want to, and if you like, it is all right to stay and see the film several times. The first performance begins at three o'clock and goes on for two hours. I watch a film about a large ape called King Kong, whom everyone misunderstands when he defends a lovely young blond woman. I like that film and want to see it over and over again. My anxious parents find me in the darkness of the cinema at half past seven that evening. In future, I have to have an adult with me whenever I go to the cinema.

Most of all, I like it when I stay at a guesthouse alone with Sarah and Pinkus, as then they have lots of time for me. If I go with Sarah, we meet many of her acquaintances and I am allowed to go with them to 'five o'clock dances'. The orchestra plays, many couples dance, some better, others not so well, some very well indeed. I watch them, trying to learn. Sarah is asked to dance but refuses if Pinkus is not there, except sometimes she dances with me, although I am only six. It is tremendous fun, and I also learn something new — it's good to begin early, then you learn better.

Sarah has a lot of acquaintances and friends all over Poland. Mrs. Orzechowska is the only one I know of to survive. When the war starts in 1939, Sarah is thirty-eight and Pinkus fifty-three. Of that generation of Jews, very few survive, and those who do are often younger. At the beginning of the war, Mrs. Orzechowska and her husband have a three-month tourist visa to the USA to go to the world exhibition in New York. It is valid until November 1939, when those with visas to neutral countries are still allowed to leave. We were to meet again thirty-one years later, when for the first time Nina and I and our children are in the States. Mrs. Orzechowska lived with her husband in Miami Beach and was to live a long time and die a natural death.

With great care, Pinkus chooses the moments for our conversations, wanting to be sure we shall not be disturbed. He is serious then, calls me Jurek, which means little Jerzy, or Josele, little Chil Josef, my Hebrew name. "Jurek" — he says — "all human beings are basically good. If people act as if they were not good, they are disturbed. The reason for that may be that something unjust and bad has happened to them, which has disturbed and changed them. You have to feel

The Maple Tree Behind the Barbed Wire

sorry for such people, for they are rarely happy, but there is no reason to hate them. There is no reason in general to hate anyone," Pinkus says to me on another occasion. "Instead, you should try to understand why they behave so badly; there is always an explanation. Understanding helps you yourself, then you don't hate. Hatred damages the person who hates, not the person who is hated." I have absorbed that and it makes my life easier. I can be temporarily agitated, but lack the ability to hate.

"Money, insurance and property do not provide security," says Pinkus. "We have invented money to make our lives easier, to make the exchange of goods and services easier. It is good to have money so that you can live decently, but it should be used. Money is no use if you don't put it to some use. Accumulating money must not be end in itself. Money has no value in itself; there are other values which are more important." We are silent for a moment, then Pinkus goes on. "What is most valuable and lasting is what you have learnt; if you learn properly, then you will always have your knowledge". That, too, was to prove right, not least during the war. Money provided no security, and knowledge was the only thing you could take with you.

On another occasion, Pinkus says: "It is a privilege to be the person who gives to those who need help". "What do you mean, help?" I say. "Any help. If you have helped someone then you will be given it back, sooner or later, and you will also be pleased to be able to help someone else." Pinkus practices what he preaches, sometimes going so far, it seems as if he wants to be exploited. This doesn't worry Pinkus. He has nothing against giving to other people, even if some may think he is being exploited.

When Pinkus talks about various philosophers and writers, I find it hard to keep up. But I realize that when he explains that Gutenberg's invention of the art of printing books is the most important of all inventions. "It makes the preservation and exchange of knowledge possible, makes new knowledge accessible to everyone who can read and wants to learn. Knowledge is the most important asset of humankind," Pinkus says.

Pinkus does not instruct. He reasons with me. Some things I learn from Pinkus by seeing how he behaves, such as he never says anything which is not true, but nor is he in a hurry to say everything he thinks.

Sometimes Pinkus takes me with him to an art exhibition. But I can't distinguish good art from bad and never learn to. Either I have no talent for that, or else Pinkus has started taking me to art exhibitions too young, I thought then, and I still think art exhibitions are boring. But I realize Pinkus knows a lot about art and that other people respect his judgment. Everyone seems to respect my father, although he has never bothered to accumulate money and he cannot write.

The Maple Tree Behind the Barbed Wire

I want to be a tailor and Pinkus wants me to be a tailor, but he says I ought to set about it in a different way from the way he has. "You don't have to have a workshop at home, for instance." No, Pinkus is right, but why does he have his workshop at home? "I have got used to it. It is always difficult to make a break and do something different," says Pinkus. "What suited me when I started doesn't have to suit you, and anyhow times have changed," he says. "But a prerequisite is that you become a good tailor, otherwise you should choose another profession. First you must go to school. You will benefit from that all your life. I never went to a proper school," he says, with no sorrow or loss. "If you want to and have time, you can certainly come to the workshop when you are free from school."

Will my children be as proud of me as I am of my father? Will I ever be able to give my family as much security as Pinkus gives us? I don't think so. I am a fairly uncertain boy when I am seven on July 26th 1932.

The Jewish people of Eastern Europe are going through a transformation, larvae developing into butterflies. After centuries of petrification owing to oppression and isolation, we are in the midst of a process of liberation. It is instructive for a little boy to live in the many separate worlds of this transformation process, the gleaming world of extravagance and artificial luxury of the Wajnapels, the simple prickly world of Maurycy, the world of Jewish mysticism of Szyja and Szprynca - already a world of the past, the rich and joyless world of Ignas Enzel - into which not even the sensuous Bela can bring warmth, so she leaves, the world of my mother — warm, making no demands, over-protective, the world of the fitting room — of the customers, with the big mirror in its gilt frame, the throbbing world of skilled craftsmen in the reality of everyday — handpicked talented men, trained with great care by a master tailor. Josek Lewenreich can be found there, a skilled cutter occasionally allowed to lay with his own hand the foundations of the next suit Pinkus has no time to do, the brothers Berel and Sam Mejerowicz, masters of the needle and thread who have a sister in Belgium, then the quiet smiling hunchback, Garbusek, whose real name is Miodownik, who with his art of pressing can bring every jacket to life, and the always happy singing Sonny Boy, he can do everything but not so well as to be the best at anything, also, Herszkowicz, who is not particularly gifted. Pinkus kept him on because he has six children, taught him to sew buttons on long threads, comfortable to button up, then Grünbaum the presser and the Glicksman brothers. They have all started as apprentices and been allowed to stay, the latest, Chaimek Rotenstein, accepted after a three year apprenticeship, and finally Heniek Moszkowicz, who came last year but will never be a good tailor.

The Maple Tree Behind the Barbed Wire

Anyhow, it does not really matter much, for only Chaimek is to survive the war and later on build up one of the biggest off-the-peg clothing firms in New York, and then Pinkus. My father survives the war and helps his wife and his two children to survive. But the whole of his world irretrievably collapses, his life changes and is fundamentally impoverished. A fragment, a shard of his existence is to remain and he is to hold firmly on to it until the last day of his life, which is to be a long one.

For all these Jewish worlds in which I grew up were all doomed to destruction, with only seven years left to live. Mein Kampf is already written, its author Adolf Hitler has won the latest election in Germany and his party is the largest in the German parliament. Adolf Hitler has already widespread and increasing support in the business world and heavy industry, to whom he promises large orders for arms. There are only a few months until January 1933 when what happens is what everyone has been waiting for, the old president Hindenburg summons Adolf Hitler to him and offers him the post of Chancellor. With that, all Hitler's predictions are fulfilled: he is to acquire power via the democratic
route in order then to abolish democracy — and "once and for all" solve the Jewish problem.

There are Jewish schools but it is difficult to get into university from a Jewish school. Sarah wants me to have a good start in life and go to the best school in our town. Zofja Wygórska Folwasinska's school is a private school with high fees and a good reputation. Sarah wants me to have friends and feel secure in Polish society, and that I shall be able to continue at a state gymnasium, preferably Traugutt's gymnasium, then, before I return to tailoring go to university.

At the end of August 1932, a week before I was to start school, Pinkus walks round the fitting room with me. It is dusk, the lights are out and we walk slowly to and fro. After a while Pinkus says: "Jurek, when you start school, you will be shorter and physically weaker than the other boys in your class. It is possible that you will also be slower at learning than the other boys — all the men in our family develop late. But don't give up, you will catch up with the others in the class." I say nothing. That I am behind my contemporaries in most things is nothing new and hitherto it has not worried me.

We go on silently walking to and fro as it gets darker and the street lights go on. I realise Pinkus has something more to say. "You see," he says after a while, "people are different, nor are any two leaves on the same tree the same either. When a cow gives birth to a calf, the calf can stand on its own legs, and an hour or two later it can already walk, but it becomes nothing but a cow or an ox. When a human child is born, it is helpless and cannot manage on its own for several years, but it becomes a human being who can learn to speak, read, write, build a house and make suits. So don't be downhearted if at first you find it all difficult to follow." This is what Pinkus says to me, who has grown up in a protected environment and in a week's time I am to be sent out into the hard world where my parents can no longer protect me.

These words of Pinkus' remain in my memory even today, and help me. Things were to turn out to be exactly as he had said. But Pinkus does not tell me everything about the reality I am to face at the Polish school. We live in a segregated society, the Christian and the Jewish worlds separated from each other. When in 1930s, they begin to meet, it seldom goes well, particularly for the Jews. Pinkus says nothing about this, perhaps not even knowing what to say, for Pinkus is like that, rarely pronouncing on things he does not know for certain.

My memories from my childhood are bright and warm. Sarah gives me unlimited and uncritical love, and everything I do is good. She over-protects me — what does that matter? She teaches me to love and to dare to show it. Nina, my wife, benefits from that. My father gives me security, treats me seriously and shares his wisdom with me, most of all on what relations between people should be like, but also about what is important in life.

We cannot choose our parents. Some people are lucky, others not. I was lucky, but there is a fly in every ointment. It turns out that there are quite a lot of flies when you are growing up as a Jewish boy in 1930s Poland and have to leave your sheltered home.

The Maple Tree Behind the Barbed Wire

An Unwelcome Guest

When I describe the world outside my sheltered Jewish childhood environment, I have problems with my identity. During my childhood, I regard myself as a Pole. When I come across the Polish - non-Jewish world — at school, I realize, at first with some confusion, then, with despair, that I am not regarded as Polish, but as a Jew, at best a Polish Jew. Everywhere, even in the school register I am given as "of the Mosaic faith". Jew in Polish is a term of abuse, of the Mosaic faith a slightly more cultivated description of a Jew. All the teachers are Roman Catholics, as are the majority of pupils; a few are Protestant - and all of them are Poles. But Jews are Jews and not Poles - not a single one of my classmates would seriously accept it if I maintain I am a Pole.

Even after the war, when I again start school in Czestochowa, the class teacher's first question to the entire class is "Wyznanie" — profession of faith. Then I no longer bother about being pointed out as a Jew.

In Poland, I have reluctantly learnt to accept that I am not considered to be a Pole. Not until I go to Sweden do I become a Pole, not a Polish Jew, but a Pole. All the time I was growing up I wanted to be a Pole - but was not allowed to be. Not until I leave Poland and go to Sweden does a Swedish policeman convince me that I am a Pole. That explains why when I write about the time when I was growing up I talk about Poles without considering myself a Pole.

I have come across the world of Poles before I start school, but only sporadically and at a distance. Many of Pinkus' customers are Poles, elegant gentlemen who often bring their ladies with them. Trousers are not made at Pinkus' workshop, but at the home of a tailor who specializes in them. He is a Pole and I meet him when he comes to fetch cloth and to deliver almost finished trousers for fitting and finishing off at Pinkus' workshop. He is still in Czestochowa after the war, and outside his tailor's business and ready-made clothing shop is a large notice which says: Previous Member of the Firm of Einhorn.

Both Jews and Poles live in the building in Second Aleja 29. All policemen are Poles and every week the local policeman comes to be given his compensation for closing his eyes to the fact that the business is shut on Saturdays and is working on Sundays. In the streets, I see soldiers saluting officers, and all the officers seem to be Poles, but I have heard that there are occasional Jewish officers. When a subordinate soldier meets an officer, he is to salute smartly and the officer is to respond with an easy, rather sloppy salute. I wonder what it feels like to be an officer and see all passing soldiers saluting.

Marshall Jósef Pilsudski, undisputed leader of the country, is a Pole. He became leader of Poland at the liberation on November 11th 1918, then stepped down voluntarily, but took over power again in an undramatic and bloodless coup in 1926, when the elected parliament turned out to be incapable of making decisions over the constant struggles between the different factions. Parliament is still elected, the president has primarily ceremonial duties and everyone knows it is Marshall Pilsudski who makes the decisions. He is a taciturn, generally respected and appreciated charismatic leader and can be regarded as just. Shortly after the liberation of Poland, he gives the Jews full citizen's right and does not wish to hear of any persecution of minorities, at least not with physical force. Some people maintain he has been married to a Jewess, others that he has a Jewish mother, which is what we Jews say about Poles who are kind or at least fair to us. When the news comes that Marshall Pilsudski has died, Sarah, Pinkus and I go to Kraków. We stand in a long queue to pay our last respects to the man lying there in state in a glass-covered coffin in Wawel, the fortress of the old Polish kings. Pilsudski, experienced as a guarantee of some kind of just state power, is succeeded by a military junta, which forms a government with the support of the officer corps and the aristocracy. After Pilsudski's death, discrimination and the persecution of the Jews increases in Poland and I experience my first pogrom.

Czestochowa is dominated by the great Pauline monastery, Jasna Góra, with its sacred image of the Black Madonna - the Virgin Mary with a long scar on her left cheek. It is said to have bled when the image suffered a wound from a soldier's saber, and the heroic defense by the monks takes up several pages in our history books. According to our school textbooks, this is the place where the Poles took the sting out of the Swedish invasion in the seventeenth century. The sacred image of the Black Madonna, the monastery of Jasna Góra and with that Czestochowa is the leading place of pilgrimage for Roman Catholics in Poland. Thousands of pilgrims come, the majority on foot in endlessly long lines, singing spiritual songs as they walk along the First, Second and Third Aleja leading to the monastery. Then they stay in Czestochowa, the majority in large tents at the foot of the monastery hill; sometimes in a religious frenzy they may smash the windows of Jewish shops and sometimes they may strike a Jew.

I have understood why people may hit Jews, perhaps not legally, but in practice. According to a statement by an early Pope, we Jews are to blame for the death of Jesus over nineteen hundred years ago and all Jews bear a collective guilt, as the priests say when they preach in the monastery.

Jews in Czestochowa prefer not to live in ground floor apartments and try to protect their premises with heavy metal shutters. When the pilgrimage season starts in the late spring and large groups of pilgrims walk through the streets of Czestochowa, many of the Jewish shops are closed. It is safest that way. The shopkeepers forego income so as not to risk losing everything they possess, including their health and lives. Insurance does not cover damage done during pogroms; these are called riots and no insurance policies cover damage done during riots. For a few days I find out what a nightmare a pogrom is.

In his sermon during Easter Communion, the officiating monk excites the crowds by saying that Jews take blood from a Christian child for our Easter bread — matzes. Pinkus says that cannot be true; our religion strictly forbids us to eat red meat. Later I was to understand that Jesus also ate matzes for seven days every year, as well as at the last supper with his disciples. But at the time I did not know Jesus was a Jew; they don't talk about that in Poland and even Pinkus does not tell me. For if I were to say that to a Pole, anything could happen as it could be taken as blasphemy.

We live on the first floor in the Second Aleja and we can hear the pilgrims' cries and religious songs. They sing as they smash the windows. Before Sarah pulls me away from the window, I have time to see excited crowds getting hold of a Jew and they don't stop beating him up although he is lying bleeding in the street. Mostly younger men, but also middle-aged men and women are running down the streets, calling out loudly, throwing stones and seeking out their victims.

In the evening, a Christian woman who lives in our building tells us that several murdered Jews have been left lying in the streets, quite near our building, too, worst of all in ulica Garncarska, in the centre of the old Jewish quarter. I see the police watching what is happening without intervening. We know it is not worth calling the police; there is no one to turn to for help. Not until late in the afternoon of the second day of the pogrom are the police given orders to clean up the streets, and they do so within an hour. Why does it take so long before the police intervene and stop the pogrom? Are we Jews not citizens of the country? Have the police no duty to protect us?

I shall never forget those two terrifying days. Long after the pogrom, I am frightened of everyone who is not a Jew. But sooner or later, I have to leave my sheltered environment and face the Polish world.

A few days before school starts, Sarah dresses me in my sailor suit with its wide collar and we go together to meet the headmistress of my future school. We are tense as we meet Mrs. Wygórska - the daughter of the founder of the school — in her office. Three pictures are on the wall behind her desk, President Móscicki in the middle, Marshall Pilsudski in his grey general's uniform on the left and Mrs. Zofja Wygórska Folwasinska, founder of the school on the right. In one corner of the room is a dark polished walnut filing cabinet with a discreet lock, on the floor a thick carpet, the visitor's chairs are comfortable, the light subdued, the thick curtains not fully drawn back - I have a feeling that the same furniture, pictures and curtains have always been in this room. The room is dominated by the headmistress' big desk, on which lies a single sheet of paper — registration for Jurek Einhorn - though here I am to be called Jerzy.

Mrs. Wygórska in a black dress, black buttoned boots, wide white cuffs and a starched high white collar, assures Sarah with great conviction in her voice that she will make sure Jerzy gets into Traugutt gymnasium. Then she looks at me. I feel small, but at the same time it feels safe with this important person promising Sarah to look after me and that all will go well.

But it does not. In future only extremely rarely do I catch a glimpse of the headmistress, and then always at a distance. Over the following years she is never to say a word to me and I am never again invited into her office. In the end, I do get into Traugutt gymnasium, but in quite a different way from what my parents had intended and without the help of Mrs. Wygórska and her school.

My memories of the four and a half years spent in the Polish school are indistinct, hidden in merciful oblivion, in contrast to my memories from the years before and after. Later on, I learnt that we human beings have a wonderful ability to forget, even deny unpleasant experiences.

All the pupils at Zofja Wygórska Folwasinska's school wear identical uniforms. We are expected to wear it not only in school but always whenever outside our homes. Although we wear similar uniforms, we are nevertheless different. I soon discover that I am a deviant, do not belong, and there are two others treated in the same way as I am. They are also Jews.

Kazik Czestochowski, Tomek Zygman and I - Jerzy Einhorn - are the three Jews in the class. Kazik and I sometimes talk to each other but we do not mix, have nothing much in common, and he also lives in a small community several kilometers outside Czestochowa, so we can't meet outside school. Kazik's parents are poor — that can be seen from his clothes and from the lunch he brings with him to school. They must have made great sacrifices for Kazik to be able to go to this fine school. Tomek Zygman hardly speaks to any of the pupils in the class and no one talks to Tomek. His parents must be wealthy, for he is fetched from school by a chauffeur-driven car when the weather is bad or if there is unrest in the streets of Czestochowa.

In my memory my school friends have no faces, and the only names I remember are Rysiek Erbel and Beate. Rysiek is the only one to have anything to do with me and he does so openly. He has been back home to us several times but I have never been invited to his home. Rysiek is one of the strong boys in the class, not the strongest, but he is unafraid and dares to behave towards me in a different way from that of the others, but he does not go so far as to defend me. Nor can anyone expect that in a Polish school in 1930s Poland.

The Maple Tree Behind the Barbed Wire

I quickly realize that Kazik, Tomek and I are regarded as less good people than any of the others in the class and I begin to accept it. I understand that all Jews are less good people; I am a Jewish boy and must be prepared to live with that. But the worst thing for an uncertain seven year-old boy is not to exist to his school friends. If they notice me in the breaks, then it is because I am being troublesome in some way.

It is unusual for things to come to blows, for this is a grand school. I once try to defend myself against their contempt. I hit back at Janek, the boy who has just pushed me. We roll round in the dusty schoolyard. A circle of boys and a few girls forms, "give him one, go on, give him a Nelson", they all cheer Janek on, although he is not usually particularly popular; not a single one cheers for me. Rysiek is standing a little way away, saying nothing. But that unconcealed contempt breaks through with brutal clarity and makes me despair. I feel alone and to my horror I begin to cry. I go on fighting, but am profoundly humiliated because I am crying. Although I have the upper hand, I give up just to put an end to the unendurable collective scorn and their collective hatred.

They all go away. I am left lying in the dust of the schoolyard, no one showing any interest in me. How shall I explain my torn clothes when I get home? No one complains about such things, either to the teacher or parents; one is simply ashamed. I hope Pinkus and Sarah will not find out; to be beaten is humiliating and yet not unnatural, for after all, I am a Jew.

Boys and girls go in the same class, but the girls mix with girls and the boys with boys. In the second and third class, when we are a little older, it happens more and more frequently that a girl speaks to a boy, but not to me. Once at the beginning of my third year, during the long breakfast break, Beata speaks to me. I flush — with pleasure. We exchange a few sentences about school and our homes, but that's enough, I fall in love immediately. Before I go to sleep I like to think of something pleasant, so I think about Beate's pale little freckled face and fantasize about us talking to each other, my semi-conscious thoughts drift into sleep and I dream we are holding hands. A boy soon to be ten needs to think about girls and who should I think about if not Beata. She has spoken to me only once, but I like to imagine she occasionally smiles at me in a friendly and encouraging way.

My mother has great expectations, the latest that I shall learn to play the violin — if Jascha Heifetz can, then Sarah's Jurek must be able to. After school I have to stay with a group of pupils who have private lessons from the school's uninterested music teacher. Worse still is when I have to go back to the school for my extra lessons in music. I play false notes, my fingers ache and I find it difficult to hold the violin under my chin, I complain, but am not allowed to give it up. It's always difficult at the beginning, says Sarah. You will soon enjoy it and when you grow up you will be grateful that you were allowed to learn to play the violin.

My torment does not cease until Sarah is to show me off to her acquaintances. I stand on a wooden stool in the living room to play Kuba do Jakuba - Brother Jacob, and I saw away on the violin, working my way through the short melody. Pinkus looks attentively at me, but without his usual gentle smile. A little while after this "concert", he takes Sarah aside and the very next day I don't have to go to music lessons. I am relieved and grateful, but a day or two later feel a stab of resentment. Had Sarah not seen how much I loathed those boring music lessons? Could Pinkus not have intervened earlier?

Over these years I must have been an obedient and easily handled child, but I have difficulty finishing up my food, sometimes sitting alone for hours at the table, still chewing away after all the others have left. My parents are worried. I am taken to Dr Kluczewski, then to several other doctors, at first in Czestochowa, then to various specialists in Warsaw. All they find is that I have a slight temperature in the evenings. A doctor in Warsaw takes out my tonsils; it hurts horribly but makes no difference. In the end Sarah, Pinkus and I go to the rabbi, a worthy elderly man with a beard and clothes like Grandfather's. I don't know if it was the rabbi who gave Sarah the relieving advice that she should stop taking my temperature every evening.

We have acquired a new radio, which does not crackle and is run on six unusual-looking bulbs in a box behind the loudspeaker, which give off a special though not at all unpleasant smell. One day we are all sitting by our radio set, listening to a man with a hoarse provocative voice; he is speaking German, but I understand what he is saying — it resembles Yiddish. He is shrieking mostly about Germany: das Reich, das deutsche Volk, but also about Jews. We are the cause of all the misery on earth, we are the greatest danger to the Third Reich, we control international capital. He yells hysterically that the Jewish problem has to be solved once and for all; it is his and the German people's task to solve it.

Is he talking about Pinkus and Sarah, about me and my little brother Roman, who is three? The man yelling on the radio is called Adolf Hitler, his name alone ominous. He has recently come into power in Germany. Neighbors and acquaintances say he is mad and will not grow old as Chancellor of Germany. But Pinkus is worried.

At the same time a stream of Jewish refugees arrive from Germany. The first group of them have lived in Germany for a long time but kept their Polish citizenship. Then come the Jews who have no valid papers to say they are German citizens, and finally German citizens who have

The Maple Tree Behind the Barbed Wire

relatives in Poland. They are all tipped out at the German-Polish border, and then chased across it into Poland. Many of them come to Czestochowa, dead poor and frightened by what they have seen. The refugees are given help by Zydowska Gmina, the Jewish Congregation, are found quarters in Jewish homes until they acquire homes of their own. There are collections and attempts made to find work and schools for the young — the new arrivals are slowly incorporated into the Polish-Jewish community and Adolf Hitler is increasingly the subject of conversation.

The school library has received a book which the entire class has been waiting for — w Pustyni i w Puszczy, "Through the Desert", an adventure story for young people by the Nobel Prize winner Henryk Sienkiewicz - everyone in the class wants to be the first to borrow it. Our teacher says the loan will be after the breakfast break and we may borrow the book in alphabetical order and keep it for four days at the most. In the break, five boys come up to me and say menacingly: "Don't you dare borrow it first. You can have it after all the others" — several more are standing at distance, looking on. This becomes the general subject of conversation in the class. Rysiek Erbel tells me it would be best if I don't borrow it first. But I very much want to read this exciting book. Why shouldn't I make the most of being first in alphabetical order and not have to wait three or four months - that's unfair.

When break is over I get the book out and am pleased that I dared, but the price to pay is to be high. Open hatred breaks out and the boys in the class threaten to beat me up. After the last lesson, the majority of them are waiting for me outside the school, not hurrying home as usual. In the distance some girls wait to see what is going to happen.

The teacher says I may not go home, that I must stay at school after lessons. She has telephoned my parents and told them not to worry. The teacher stays with me, but after an hour, she says she must go home and that the caretaker will look after me. I stay there until the evening and my classmates have all left the street outside the entrance to the school — only then do I dare go home. But I have the book and am looking forward to reading it, still feeling proud of my courage and say nothing about it to my parents. That is my last memory of Zofja Wygórska Folwasinska's school — of my visit as an unwelcome intruder among children in a Polish school.

I meet Rysiek Erbel on one more occasion when he is on a visit to Sweden twenty-eight years after the end of the war. He tells me about the difficulties my previous classmates have had during the war, but also that everyone in the class has survived, everyone except Kazik and Tomek.

Back to Fellowship

I am ten; Roman just four — two rooms and kitchen behind the workshop are now too small for our growing family. It is cramped in the tailoring workshop too, and we can afford a larger apartment. In the autumn of 1935, we move from Second Aleja 29 to the larger and more comfortable apartment in Aleja Wolnosci 3/5 - Freedom Avenue.

In connection with our move, I have a stomachache. At first our felczer - Mr. Feldman - is summoned, a doctor's assistant with some surgical training, a middle-aged, thin-haired, quite powerful man who seems to have a lot of practical knowledge acquired from long experience and who radiates human warmth as well as conveying confidence.

Mr. Feldman questions Sarah and then feels my stomach, frowns, says worriedly that I will be examined by a surgeon. The young surgeon, Dr Szperling, questions me, feels my stomach, takes my temperature, shakes his head and summons an older surgeon——two doctors are to examine me at the same time. This seems increasingly worrying. The older surgeon asks the same questions, again feels my stomach, and finally says it is not inconceivable that I have appendicitis — he is not entirely sure, but one should not leave it too long. The two doctors and my parents then leave the room to carry on their deliberations and no one explains anything to me, for I am only ten. I lie there fantasizing, starting out from what I have heard them saying, but also from what I have previously heard about others who have had appendicitis. What does an appendix look like? Is it short or long? Why do we have an appendix? What happens if it is removed? How do they remove it? Do they have to cut up my stomach? I lift up the bedclothes and look at my smooth stomach, then start feeling it, but feel nothing except a slight tenderness down on the right hand side.

A few years back, a boy at our school had died from a burst appendix. The year before, a girl had recovered, but had had to stay in hospital with tubes in her stomach for several weeks for all the pus from the burst appendix to run out and the hole in her stomach could be sewn up. A tube in your stomach for several weeks? My fantasies become more and more terrifying. I can feel my appendix swelling up and bursting, the pus running out into my stomach and settling round my intestines. Every possible alternative seems threatening, an operation or a burst appendix, or both. In a cold sweat, as I lie there on my sofa in our big living room, I try to calm myself by studying the details in the big Wilenski picture of a whole lot of old trees in a forest on the wall opposite my bed. I try to read my book — but that does not work very well.

The Maple Tree Behind the Barbed Wire

In 1936, a burst appendix and peritonitis were serious ailments, often with fatal consequences. We have not yet learnt to produce penicillin, and sulfa drugs had not been invented. Without the help of modern medicine, the body has always found it difficult to deal with pus in the abdomen, and many young and old died a painful death. So doctors were keen to operate — removing the appendix even with only faintly suspected appendicitis. But they were not so keen on explaining, least of all to children. In cases of severe illness, they often did not even inform adults, only relatives. This was comfortable for the doctor, but cruel to the patient, who is then isolated, handed over to his fantasies and through lies shut off from seriously discussing his condition and his anxieties.

There is nothing more instructive than one's own memories and experiences, as long as one has the ability to remember and empathize with other people's feelings, so realize that they may feel the same way. I think and hope that the paralysing terror I experienced as a boy during those days has influenced my attitude as a conveyer of knowledge to my patients when after many years I myself become a doctor.

A few days later we go to the hospital and I am operated on without being told much more. It is frightening, but not so horrible as I had thought it would be. When I come round after the operation, everyone is tiptoeing round and being very considerate to me. I may not drink and several days go by before I can take any solid food or be allowed up for a while. I am not allowed to leave hospital for nine days, after they have taken out the last stitches. I must not exert myself, they warn me, nor go to school for several weeks. That's what happened to patients who had had abdominal surgery in the 1930s.

But I soon recover and go out to play in the courtyard. Aleja Wolosci 3/5, which I am beginning to get to know for the first time, is a gigantic building with a large inner courtyard divided into two, where the children play and I meet Maniek Rosen.

In Czestochowa there are two Jewish schools, Zydowska Buda - the Jewish School - run by a foundation with several good schools all over the country, and the private school, Axera, largely for girls. At the Polish school, I hear occasionally that the boys would gather together after lessons to go out and fight the boys at the Jewish School. It sounded tough, although I realize that they were mostly teasing. For that matter, are Jews allowed to hit back?

Maniek Rosen goes to the Jewish School. He has thick wild black hair, calm dark blue eyes, he moves in a leisurely way, is strong and confident, and I find it's all right to wrestle in Maniek's good-natured way; we can do that to test out our strengths without starting to fight seriously. He is like a friendly bear cub and can afford to be like that because he is so strong — just think that there are such Jewish boys.

The Maple Tree Behind the Barbed Wire

Maniek is in the fourth class at the Jewish School, in the same class as I am. One day, Maniek takes me with him to his school and we go into his class when the long lunch break begins. Several of the pupils talk to me openly, as if with an old acquaintance although I am only visiting. Even the girls talk to me, looking me in the eye and laughing. All of them have faces, friendly faces, all of them have names, which I find easy to remember. It is obvious I am accepted among these Jewish boys and girls, with no fuss, in a natural way. I am one of them after only thirty-five minutes in break between lessons.

No one tries to persuade me to change schools, for no one needs to. When I get home I say to Sarah that I refuse to go back to my old school, not even once, not even to fetch my books; I never want to set foot in it again.

Sarah hesitates but does not object, which I appreciate. It is clever of her not to try, as that would have been no use. What is wrong is that I had not known beforehand that there was any alternative, and that I had been so oppressed. In the middle of the school year, I change schools and register at the Jewish School without even meeting the headmaster, for there is no need to.

We are two to each desk. I sit next to Heniek Ufner in the last row but one, nearest the door. Behind us in the back row are red-haired Wladek Kopinski and Edzio Zandsztajn with his hair plastered down with water, in front of us two girls, Pola Schlesinger and Rózyczka Glowinska.

I quickly adapt, wanting to make up in a short time for all the comradeship I had missed previously without knowing it was so near and so easily accessible. Now I can go up to any group — no one falls silent, no one turns his or her back on me. My classmates come back home with me and I go home to them. We play the popular game of Tiddlywinks. I am fairly good at it, for I am a tailor's son with a large selection of buttons. I begin to take an interest in girls and like to think they are interested in me. I like it all.

Perhaps you have to experience being frozen out and a deviant to be able to appreciate what the majority take for granted — to be accepted and included in their fellowship.

I have fallen behind with schoolwork because of being ill and have a lot to catch up. I also have to take up new subjects - Hebrew, the history of the Jews, the Bible and religious knowledge. Despite this, I behave lightheartedly. During lessons I mostly sit thinking and I have no time for homework, so I get poor marks. Sarah is troubled after every visit to the school, but I am not. I am beginning to gain more self-confidence, becoming aware of what I really want to do, I also do it.

The Maple Tree Behind the Barbed Wire

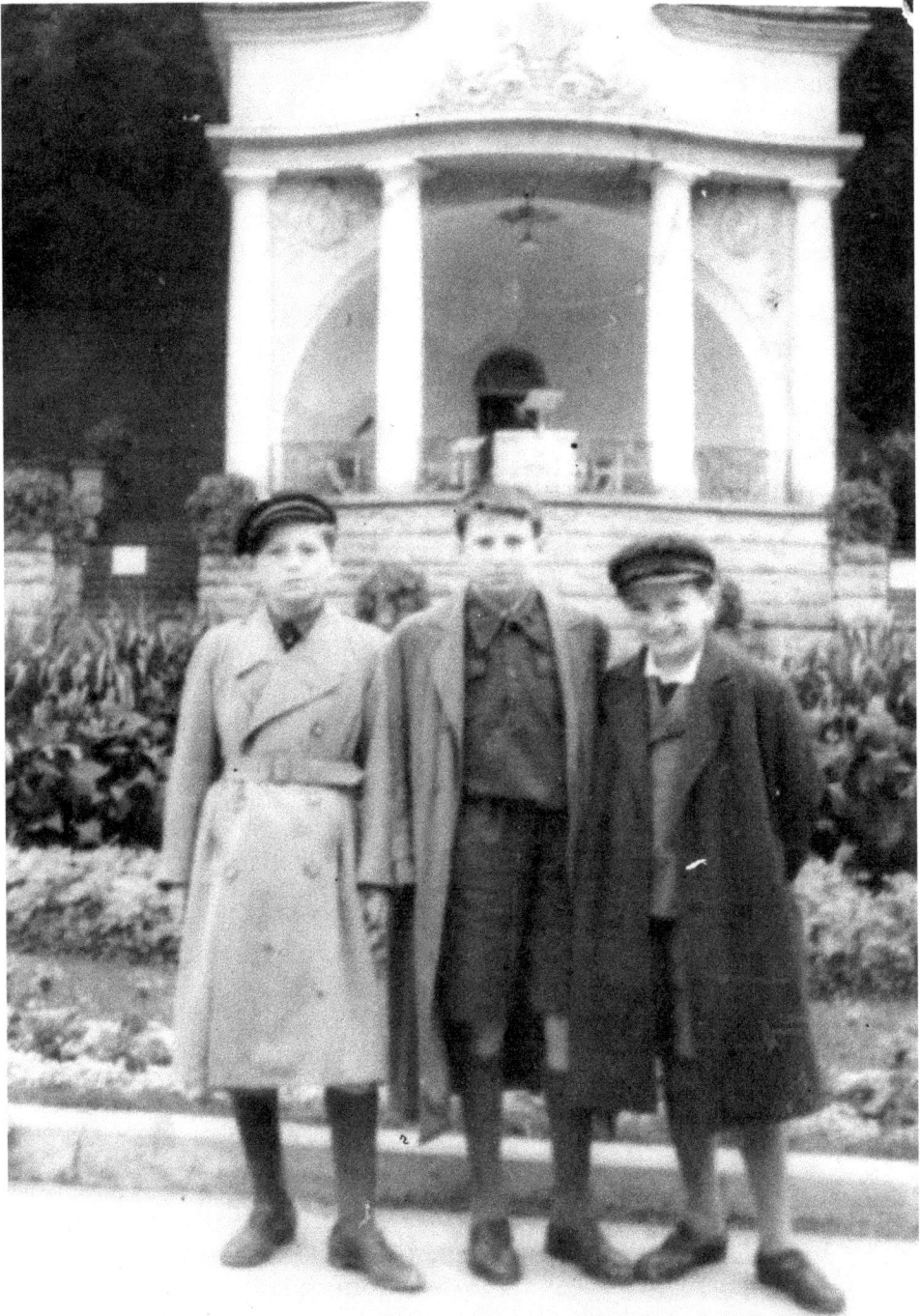

When I go to the Jewish School, in a very short time I am to make up for all the comradeship I lacked at the Polish School. I have grown and am no longer one of the smallest boys in the class

The Maple Tree Behind the Barbed Wire

Time passes, happy-go-lucky months and years. I meet my friends, am mostly with girls and like their company, and I am often the only boy among them. There is domineering Doska Ferenc, gentle Stusia Najmark, silent Rózyczka Glowinska, powerful Pola Schlesinger, beautiful jolly Bronka Mass and beautiful serious Hanka Bugajer - opinions are divided among the boys as to which of these two is the most beautiful in the class. One evening Dóska and I are kissing — she is the one to take the initiative — but I fall in love with gentle, always friendly Stusia Najmark. We meet every day, sometimes I kiss Stusia behind a cupboard — an innocent childish love affair.

I still have no time to do my homework. It has gone so far that our kind flat-footed geography teacher, Professor Schaffer (all schoolteachers in Poland are called professor) summons me up to the map hanging on the wall - Einhorn, Einhorn, come here and I shall question you and you can display your usual ignorance and be given a two. I manage to get into the gymnasium by the skin of my teeth with threes in all subjects — the lowest marks to pass. But I go on at the same school and keep the same school friends, the same fellowship.

There are two entrances to our apartment, one through the main entrance on the street and up to our first floor apartment via the wide stairway, then first into a large hall. Straight ahead is the door to the fitting room, on the left a door to the big workshop and on the right two doors to Roman's and Rózia's rooms. From the inner courtyard's narrower stairway, you go straight into the kitchen and our other rooms — the living room and my parents' bedroom. We no longer have to go through the fitting room to get to our living quarters. Roman has been moved from my parents' bedroom and has a room of his own. I am still sleeping on the sofa in the living room. Rózia - Sarah's next to youngest sister — has moved in with us, and the youngest, Karola, periodically also lives with us, sharing a room with Rózia.

Rózia and Karola are the only unmarried ones of the large crop of siblings. Rózia has straight, smooth black hair, large moist brown eyes, faultless light skin and a nasal voice. She is slightly plump and never goes to a hairdresser — she does her hair herself and does not dress all that smartly, although Sarah tries to help her, and she usually wears low-heeled shoes. Rózia is serious, gentle and kind, but not as beautiful as the other sisters. She has no beau courting her and seldom goes out. Karola is also unmarried, but she is younger, jolly, extroverted and flirtatious. Several young men are courting Karola, but she hopes for Heniek Epstein, the dark-haired bookkeeper in Pinkus' workshop.

I am pleased when Karola comes to Czestochowa. I try to get her to come with me for a walk in the deptak — the promenade stretch for

The Maple Tree Behind the Barbed Wire

schoolchildren on the wide Second Aleja. Young Jewish people promenade on the right hand side of the Third Aleja, where the big Pazderski clock hangs above the entrance to the apothecary with the same name, and young people from the Polish schools promenade along the left hand side — no one would even consider walking on the wrong side of the street. The adults stroll along the middle stretch beneath the shade of the trees, and mothers with their small children sit on the comfortable green wooden benches the local council puts out in the spring. I am proud when I am able to show myself under the Pazderski clock with the slightly older, elegant, merry and beautiful Karola.

I like Rózia, although she is so quiet. It is Rózia who looks after us in the evenings when our parents go out. When Roman has gone to sleep and I have gone to bed with a book, Rózia may come in to the living room, sit down on my sofa and comb my untidy light brown hair. We say nothing on these occasions, but I like her standing beside me or sitting on my sofa combing my hair before she goes in and closes the door to her room. Sometimes I fantasize about touching her, thinking about what she looks like under her clothes — on one occasion I have seen Rózia coming out of the bathroom in a short white, partly unbuttoned bathrobe and she was naked underneath the bathrobe. I never think like that about Karola, or about any of my girl friends of my age.

I am often in the workshop, even more often in the long holidays when I don't have to go to school and my school friends are away. Those who work in the workshop also have more space now; in fact nothing very much has changed otherwise — the same robust, friendly and professional atmosphere. They talk about what is happening in Germany, about Adolf Hitler and the Jewish refugees he has chased out of his country, about the many Jews going to Palestine, but also about there being mostly stony desert and marshy land there, malaria and that it is very hot. Yet the country attracts many young Jews, halucim — pioneers, usually young boys and girls, who go to the Promised Land in large groups, the land the Jews had to leave almost two thousand years ago. They cultivate the stony ground, drain the marshes, build and arm rural villages surrounded by palisades — kibbutzim — where they share the work and their limited assets equally.

Pinkus again spends more time teaching me tailoring. He is pleased I am often in the workshop. He asks his various assistants to teach me their specialties, but I am still too small for Garbusek to show me how to press a jacket. I am often with Pinkus in the evenings, when, alone in the workshop and undisturbed by other duties, with great care and concentration he cuts the cloth for suits that are to be made — he usually does the cutting himself. "It's strategically important," he says to me. "It's at the cutting table the suit is shaped. If you don't get it right from the beginning, it is difficult, sometimes impossible, to correct it later.

Pinkus also talks about Palestine. We can't go there ourselves. It is too hot. Pinkus says he can't work where it is hot. And anyhow, for whom would he make suits for in Palestine. The clothes Jews wear there are shirts and trousers, the Arabs wear full length gowns, and what would happen to his assistants — he knows a lot about the private lives and troubles of his employees.

There is a lot of talk about Palestine at school as well, about hachsharah, the special preparatory camps for the halucim who are to go there, about life in the Jewish settlements. A special organization collects up money to help the settlers buy land they can cultivate, and plant trees to make the country more habitable — the organization is called Kerem Kajemet. In every Jewish home — rich or poor — there is a characteristic Kerem Kajemet blue and white metal box into which money can be put. Sarah puts in a coin every time she has been shopping. When acquaintances come visiting they put in a banknote instead of buying flowers, and when they play cards they put their winnings into the blue and white metal box. Every six months, a young woman comes and empties the box with a special key, counts the money and leaves a receipt - Sarah adds one or more banknotes if she thinks it is too little. Pinkus also signs for a larger contribution to the annual collection for a newly formed organization — the Jewish Agency, or Keren Hayesod -- which helps Jews to leave countries where they are threatened and persecuted, now mostly from Germany.

That is what we can do — collect money — the halucim who go there are the real heroes. In a single day they have to build up the core of the settlement surrounded by a fortified palisade so that they can defend it when night falls. Imagine armed Jews? Possessing arms and owning and cultivating land have been forbidden to Jews in Poland, Russia and other countries for hundreds of years. The new heroes are emissaries from the Jewish Agency. They are Jews, the majority already living in Palestine, who are sent out to countries where there are persecuted Jews and their task is to help them escape.

Why do we cling to this bit of land where almost no one wants to live? We discuss this at our school. It is the only soil we Jews can be thought to have any historical rights to, the only land to which we can maintain that we return, even if that happens after almost two thousand years. Once upon a time we were driven out of our land to Babylon and we managed to return, so perhaps we can succeed once again. Then we were chased out there by the Romans - by Vespasianus and Titus, both of whom became Roman emperors — because our forefathers wanted to adhere to their religion and their traditions. They rebelled against images of alien gods being put up in their temple. We are not allowed images of our own god — that is

The Maple Tree Behind the Barbed Wire

forbidden according to our religion and tradition — so even more difficult to accept images of alien gods in our temple.

In the Diaspora, we go on clinging to our religion and our traditions, with no country of our own, scattered and persecuted all over the world since Masada, the last of our fortresses in Judaea, fell in AD 73. In our prayers, ever since then we pray twice a day that we shall be allowed to return. Though I don't pray, nor does Pinkus. Sarah prays every Friday evening, a short prayer while she lights the traditional candles as a Jewish housewife is to do before the Sabbath dinner — though I think she mostly prays for her family and not for us to be allowed to return to Palestine. Sarah is rather scared by the thought of Palestine.

Meanwhile, black clouds are gathering over happy-go-lucky Europe. You can feel in the air that there will soon be an explosion, but where will the lightning strike, and who will be affected? Apart from Adolf Hitler, new names keep cropping up: Hermann Göring, Joseph Goebbels, Rudolf Hess. Hitler's speeches become increasingly hysterical, shriller than ever in tone, and whatever he is talking about he finally comes to us Jews. The newsreels at the cinema show German troops marching into the Rhineland, which is worrying, but perhaps reasonable as they have a right to rule over their own land. Hitler wins the election in the Saar and he and his party are clearly popular — the Saar is then incorporated into Germany. Then it is Austria's turn. Hitler shrieks that Austria is part of the German Reich and he himself is Austrian. New names are mentioned in the papers and heard on the radio — first Dollfuss, who is murdered, then von Schuschnigg, who bravely makes a stand in Vienna, but in vain. He is given no help and hardly any encouragement from other countries. Hitler's tanks roll on and heavily armed German troops march into Austria, to be greeted with enthusiasm by those who go out on to the streets. The others sit silently in their homes, perhaps frightened, but they are not mentioned in the papers, nor are they visible on the news reels. The world looks on, but does not react, except possibly with a sigh of helplessness. The only one to question the annexing of Austria is Benito Mussolini, Italy's fascist dictator, but Hitler gets him to accept being a neighbor of Greater Germany.

Hitler speaks again — he now thinks the Sudeten Germans have been treated badly by the Czechs, and he cannot tolerate that. Once again the radio, the newspapers and the newsreels are filled with new names - Edvard Benes, the Czech Prime Minister in Prague, who resists. It is not so easy with Czechoslovakia. The country has the sympathies of the entire free world, but most of all Czechoslovakia's farsighted people and government, in contrast to the rest of Europe, have built up a strong modern defense system, mobilized its small but prepared for action army, its air force and tanks. The country also has a binding defense treaty with one of the great powers, with France.

The Maple Tree Behind the Barbed Wire

Hitler shrieks and threatens, the British Prime Minister, Neville Chamberlain, appeals to him from London, but Chamberlain has to take the trouble to go to Germany himself if he wants to talk to Hitler. And Neville Chamberlain - prime minister of the leading great power and the British Empire - goes, bows to Hitler and gives away Sudetenland, and with that an allied country - Czechoslovakia.

When Hitler begins to arm, Czechoslovakia has also switched its high-tech heavy industry, primarily the Skoda and Tatra works, to arms production. The country has built up modern defenses with tanks, planes, well-trained and motivated soldiers and a well-educated command. Apart from Germany, Czechoslovakia is the only country in Europe with modern defenses — and, in the Sudeten mountains, a strongly fortified, difficult to penetrate border to Germany. With what right does the British prime minister — for a piece of paper, for an empty promise he calls "peace in our time" — give away another country's territory? Hitler assures Chamberlain that apart from Sudetenland, he has no other territorial claims in Europe, and as long as he has that, he will be satisfied — if he is left in peace and is not provoked, Hitler stresses. All he wants is Sudeten Germany, that natural, strongly fortified wall of defense, the best equipped, highly industrialized country in Central Europe.

Josef Stalin, leader of the Soviet Union, says from Moscow that he does not think anyone should give way to Hitler's threats and betray Czechoslovakia, and he undertakes to send planes and troops to support the country's own defenses. But the Polish government reacts in return by Poland not allowing Soviet troops or Soviet planes to cross Polish territory to get to Czechoslovakia. And Chamberlain has no desire to speak to that red Stalin. He relies more on Hitler. The greatest betrayal of pre-war days takes place with the curtain up and the whole world can follow what is happening day by day - Central Europe's only democracy is betrayed and abandoned to an aggressive dictator.

Hitler graciously shakes hands with Chamberlain and even manages a stiff smile, but all the same, a smile — we can see it on the newsreels. Chamberlain goes back to London, deeply moved, tears of happiness in his eyes as he waves his bit of paper — "Peace in our time". At the same time, German troops march into Sudetenland and on all the well-produced news reels, we can see them again being greeted by enthusiastic crowds — of those who go out on to the streets.

But the German troops only stop for a moment on the new border. Hitler howls again, demanding Benes' resignation - Edvard Benes, one of the leading European diplomats between the wars, the author behind the 1924 Geneva convention that was unanimously accepted by the League of Nations, and also an initiative taker in the prohibition of war of aggression, of arbitration procedures and if necessary sanction procedures in the case of disputes between states. Hitler maintains Benes and what is left of his country is provoking the great German Third Reich - Benes refuses to disarm and demobilize his country's army. This is provocation, Hitler says, do the Czechs not believe in Germany's and Hitler's promises to Neville Chamberlain? Hitler cannot tolerate this.

Neville Chamberlain and now also Edouard Daladier - prime minister of France, Czechoslovakia's closest ally — put pressure on that little country and its democratic leaders: we won't help you if you don't do what Hitler says. Hitler has said to Chamberlain that he has no further territorial claims, but he has also said this is only on condition he is not provoked. Czechoslovakia has to take a stand and make its contribution to peace in Europe. The Czech national hero, the strong Benes, gives up and is succeeded by a puppet, the weak Hacha, and the Czech army and air force are demobilized. But even this is not enough - German tanks again roll and the infantry marches on. Again, without a shot being fired, Hitler takes the whole of Czechoslovakia - Karpato-Rus and the Cieszyn enclave are given as bribes to Hungary and Poland, Slovakia becomes a subject state of Germany. London and Paris hand in a formal but lame protest — they have chosen their way and have no desire to provoke Hitler. Benes and Czechoslovakia are forced to make their contribution to the assiduous efforts of the European great powers - Great Britain and France - to test Hitler's goodwill to the extreme and through that preserve peace in Europe.

But what peace and at what cost? The Soviet Union is the only country to say it is prepared to take a stand in support of Czechoslovakia. This should be remembered when the coming non-aggression pact is signed between Germany and the Soviet Union, which their foreign ministers Ribbentrop and Molotov have put their names to.

But Western Europe's two great democracies have to pay a high price for the naivety of their leaders, and not unexpectedly they become isolated. It is clear that Britain and France cannot be relied on. Hitler's position on the other hand is strengthened all over Europe, particularly in Germany.

Even passive resistance to Hitler ceases in Germany. More and more are carried away by the national euphoria, not least the officer corps and the army leaders who have hitherto been hesitant in face of Hitler's advances, but now allow themselves to be convinced. Hitler is successful in everything. He has given back to Germany her position of power, her reputation and international influence. He has made the Germans into lords of their own country and other countries, without losing a single German life. Everyone in Germany has work, there is practically no inflation and the Germans are respected everywhere in Europe. The German legations are the most sought after in all European countries, many, even well educated men and women from all the countries of the world go to Germany to study the German miracle.

One country after another declares itself neutral or friendly towards Hitler's Germany. The business about Jews and gypsies is rather troublesome — why is Hitler so malignant towards them? But perhaps he is right in that respect. He has been right in everything else.

No one and nothing has helped Adolf Hitler so much as Britain and France in the inter-war period. I hope we do not have war trials for revenge that we have them to learn from history and through that reduce the risk of repeating the mistakes. So Chamberlain's and Daladier's responsibility and guilt for what happened should have been analyzed and clarified, and the knowledge of the results of that analysis is accessible in the history books. Perhaps the most characteristic of their indefensible ingenuousness was that they did not even exploit the respite they themselves had acquired — by giving away two other peaceful countries — when faced with the inevitable reinforcement of their own defenses.

In Poland there is jubilation in the streets, great gratitude and sympathy increasing towards Germany when Polish troops march into Czech Cieszyn. The newsreels show Polish soldiers pulling down the border barriers, and the general leading the Polish entry into the defenseless enclave becomes a national hero. The whole country can follow on film, in the newspapers and on the radio how on a white horse at the head of his cavalry force, he proudly crosses the border. Hungary and Poland collaborate over this butchery by Germany of a friendly peaceably minded brother-country. How far can this go?

But our lives are not changed. Roman has started in my school. We occasionally see each other in the breaks, in the school corridors or out in the schoolyard. I grow and am no longer one of the smallest boys in the class. When my parents go out in the evening and Roman has gone to sleep, Rózia stays for longer and longer spells by my sofa in the living room, combing my hair. We say nothing and I lie there pretending to read my book, thinking it pleasant and slightly exciting.

I have stopped idling and started working harder, so have decent marks at the end of term in 1939. Pinkus and Sarah are satisfied, and neither they nor I know that these are the last marks I am going to get from the Jewish School.

No one at school is aware that this is our last end-of-term, that shortly our school will be obliterated, just as Axer gymnasium and all the other Jewish schools in Poland are — schools, which after several

The Maple Tree Behind the Barbed Wire

centuries of education in the Chaiders and Yeshivas of the ghettos, have fostered a first generation of Jews who did indeed grow up in a still segregated community, but nevertheless could have a perfectly satisfactory school education, young people not burdened by the ghetto mentality, speaking the country's language faultlessly and no longer just Yiddish. It is a matter of sorrow that only a few of that generation are to be allowed to live. We were so eager and wanted so much. We will never know what contribution to the culture and development of the world our generation would have been able to make.

Adolf Hitler speaks again, and the world begins to realize that his ambitions have no limits, but it is too late to put a stop to what is now inevitable. The wheels of destruction and extermination can no longer be stopped, are rolling mercilessly on, not just towards the destruction of the Jews, but also towards the destruction of a great number of towns, villages, families and cultures, in the end also towards the annihilation of Hitler and all that surrounds him. But a great deal is to happen before that, many more magnificent victories and ignominious defeats before the vicious circle can be broken.

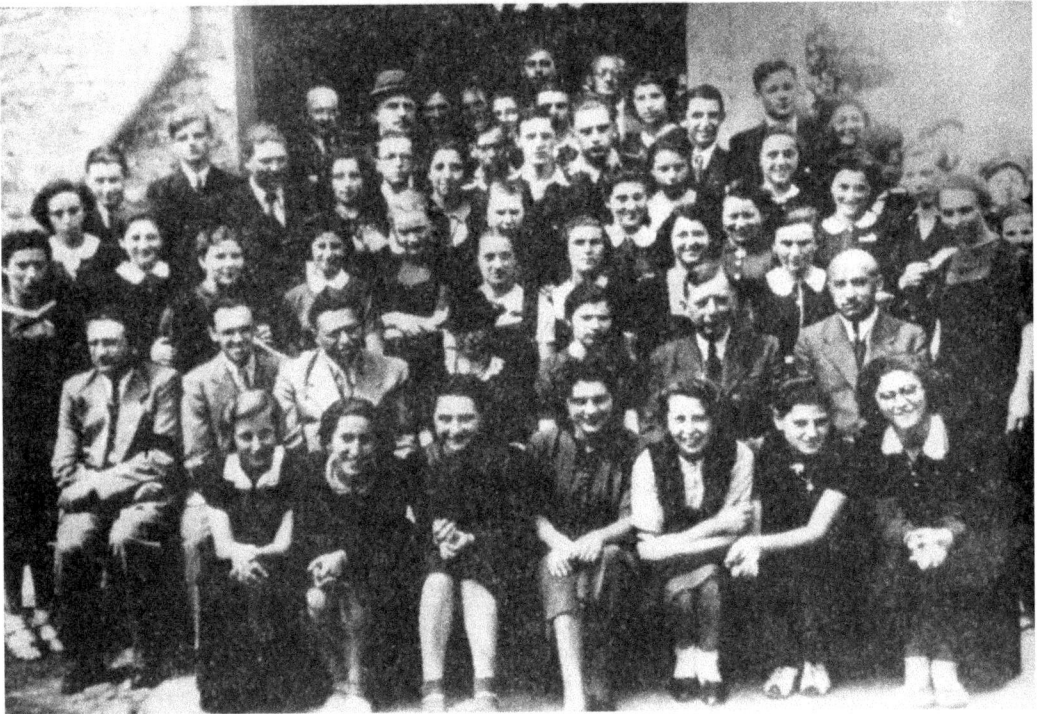

At the end of term at the beginning of June 1939, class IIB at the Jewish gymnasium assembled for a group photograph. Not one of us knows that this is our last end-of-term, that our school will soon be obliterated, and only a few of the pupils in our class are to survive the war.

The Maple Tree Behind the Barbed Wire

The Beginning of the End

At the beginning of the summer of 1939, Poland is bathing in magnificent greenery - the flowers are out, the birds twittering, butterflies straying into the towns. Women have put on colorful light summer clothes, the men summer shirts and light-colored trousers — people seem to be untroubled, and I am soon to be fourteen.

In his latest speech, Hitler has said he must have a corridor of land through Poland to his East Prussia. He draws up the corridor on the map of Poland, a wide area of land, which divides the country. A six-lane autobahn and a railway line are to be built on this land, and there has to be space for storing goods, houses for the Germans to be responsible for the maintenance and defense of this land-link, while in practice the corridor cuts Poland off from the country's Baltic ports. In addition, Hitler is to have the town of Gdansk, for a great many Germans live there.

The military government of Poland reacts swiftly, logically and determinedly. We shall not give up a centimeter of our territory, not a single centimeter. Chamberlain and Daladier say that this time they will make a stand, and they give Poland guarantees, which they say are binding. Opinion in Poland, hitherto fairly understanding towards Germany, swings radically — we shall defend our country to the last drop of blood.

Poland with her 36 million inhabitants is one of the largest and most thickly populated countries in Europe and has a large and strong army — it is thought. No one is afraid of provoking this hitherto successful neighbor. Poland mobilizes — at first surreptitiously, then more and more openly, and the whole country hums with enthusiasm and national pride. On the radio, military marches are played, proud declarations are read out and speeches made — not a single centimeter of our Polish land — it is accepted that the Jews share this swelling national euphoria.

Poland has a tradition of mounted troops on which the whole of Polish defenses are built. Soldiers in large numbers can be seen in the streets - Uhlans with white bands on the characteristic square caps of the Polish army, the cavalry with red bands, and the dragoons with yellow. The artillery is also horse-drawn, but many infantrymen can also been seen in the streets with their more ordinary dark brown cap-bands — the army's picked troops. Podhalanczycy - the mountain commandos — wear broad-brimmed hats with one side boldly turned up, and cloaks over one shoulder, held together by a broad buckle on the chest. Naval sailors have light blue uniforms, but very few soldiers from the motorized units are seen with their menacing black berets. We have an air force, but I don't know what their uniform looks like, as I have never seen one.

The Maple Tree Behind the Barbed Wire

Customers come and go as usual and I am often sitting there. Although Pinkus says nothing, I can see he is finding it hard teaching me the difficult art of being a good tailor. Pinkus gets hold of a special teacher for me, an older experienced French-Jewish cutter who tries to instruct me in the evenings. I wonder whether it is going any better.

Friends and acquaintances as usual come in an even stream, for we constantly keep open house. When the Wajnapels are staying with us, it is festive for several days, for Sarah is a hospitable and generous hostess, and also a fantastic cook.

It is quite late in the afternoon and I am in the workshop sewing on the lapel of a light-brown jacket with thick brown thread of a slightly darker hue than the light-brown worsted of the jacket. I have noticed recently that Pinkus is observing me more often and for longer spells of time when I am working — without correcting me, as before. Perhaps he is not satisfied with what I do, but I am young and have time to learn. I see Pinkus looking at me standing by the table where he is fine-pressing a dark blue jacket, but I am not worried. Jolly Sonny Boy has been away for quite a long time, is now back in the workshop and telling a funny story. I laugh; perhaps more than the others do, and stop sewing to try to comment in my not yet perfect but improving Yiddish. Pinkus listens and does not laugh. After a while, he calmly comes over to me, carefully takes the jacket out of my hands, pats me lightly on the head and says: "Jurek, go in to your mother." Silence suddenly falls in the workshop.

At first I don't understand what is happening and am confused and miserable, but I go in to Sarah, who is cleaning the bedroom. Sarah sees that I am near to tears and is cross, as usual when someone hurts me. She goes in to Pinkus in the workshop and says in a louder voice than usual: "I must speak to you." Pinkus seems to be prepared for this, puts aside the iron and follows Sarah out to the living room. I am sitting at the back of the room, so they must be aware that I can hear what they are saying.

"Why have you made Jurek so miserable," says Sarah, reproachfully, but uneasily. Pinkus is troubled and says dejectedly but in a firm voice: "Sarah, I don't think he ought to be a tailor." Sarah is appalled and wants to know why. "You know I've tried," says Pinkus - they must have talked about this before, "but he'll never be a good tailor." "What will he be then?" says Sarah, despair in her voice - I've never before seen her so downhearted? "If he becomes a bad tailor, he'll have a miserable life," says Pinkus, and I am listening. "I don't want that, and nor do you. It's better that he's miserable now than being miserable all his life," he says. Pinkus has clearly thought all this through properly, and dejectedly, I realize that. "What will become of him?" Sarah says again. Pinkus has to think a while before he knows what he has to say, and he says: "I suppose he will have to be a doctor or an engineer. They always get by."

The Maple Tree Behind the Barbed Wire

Sarah's head and shoulders droop. Pinkus does not know how to comfort her and goes back to the workshop. In a quiet and less certain voice than usual, Sarah says to me: "Don't be miserable, Jureczku, things will work out."

I go on being in the workshop and the fitting room and Pinkus raises no objections. But we know that I will not become a tailor. I am downhearted, insecure and fumbling around. Perhaps I didn't try hard enough, or was I too young when I started? I envy Roman, still too young, not even eight yet, but who still has a chance, a possibility of setting up the workshop and shop for quality clothing, which Pinkus has so often talked about.

The message I have received is clear, and I realize Pinkus must be right. He does not want anyone miserable, least of all his son Josele. It must have been a difficult decision for Pinkus, for it went against all his hopes, perhaps even more for him than me.

One evening when the parents had gone out and Roman was asleep; Rózia comes in to comb my hair. I am reading my book. Rózia doesn't say a word, just combs my hair with gentle slightly lingering and caressing movements. She is in a gleaming black satin housecoat and I catch a glimpse of the white flesh on the inside of her plump thigh — but perhaps I am imagining it.

She stands close to me and goes on combing my hair. After a while, as if by chance, I happen to brush that soft flesh of her white thigh. Rózia doesn't seem to notice, but moves so that my fingers land on the warm inside of that plump thigh. I am more and more excited and cautiously move my hand upwards and suddenly come to that triangle of hair — she is naked under her black housecoat. We are both silent, pretending that everything is happening by chance. Rózia goes on combing my hair, I look at my book without reading, the hair between the soft plump thighs is rough, but underneath it are wonderful soft secrets. I am not driven by curiosity, but by a violent, urgent excitement with this mature woman at last allowing me to touch those secretive forbidden places I have scarcely dared dream about — a fantasy dream being fulfilled. I am dizzy with excitement and Rózia lets me, stops combing my hair, moves lightly and is breathing more quickly before backing away, perhaps rather annoyed. It does not enter my mind that what is going on between Rózia and me could be anything shameful.

Even today, with memories and experiences of a long life, I can still feel excitement as I try to describe what happened between Rózia and me that late evening.

Aunt Bela at last divorces the rich Enzel. Their constant quarreling has become dogged mutual hostility. Sarah says that Bela's husband hits her, but Pinkus does not believe that. Bela marries again, a

The Maple Tree Behind the Barbed Wire

Belgian Jew this time — a skilled diamond-cutter. After a while, Bela does not want to go on living in Belgium. She doesn't like it there and they move to Poland - this was to turn out to be disastrous for them both, but her husband does, as Bela wants.

Towards the end of the summer of 1939, Sarah manages to persuade Pinkus to take a holiday with his elder son. In the middle of August, Pinkus and I, just fourteen, go to Swierk - a holiday resort in southern Poland in a gentle hilly area, Podkarpacie, before the steep Carpathians further south take over. At our departure, on the railway station Sarah says I am to keep an eye on Pinkus for her. She is joking, but means it at the same time. Sarah is rather jealous of her handsome Pinkus. They are a handsome couple and show great consideration for each other, and they clearly get on well together.

In Swierk, Pinkus and I stay at a guesthouse. There is no radio there, no workshop, so Pinkus has a lot of time to spend with me. We go for walks and talk a bit, he in his elegant light summer clothes, which I have never seen before. It is clear that several lone ladies are interested, but he is not.

He is really handsome, my father. He is quite tall, with broad shoulders, and he moves slowly and self-confidently, always holding his head high. His eyes are calm but watchful, his mouth softly smiling in his clean-featured face beneath his mane of hair with its sprinkling of grey. When he is wearing a short-sleeved shirt, or is undressing on the beach, you can see how muscular he is, although he neither trains not takes any exercise. He possesses an inborn calm and an innate strength.

Pinkus tries to relax, often sitting on a bench on a slope with a lovely view across the village hidden in the trees, thinking - I realize he wants to be left in peace. On one such occasion, one early afternoon, I climb up to the top of the hill and start running down. It goes quickly, then too quickly and I can't stop, can only go on running faster and faster, my legs can't keep up and I am very frightened and scream — papa, papa, —papa in a tearful voice. Pinkus looks up and with two long strides he puts himself in my way and waits. I am approaching at headlong pace and he catches me in his strong arms and holds me pressed hard against his chest until I have calmed down. It is just as it had felt when I was four and he lifted up that heavy gilt-framed mirror that had fallen over me and picked up his son unhurt among all those sharp pieces of glass and calmed me down by pressing me to his chest. But when he holds me like that now, I am aware that this is a moment I will always remember, the safety in the arms of my father, in whom I have unlimited confidence — he can manage everything. I really don't want to grow up and have to take responsibility myself, and would prefer to halt time and always have things as they are now.

The Maple Tree Behind the Barbed Wire

This was to be the last time in our lives that my father and I were alone together, feeling a common security — at least, I felt it.

For while we are in Swierk, Stalin and Hitler come to an agreement, their foreign ministers - Molotov and von Ribbentrop - sign an unconditional non-aggression pact. They will not attack each other whatever happens. In practice, this means they give each other the freedom of action to attack other countries. There are rumors that the pact contains more than what has been made public and that this addition concerns Poland.

Hitler - protesting that he is a man of peace and only wants Gdansk and his corridor of land through Poland - gathers large forces of tanks along the Polish border. Poland responds with general mobilization and horses and lorries are requisitioned from the civilian population. Britain and France confirm their guarantees, now in the form of an ultimatum — an attack on Poland would be regarded as a declaration of war against them. Pinkus talks on the phone to Sarah several times a day and in the end says we must break off our holiday. We pack that evening and early the next morning, we take the train back to Czestochowa. At home, Sarah has already begun to pack. We are to go to Warsaw.

It may be all right about "not a centimeter of Polish land", but we live no more than fourteen kilometers from the German border and suppose they start shooting? Pinkus phones his brother in Warsaw. Maurycy says we are welcome. People in Czestochowa are hoarding sugar, tea, coffee, flour, potatoes, razor blades, serviettes, after-shave — everything. Pinkus sends money and asks Maurycy to buy food. Maurycy thinks Pinkus is exaggerating, but promises to buy in food, which, unfortunately, he doesn't.

After only two days in Czestochowa, we set off in an overcrowded train. A lot of people are fleeing. People are standing and sitting everywhere, on their cases, on rucksacks, on the floor, the guard can't get past in the corridors of the train to check whether we have tickets. The train is slow and very much delayed. Through the window, we see large columns of military going in the opposite direction — towards the border — small and large military units on foot, on bicycles, horses and lorries. It feels safe to see all these military men on their way to the border to defend us.

We arrive in Warsaw very late in the evening of August 31st, 1939, and even later at Maurycy's home, for it's hard to get a taxi or a cab at the railway station in Warsaw.

When you are a refugee, you are not so warmly welcomed as when you are invited as a guest for a short visit. Maurycy has not bought any food, as it was too late to do that when Pinkus phoned. It is night and I go to bed. Although our parents and Rutka go on talking in the next room, I fall into the deep sleep of the exhausted.

The Maple Tree Behind the Barbed Wire

This is to be the last night of peace for a long time. On my next night in peacetime I am a grown man and the world will never again be the same as it was when I went to bed that night in Warsaw. When the Second World War is over, there are very few Jews left in Poland, Czechoslovakia, Hungary, Yugoslavia, Greece, Latvia, Lithuania, Estonia, Austria or Germany. Hitler is to succeed with at least one of his aims: to make Eastern and Central Europe Judenrein - free of Jews - and to decimate the Jewish population in several west European countries. The entire flourishing Jewish culture — that inexhaustible source of Jewish craftsmen, workers, beggars, scientists, businessmen, writers, poets, artists, musicians and Jewish thinkers — are to be annihilated. Old, young and children, men and women, those who maintain their Jewishness and those who try to assimilate, those who abandon their religion and allow themselves to be baptized to Christians, those who marry and have children with Christians - they are all to be exterminated. Rich and poor, the educated and the uneducated, those who speak Yiddish and those who speak Polish, the sick and the healthy, the beautiful and the ugly, the gifted and the less gifted, those with good and those with bad marks from school — all are to be exterminated.

What have we done? How can every single one of us, a whole people, have deserved this collective death sentence? Of what have I, my brother, my father Pinkus and my mother Sarah been guilty? Of what are all my classmates, all the Jews who tried to go to Polish schools, and the many who did not have any schooling guilty? Nothing helps, it does not make any difference which way a Jew has chosen — we are all nevertheless to be eliminated.

Adolf Hitler has spoken. Early in the morning of September 1st, 1939, German panzer troops and heavy tanks begin to roll, his air force start up the fighter plane engines and take off — towards the approaching destruction of Europe and Hitler himself. Why couldn't he be content with what he had already achieved?

Adolf Hitler has failed in everything he has undertaken in his life — he is also to fail as a statesman, dictator and warlord, and take with him his great people in the fall. But this is to take five long years, eight long months and a week, during which time hundreds of millions of soldiers and civilians are to die unnecessarily. The map of Europe and the world is to be redrawn, empires fall, his native country devastated, his people impoverished and he himself to commit suicide when there were no longer any German children and old people left to mobilize to bear his arms, his sick ambitions and his hatred. But one thing he did succeed in doing -— exterminating the gypsies and Jews of Europe - at least almost, for a few of us are to survive. By chance - I am one of those few.

CHAPTER II

WAR BREAKS OUT

The Siege of Warsaw

When I wake up in Maurycy's apartment in Warsaw on the morning of September 1st, 1939, I hear voices coming up from the courtyard. Although it is early in the morning, they are loud, but I can't hear what they are saying. I get up and go into the kitchen in my pajamas. My parents, Maurycy, his wife Magda and Rutka are already dressed. It is war. The Germans have attacked Poland.

At breakfast, Pinkus asks Maurycy about the food he was supposed to have bought. Maurycy is annoyed, as people often are when they are in the wrong. He has not bought any food with the money Pinkus wired to him from Czestochowa. He considered that unnecessary and anyhow he hadn't the time. Pinkus says nothing. He doesn't usually come up with meaningless reproaches. I have never heard him say, "what did I tell you?" or "why didn't you do it?" when it is already too late to do anything about the matter. Perhaps his influence in this respect is why I have never even felt the need to ask my patients meaningless questions such as "Why didn't you come earlier" - a cruel question to a cancer patient.

Pinkus and Sarah are to go out to buy food and I am allowed to go with them, while Roman has to stay behind. They are thinking of buying a lot, and then Roman may be troublesome. Roman does not protest. He is alone at the table, his feet not even touching the floor. He isn't usually allowed to sit at breakfast in his pajamas.

It is a lovely pleasantly cool autumn day, cloudy but not oppressively so, the sun occasionally appearing and the atmosphere in the streets elated. Strangers speak to each other. "We will give it to them. France and England will come to our aid. They have already issued an ultimatum." During the past few days, the cinemas have been showing a short film "Francja czuwa", France on guard, with heavily armed French troops marching, French fighter planes, the impregnable Maginot Line.

Every Polish soldier who happens to be passing is treated like a hero, and he easily puts up with that - Polish people have always admired their soldiers. I am infected by the atmosphere and think it exciting — we'll show them! My father was clever to arrange it so that we could go to safe Warsaw and would not have to be near the border where there might be shooting.

But in the shops there is almost no food to be bought. Only a few ordinary items with limited keeping quality are left on the shelves —

bread, milk, and fresh pastries. Flour, potatoes, even butter, margarine and meat, everything that will keep has already been hoarded by the inhabitants of the city. Since the previous week, when Poland politely but firmly rejected Germany's demands, it has been reckoned that there might be war. What has not already been hoarded, the shopkeeper has tucked away for his regular customers or for bad times to come, as food supplies during wartime may well be difficult. These small grocery stores with personal service across the counter have no desire to sell to us, who are not regular customers, and the days of the big stores has not yet come. Self-service is an unknown concept in Poland. We go back home with what we have managed to get hold of — and that is not much. Magda thinks that we have gone to a lot of unnecessary trouble, but she nonetheless takes the food.

Loudspeakers have been put up in the streets so that the population can be informed, motivated and warned. The radio adds to the atmosphere, broadcasting cheerful marches interspersed with news bulletins — all of them about the war, mostly statements from the leaders of the country. Since liberation, Poland's government since 1918 has consisted of civilian politicians and senior military men, the military dominating, without anyone I know complaining or questioning the fact. After the death of the father of the country, Marshall Jósef Pilsudski, another general, Edward Smigly-Rydz, has become the leader of the country. But he is not seen very much and could never be as popular as the morose, but self-assured and safe Pilsudki.

The radio informs us of various regulations — the blackout at night, sirens, alerts and all clears — and reports on what is happening in other countries, less on what is happening at the front. Military headquarters reports from the front are primarily details, not particularly worrying, but fairly non-committal. Everyone is waiting tensely for the message that Britain and France have declared war, as they had promised, and they are now attacking on the western front — while the German army is busy in Poland. A rumor goes round that French fighter planes are on their way to Poland.

Another day has gone by and France is in no hurry. Britain is still cautious, and notes are still being exchanged. Despite this, the atmosphere in Warsaw is quite elated. It doesn't matter; we will settle him, that madman Hitler. I see that my father is worried — that must be because we were unable to buy any food.

A few days later, France declares war on Germany, then Britain does, but it is only a declaration and they do not come and help. It is said to be quiet on the German western border. The Allies do not send any planes and the rumours of French planes being on the way turns out to be false.

The Maple Tree Behind the Barbed Wire

Instead, several countries declare their neutrality, among them Belgium and Holland. We thought they were our friends, and friends of France and Britain, but they did not want to get involved in war. They wanted to be left in peace whatever happened to us in Poland. On the other hand, there is a rumor that Soviet troops have moved into Poland, but that surely could not be true. Our government has said we do not want their help. Or are they doing the same thing to us as Poland did to Czechoslovakia, stabbing us in the back? All good news is true how ever shaky its basis. All bad news is malicious rumour.

The loudspeakers in the streets of Warsaw warn us about spies and saboteurs — don't talk to strangers, don't talk about our industrial plants and where they are, don't talk about trains, roads and other communications, and certainly not about anything concerning our defenses, which units have been seen, where relatives know mobilized soldiers are. If any stranger is inquisitive, report it to the nearest police station.

Civil defense wardens appear on the streets with armbands on their right arms. They are to make sure the blackout works that not a slit of light comes from any window. As if that meant anything. Don't the Germans know where Warsaw is? Wardens are appointed in every building to show us the shelters we have to go down into when the air raid siren sounds. There are practices so that we recognize the alert sirens that tell us to go down into the shelters, and sirens that sound the all clear, which mean the danger is over.

The first real air raid warning goes off and the first bombs fall on the third day of the war. On the fifth day, Warsaw is surrounded and we are cut off from the outside world — the radio the only remaining communication link.

It takes the German army and the German air force five days to crush the Polish defenses. With the swift advance of the blitzkrieg, the invincible tanks in the battle of Kowno mow down the brave Polish cavalry vainly attacking with their sabers, and the Uhlans with their long lances. Poland's insignificant air force is destroyed on the ground, and the dive-bombing drives the civilian population out on to the roads — where they prevent the re-grouping of what is left of the strong Polish army — then the capital is surrounded.

Neither the loudspeakers in the streets, the newspapers nor the radio inform the population of the capital that the president, the entire government, every single Member of Parliament, the senior administration and practically the entire military leadership have fled to Romania, to a safe but scarcely honorable existence beyond the dangers of war. This is revealed to us when Starzynski, Warsaw's brave mayor, steps forward as the spokesman for the civilian and military leadership, and for Poland. He seems safe and honest. Under his leadership, what is left of the capital's garrison refuses to

The Maple Tree Behind the Barbed Wire

capitulate. In peacetime, Poland has been led by the military, and when it is war and the capital is to be defended, the leader is a civilian mayor.

The air raid sirens sound more and more often and last longer. We have learnt how to go quickly down to the shelter, how to arrange life in the cramped space, what to take from the apartment to be able to sleep and eat there — and what we don't need and don't take with us.

But we find it hard to sleep. We have learnt to distinguish between the sound of shells from heavy artillery and diving Stukas - those effective German air force dive-bombers, the sound of falling bombs and that the silent incendiary bombs are dangerous. It can be imagined what it sounds like and what it feels to be in a small enclosed area in the middle of a besieged city, what it is like to have nowhere to go, nowhere to flee to. Can you imagine how a child — like my little brother — or a teenager at the beginning of life — experiences this? Or how parents with their inborn instinct to protect their children — like Sarah and Pinkus - experience it when they have no possible chance whatsoever of protecting us, not even with their own bodies? You know that shells, or bombs, will soon land, but you don't know where. You know that very soon, in a few seconds, there will be a huge explosion but you don't know how close it will be to you — whether this time it will be a hit which you don't have time to hear because it will hit just you, whether in the next few seconds you will be still alive, dead or injured, but with no chance of getting to a hospital or any proper help at all. You have nothing but your shelter, not much of a shelter, but you have nowhere, absolutely nowhere to flee. Whether you are allowed to live depends on when the pilot starts diving and the bomb-aimer releases the bomb, which way the crew of a heavy artillery piece will direct their gun this time — a few centimeters to the right and you and your nearest and dearest are dead, a few to the left and you escape, for this time. But many more shells and bombs fall, in a few minutes, tonight, tomorrow, never ceasing, and there is nothing you can do. You belong among the unarmed, defenseless and pushed-around civilian population, the most exposed victims of modern warfare.

If you belong to the civilian population, in practice you have no rights during wartime. The proud declarations worked out in peacetime and the conventions that are to protect you, in wartime are worth less than one single pistol. For you can imagine that a pistol, a bayonet, a gas mask perhaps might come in handy, at least offer you a false sense of security, a feeling that you have something with which to defend yourself. But after a day's indiscriminate bombardment, no one so much as mentions the detailed Geneva Convention on the duties of countries at war to protect the civilian population. Nothing of all that had been said, written and after long negotiations decided upon for civilian populations during peacetime applies now. For it is

The Maple Tree Behind the Barbed Wire

war, you are in the reach of foreign troops, and you have no rights. It is surprising that clever people spend so much time, work and money on negotiating such naive, meaningless and unreal documents. Everything that happens during this war confirms that such conventions are not worth the paper they are written on. War has to be prevented, cannot be won or lost, for after a war there are no winners, only losers.

You try to do the little you can to protect yourself and your nearest and dearest. When the sirens wail, you run down to the air raid shelter, in our building a simple cellar. You hope it will protect you, not from a direct hit, but at least from the sharp bomb fragments that whistle through the air after every hit. You know the projectile has been made in another country, by workers you will never meet, that it has been fired by anonymous men in uniform strapped into their seats in their planes, that the intention is to hit you or someone else in this besieged city. The projectile is insensitive, relentless, its function to destroy indiscriminately everything it hits. When a bombardment is going on, you think that whatever happens, if only it would stop, now, immediately, and when it has stopped, you know that it will soon start again. This is a war on the civilian population, on children, old people and women.

Only those who have experienced a besieged city from the inside can understand what it is like for people in other besieged, defenseless and bombed cities. I understand what people went through in the siege of Sarahjevo by the Serbs, in Knin ruthlessly bombed by the Croats, and in Baghdad bombed by the Americans and the British. But in Sarahjevo, the besieged knew some people were trying to help, were disappointed they did not do more, that was natural, but it was known that someone was trying. In Warsaw no one tries to help, and we are painfully aware that we can expect no help at all.

We listen to the radio, and several countries declare their neutrality, thinking that is significant. It is not if it does not happen to suit the aggressor, for it is the aggressor who decides which countries are to be allowed to remain neutral.

No one repeats or any longer believes the rumors about help being on the way. Many cheer, others weep with joy when during the first days of the siege the last Polish fighter plane takes off to defend us. The pilot, Lieutenant Palusinski, was our last war hero. Now his plane has also been destroyed — on the ground. We have no war hero to look up to or hope for. The Polish anti-aircraft guns are heard more and more infrequently. They helped us keep up our courage, although they were fairly useless. We have heard of only one German plane shot down at the beginning of the siege and people trek off on a pilgrimage to look at the burnt-out wreckage. Now they can torment us without any danger to themselves.

The Maple Tree Behind the Barbed Wire

When the air raid stops late in the afternoon, and before the evening artillery has begun, hunger comes. For the first time in my life I feel hunger and realize what real hunger means. Hunger isn't just that longing in your stomach for something good. Hunger is — hunger — a constantly present longing for almost anything that can still it. For the first time I feel my life threatened, for the first time I realize that human life is frail and can be abruptly crushed. For the first time I realise that life is not something I can take for granted, but a wonderful gift that can be taken away from me at any moment. This comes to influence my attitudes and values for the rest of my life — if I am to be allowed any remaining life.

With us in the shelter is a middle-aged, rather silent, rather dignified and determined lady with greying hair and a sharp but occasionally wild look in her grey eyes. Her husband, who is no longer alive, had been an officer in the German army in the First World War. He left behind him an old German spiked helmet and an equally old rifle. To her, it is more important to have this long clumsy weapon in the shelter than a warm blanket, a mattress or a pillow. The rifle is her pride and the helmet her security, a reminder of other times. All of us in the shelter understand and respect this, and it is touching that it is a German rifle and a German helmet. One day, in the middle of a raid, just as we hear the bombers diving, she takes her husband's rifle, goes with calm determined steps out of the shelter, the guard not stopping her, although a raid is on. With the helmet on her head and the long rifle in her hands, she stands in the entrance and aims composedly up in the air and fires at planes in the air. We can all hear the sharp bangs from the old rifle. We know this is useless, but no one laughs. We hope all the same that she will hit the pilot, that the bullet from her rifle will at least drill a little hole in one of the planes so that even those tormenting us become a little afraid.

The air raid alert has gone on for several days and we spend all day and night down in the cramped shelter. Sarah talks about the things she should have brought with her from the apartment, but Pinkus says she must not go up as long as the alert is on. Roman is asleep with nothing but Sarah's summer coat between him and the concrete floor, and Sarah says that next time we can go up, we must fetch the thin mattress from their bed so that the children can sleep more comfortably — she doesn't mention herself, only the children.

The water we have in the cellar in two big pans is enough for drinking, but not for washing yourself or your clothes. Nor do we change our underclothes. It's all right living like this, especially as it is the same for everyone. Things, which were important before, are suddenly uninteresting — it's a question of survival.

The Maple Tree Behind the Barbed Wire

After ten days of siege, we are tired, frightened and hungry. Not just Roman, but I also complain of being hungry — children are ruthless. Our relationship with Maurycy and his family has not improved. Sarah says they eat when we aren't looking. One morning, Magda asks whether we would like a piece of salami, which is slightly moldy. Sarah tries to cut away the mould and she keeps cutting until less and less remains. We - Pinkus, Roman and me — look on. In the end Sarah says we must not eat the salami however hungry we are.

Pinkus has heard from a man in the shelter that there is a horse that has just been killed in our street. The bombing goes on, slightly less intensively, but we can hear bomb splinters flying through the air. Despite this, Pinkus leaves the shelter and goes out on to the street. I follow him, but stop in the entrance.

It is a lovely fairly warm September day. There are no signs of planes in the clear air, but I can hear explosions in the distance. Fires are burning in several places and I can see grey smoke, but not the buildings that are burning. I hope no people are still in the buildings — how awful it must be to be shut in a burning building. Can you get out of a shelter when a building is burning?

I see that several buildings have collapsed and in their place is nothing but ruins, some with nothing but the ground floor left. One of these is quite near ours. That must have been hit when earlier on in the day we had heard a huge explosion and the whole shelter shook. After the explosion came the horrible sound of collapsing walls and stones — no one could have escaped that. A little further away, on the other side of the street, there is a house with its façade quite gone. I can see into several of the rooms — at a distance they look quite undamaged. I can see cupboards, tables and chairs in their usual places, a tiled stove in the corner, pictures on the wall and rugs on the floor. As good as all the windows have gone, some patched over with paper or blankets. Further down the street is the body of a young woman in a black skirt, a dark red floral blouse, and hair brushed back; her still beautiful and glossy dark hair is spread out on the pavement.

Fifty meters away from our building, perhaps not so far, in the middle of the street, is a big grayish-brown dead horse, its lips drawn back and large yellow teeth exposed, almost as if it were laughing. Several men are standing round the dead horse, cutting off bits of flesh. Pinkus goes close to the horse's long tail and starts cutting into the hindquarters above its hind legs. He is doing it with a sharp knife he has borrowed from a man in the shelter, and he seems quite calm and composed, but he is in a hurry. It takes quite a while, perhaps over quarter of an hour, before he has finished. Sarah is worried about me standing in the entrance of the shelter and calls to me, but I don't want to come. She comes over and says agitatedly and pleadingly that

The Maple Tree Behind the Barbed Wire

I must come back in immediately. "Isn't it enough that your father is risking his life?" But I, who always obey my mother, stay where I am, watching. Pinkus comes running back at last. I have rarely seen him running, and he has a large piece of horsemeat with him.

Sarah shares it with the family who lent Pinkus the knife and asks Maurycy if he wants some, but Maurycy peevishly says he doesn't.

In one part of the cellar it is possible to boil water or cook food on a large spirit stove. Sarah does just that. She cooks a meal of fresh horsemeat with the spices she has brought with her and others she has got from the same family who lent Pinkus the knife.

I have never eaten horsemeat before. What I eat in that cellar beneath Maurycy's apartment in Warsaw is rather tough and sweetish. Not until then do I realize that hunger is really the very best spice. I have never liked meat, except possibly minced or as sausage. But never has meat tasted so good as that horsemeat, but then never have I ever been so hungry as I am now.

The meat dish Sarah had made is more than enough for us four. Sarah shares it with the others in the shelter. For the first time during the siege, we have food we can give to other people.

Before darkness falls, the dive-bombers are back again, the terrible Stukas. Again I hear the whistling sound as they dive, and know they let their bombs go as they come out of the dive and start upwards again. The militiaman in our building tells us that nowadays they carry five hundred kilo bombs, which leave nothing but ruins and no survivors wherever they land.

The air raid goes on until dusk, then — after a brief pause — the shelling from heavy artillery starts. But we children have fallen asleep. We are full for the first time for ages. As I slide into sleep, I think about what a fantastic meal it had been. A family next to us had some rusks left, another tea, even sugar, we have shared everything, and we too have had something to share — but Pinkus had risked his life for us to have it.

Three days later, two weeks after the siege had begun, the militiaman tells us there has been a temporary cease-fire to attend to the injured and to bury the dead. Some of the men are taken out to do this, but not us. Pinkus is fifty-five and too old. I am fourteen and too young. We go up to Maurycy's apartment, as we have nowhere else to go. The apartment is undamaged, but there is no running water, no electricity and no gas in the stove.

There is wood stacked in the dark storeroom, the bath has been filled with water, but there is no food.

The atmosphere between Maurycy and Pinkus is tense, even worse between Sarah and Magda, and we hardly speak to each other. I have to admit that I don't really grasp why, but I realize that in the household garbage Sarah has seen fresh remains of food, from sardines in oil, skins from salami sausage and crumbs from hard-baked scones.

Sarah can't let it go — she tells Magda she knows they have food. Sarah asks if the food has been bought with the money Pinkus had sent. Maurycy brings up old events he has considered injustices. Pinkus says nothing, but nor does he do anything to make the situation any better. Perhaps it can't get better? Of course my undivided sympathies are with my parents, yet I do wonder whether it is necessary for things to be like this between two brothers, but I say nothing.

We are hungry, have nothing to eat and we must get hold of some food somehow. We have to make use of the cease-fire to go shopping. Sarah says she is best at that, and Pinkus has to agree. Sarah has some money on her and Pinkus also gives her what he has got. No one knows what the food may cost. Sarah gets smartly dressed and goes out alone. Someone has to stay with Roman and me, and they don't want to leave us alone. Pinkus stays with us.

After Sarah has gone, we try to tidy up, then feel what it is like to lie in real beds, look out and go down on to the street. It looks just as it did three days ago, but the dead woman and the horse have already gone. There are a lot of people, but not a single soldier, only the militiamen and the blackout wardens with their armbands. Where have all the soldiers gone?

The weather is still quite sunny and pleasantly warm, a lovely late September day in 1939. The patches of grass in the area are still there and the leaves are turning yellow. Everything seems calm, but we don't dare go far away from our building.

Three hours go by before Sarah comes back. She is pleased. She has some potatoes, a little cooking oil and chicory — before the war the substitute for coffee for the poor, the sick and now the besieged, which is all she has managed to find.

Sarah tells us trading is mostly going on in the market square closest to us. That's as far as Sarah has gone, and it is quite a long way to walk in a city the size of Warsaw. People are exchanging food for other things they want, mostly food for food, but Sarah had nothing to barter with. Sarah says she should have taken her fine grey Persian fur with her to Warsaw - a good fur is a very desirable object for barter. But the fur had been left behind in Czestochowa, for it was summer when we left. No one wants money; at least not Polish zloty, although she had been prepared to pay anything to be able to buy a little.

Sarah fails to buy anything at the market, but she does get some food from a peasant woman standing on the street with a sack of potatoes and other things she has to barter, though not for money. The woman had taken pity on this grandly dressed lady who had desperately gone around without having anything to barter with.

The Maple Tree Behind the Barbed Wire

Sarah tells her she has two children at home who are hungry, and she is allowed to barter her ruby ring for a few potatoes, a small bottle of cooking oil and chicory. In besieged Warsaw, ruby rings are not particularly high on the list as barter goods, at least not when you want food.

Sarah cautiously peels the potatoes so as to remove as little as possible, then mashes them and fries thin little crisp potato pancakes. Roman and I begin to eat — they the best potato pancakes I have ever eaten. Sarah eats one and gives one to Pinkus. I ask her whether she wants another one, but Sarah says she isn't hungry, and we boys are to eat. Pinkus isn't hungry, either. Pinkus and Sarah drink chicory coffee, with no sugar. Roman and I eat up all the remaining potato pancakes.

When I recently met Roman at his home above Lake Ontario in Burlington, Canada, he says he can't remember the potato pancakes. He was only eight. I am ashamed when
I think how selfish we were. Nowadays, my brother and I often talk about what fine parents we had. But perhaps many parents did, and do, and even in future will do just as they did -when there is a war on.

Warsaw sticks it out for another week. Then everything runs out, food, water, ammunition and courage in the defenders. One could rightly say that the defense of Warsaw was meaningless. In the history books, there will be a footnote on the courageous defense of the city, and how it took a whole month to conquer Poland. The price for those lines, however, is high, and it is the civilian population who have to pay it. But the civilian population has no say in the matter when it is war, they are not asked, democracy — government by the people — is a word that sounds strange when there is a war on.

Yet I do wonder whether some of us, perhaps many of us — if a referendum had been arranged in Warsaw in September 1939 - would have voted for defending ourselves, not to give up before we had to. I wonder how my father would have voted. I guess — when it was obvious that no one was to come to our rescue — he would have voted for an earlier capitulation. I think my father, a self-taught humanist, would have said that human lives are more important than a footnote in the history books.

But what is right and what is wrong? Are those responsible for the defense of a defenseless city against a ruthless aggressor heroes or felons against their own civilians? Is there any right or wrong in war? Perhaps it was right after all to hold out for so long, considering the unfathomable crimes the German people during the Nazi regime were to commit between September 1939 and May 1945.

Wars seem to be inevitable. They seem to be part of man's nature and of the history of mankind, in all times and all cultures. Humanity lives in a vicious circle of threat and fear, war and, in the pauses

The Maple Tree Behind the Barbed Wire

between them, arming for war — if you feel threatened then you must arm. I know that is so, but I find it hard to understand why it has to be so. Is mankind doomed to constant wars, until the end of the world?

German troops march into Warsaw, frightening in their steel helmets, their tramping boots and armored vehicles, but not the monsters we had imagined. If you manage to imagine their faces without the steel helmets, they look like human beings after all. Is it the weapon in his hand, the steel helmet on his head, the greatcoat, the riding breeches and the boots that change a human being? Or is it the propaganda from the loudspeakers, or that unlimited power over other people's lives?

In contrast to other Polish towns, Warsaw it not exposed to any terror actions. The population is probably judged by the occupying forces to be sufficiently terrorized, frightened and subdued already. The German war machine's powerful Oberkommando judges that no more is necessary. We are given a temporary breathing space, but the worst is still to come.

The Maple Tree Behind the Barbed Wire

Back to Czestochowa

The war is not over, has only begun. But Warsaw has fallen, and with that warfare in Poland is over — only the naval base on the narrow little sandy peninsula of Hel holds out for a few more days. Many people are dead, even more injured — invalided for life. We are all right, and we want to go back to Czestochowa as soon as possible. But first we are to pay a visit to our friends the Wajnapels. We pack our cases; say goodbye to Maurycy, his wife and Rutka - all of us doing our best to make our farewells not too chilly — and we set off for ulica Marszalkowska, where the Wajnapels live.

All kinds of vehicles have appeared on the streets, horses the army has not requisitioned hauling cabs or adapted carts, a few ramshackle taxis the military have rejected, even a few lorries and various types of homemade vehicles pulled by bicycles or human beings. Necessity is the mother of invention, and the individual's ability to innovate great when new everyday problems have to be solved quickly. We find a horse-drawn cab, which will take our cases and us to the Wajnapels.

The building in ulica Marszalkowska is still standing and the Wajnapels welcome us warmly. But they are not the same people as when we last saw them. They are bewildered, depressed and are finding it hard to adapt to this new situation. The youngest son is still in Paris, where he is reading medicine. Lucky him. The governess is still there, but the festivity, the laughter and joy have gone, and the luxury has lost its luster.

The trains are not running and no public transport is functioning, but at the Wajnapels we find out there is a hauler who collects up passengers and takes them by lorry to various places. This suits us perfectly. The hauler in question, whom we go to see, turns out to have a lorry going to Czestochowa. It is already rather full, but he says he can squeeze us four on to the back. We stay overnight with the Wajnapels and the next morning we load our luggage on to the back of the lorry and set off on our journey to Czestochowa.

It is early in the morning of October 4th, 1939. The hauler and his driver have made it fairly comfortable for his passengers on the back of the old lorry and it is not at all cramped. Most of our luggage has been stowed away up at the front, the rest in between the specially made low sturdy benches with backs to them, where we are to sit during the journey. Brown blankets are laid out on the benches, and there are also some big black umbrellas — should it rain, but we never have to use them. It is pleasantly warm, the sun covered by white clouds and there is practically no wind.

The restaurants along the road are closed. We have thermoses of hot tea and bottles of cold water with us, and those who had some food left, or have been able to buy some, have packs with them. Everyone shares with everyone else during the journey. We have a good view — you see a lot from the back of a lorry — and at first we have to make our way through the bombed-out capital city.

Clearing rubble and repair work have already started, although it is early in the morning and only three days since the capitulation. Poles and non-uniformed Germans are supervising the work. We see blue-clad Polish policemen directing the traffic, but only a few German soldiers are to be seen on the streets of Warsaw.

There is a new kind of poster on the walls of buildings — white with thick black frames, German text in menacing Gothic lettering and the same text underneath in Polish. At the bottom is the rubber stamp — the typical German eagle with its wings outspread, perched in a black circle with that crooked swastika. They are here with their swastika. When the lorry stops at a crossroads, I can see the posters are about various prohibitions, all the things the inhabitants may not do, and if anyone disobeys the orders, the punishment is death. Death seems to be the standard punishment for infringing the orders of the occupying powers. Do they really mean it seriously? Will they shoot people, or do they just want to frighten us into obeying their orders?

We leave the centre of the city and drive through the suburbs. Only a few of the buildings are damaged and there are hardly any of the deep craters there are in the thickly populated central part of the city.

It is just about two hundred kilometers to Czestochowa. We drop off some of the passengers at a couple of places along the road, like a train stopping at stations. The luggage stowed between the benches is theirs.

We are driven along the main roads of the country, but despite this, there are only two lanes and they are not wide. There are a great many civilians on their way to or from the capital — cars, lorries, horse-drawn vehicles, bicycles and pedestrians. Several people are carrying large clumsy sacks on their backs. The lorry makes good speed cruising ahead in this crush of vehicles and people in constant motion.

Sometimes a German military column passes, always motorized — not like the Polish army on foot or mounted. Each major column is preceded by military police — soldiers in thick green outer clothing on big noisy dark green or camouflaged motorcycles. They stop at every crossroads, look around, firmly stop all crossing traffic and supervise the passing of the military column.

At first comes a camouflaged car containing a few soldiers, clearly officers, in green or sometimes brown leather coats or some material resembling thick rubber. The following vehicles are usually tarpaulin-covered trucks, sometimes single armored vehicles with heavy machine guns. Protruding from them. But we see no tanks.

Whenever a military column approaches, we all have to make way to one side and stop until the column has passed. Then the military policemen leave the cross-roads and the colorful many-headed civilian traffic gets going again, until the next advancing column, then all civilians have to get off the road. It is slow going for the civilians, but fast for the German military. The Germans do not allow civilians to hold up military traffic, and they are very efficient.

At major crossroads, some motorcycle military police are standing around, often with an officer, waiting for the next troops to pass. I see an officer in a full-length leather coat standing in the middle of a large crossroads, directing the military traffic and shouting Schnell! Schnell! when he thinks it is going too slowly. Army couriers on heavy motorbikes ride back and forth along the long Germany military columns. We think it is perhaps not quite so stylish as our handsome cavalry, like the mounted Dragoons or Uhlans, but much more efficient. Orderliness and control prevail in everything the Germans undertake, and they do not seem unfriendly.

As we near Piotrków, a long military column is passing. We stop at the side of the road and the driver and the two women with three children sitting up front with him get out of the big cabin, while the rest of us stay sitting or standing on the back of the lorry. It is difficult getting down, and it takes time to get back up again when we are to go on.

An older German soldier comes over to our lorry. He is in the typical grey-green uniform of thick cloth, his forage cap in the middle of his head — not at a slant like on many of the younger soldiers — no badges of rank. An ordinary Werhmacht soldier, no medals or other distinctions, neither SS nor a party member. He seems ordinary and good-natured, has a bayonet hanging at his side, but otherwise is unarmed — no firearms. He is fairly short and we are not afraid, just curious. The soldier looks up at us sitting on the back of the lorry — it is the first time I have seen the face of a German soldier at close quarters. He asks a question. Gibt's einige Juden im Auto? Are there any Jews in the vehicle?

I want to show that I understand and can answer when a German soldier addresses us. Yes, I say, holding up my hand. He looks at me and says good-naturedly, with no aggression but quite firmly: "We've come here to solve the Jewish question once and for all." Just that, nothing else. That is the first German I have ever spoken to — a friendly, private soldier, no party man — and his statement is a calm affirmation of a fact he himself accepts and clearly approves. He turns on his heel and saunters leisurely back to his group of other older soldiers taking a rest on the roadside.

Pinkus is horrified - I think not so much because of what the soldier had said, but because of my stupidity. I am not afraid at all, but somewhat shaken and mystified. I have not done him any harm and he is just repeating what his Führer, what Hitler had said on the radio. To Pinkus I say a little remorsefully, nothing has happened to us, nothing to make a fuss about.

After we have been on our way for several hours and start getting away from the proximity of Warsaw, the traffic thins out and our lorry gets up speed. We go on towards Czestochowa one experience richer. I have spoken to my first German soldier and heard what he had to say.

There are no controls along the entire long way from Warsaw, none except the one when the older soldier had spoken to us, wanting to know who we were. It is evening and still quite light when we arrive at Czestochowa. Nothing seems changed, nothing has been destroyed, no ruins, no damage to the buildings. Everything looks peaceful — except those black and white posters and the green-clad German police in charge of law and order with their strange high helmets. The new German civilian administration has already settled in —Czestochowa.

The driver puts down his remaining passengers at various places along Aleja, the main street in Czestochowa. We get down at Second Aleja, on the corner of our street, only one block away from home, Aleja Wolnosci 3/5.

The door to our apartment is locked, just as we had locked it when we had left. Sarah opens up with her two keys — one for each lock — we go inside with our cases and look around. Everything looks just the same, just as we had left it, everything untouched, and it feels safe.

Roman goes to his room and his toys. Sarah unpacks and starts preparing food. There are some tins, some dried food and potatoes in the cold cellar, where food keeps best when you can no longer fill the icebox with ice every day. There is plenty of wood for the stove. I wonder whether it had been necessary to go to Warsaw and go through the siege. Pinkus goes over to some neighbors to find out what has been happening. He always wants to know what is in the wind — listen to the Jewish Najes news. From him I have learnt that it is good to listen to the radio, to be interested in the news, to know what is going on.

After a while, Pinkus comes back with our neighbor, Herr Frank. Herr Frank is quite strong and always wears dark clothes. He lives on the ground floor in the rear courtyard and has a friendly round clean-shaven face. His wife is clever at sewing corsets and has two employees. I don't actually know what Herr Frank does, or whether he has any work at all. Pinkus likes talking to him, as he usually knows what is happening and is a constant source for Najes as well as a good storyteller.

Frank tells us that on the very evening of September 1st, the day the war started, the Polish military and the administration had silently slipped away, leaving Czestochowa with no defenses. Many had wanted to go with them, but not many had succeeded. On September 3rd, the Germans marched into town early in the morning, and the next day they carried out their first terror action. The intention must have been to gain respect quickly and effectively, to show who decides things now, to frighten the people and get them to obey. This was just what their leader Adolf Hitler had promised them, had said to them and had written down. He has promised he will bring in a thousand year reign of terror if he comes into power. He has promised his people, the German people, as Herrenvolk, superior to other people, under his leadership, are to lead this reign of terror and that is what they are doing now — just as they have been promised.

The terror action was started in ulica Nadrzeczna, in the middle of the area mostly inhabited by Jews. Uniformed Germans went from house to house, banging on every apartment door, hounding out the men with blows, yells, lashes and threats. The first were hustled into the big courtyard of the Craft School in ulica Garncarska in the Jewish quarter, then made to throw themselves down on the ground, face down, and they were forbidden to look up. When the courtyard was full, others were hustled into the empty old Polish 27th Infantry regimental parade ground. When that was also covered with prostrate men, the rest of the men, Poles and Jews, were hunted down round the town streets, through Nowy Rynek, Katedralna, Narutowicza, First and Second Aleja, the Germans mostly shooting up into the air, but occasionally also into the running crowds of people. Several wounded and dead were left helplessly lying in the streets.

Some were chased into Holy Sigismund church, but most were assembled in the open space in the middle of town, in front of the Magistrat - the town hall. They also had to lie face down and were forbidden to raise their heads. The Germans fired machine-guns over their heads, and anyone happening to raise his head, or an arm or a leg, was either wounded or killed. Sometimes they fired a salvo slightly lower, so some of those lying flat and quite still were hit. This went on for varying spells at different places. The Germans had begun in the Jewish quarter, and then went on to other parts of the town. It was random killing, just as it usually is in terror actions — no one was to feel safe and everyone was to feel threatened.

On September 6th, the action was completed. At first, people began to bury their dead and help the injured still lying in the streets and squares, most of them having been there without any help for up to two days. When the action was over, four hundred people were dead, three hundred of them Jews. Many more were wounded, men of all ages, young boys and seventy year-old men, no one knows how many. The wounded were still in hospital, though others did not want to go to hospital — or their families did not want to send them there, so tended their wounded at home. Many had also been taken away, mostly young men, Poles and Jews. It was said that it might be three thousand men, or more, and that they had been sent to forced labour camps, but no one knew where, or even if they were alive, or whether they would ever come back.

The Maple Tree Behind the Barbed Wire

This is the beginning of the promised thousand-year reign of terror, but actually it had been started several years earlier — on the Kristallnacht, the Night of the Long Knives. Though then it was thought to concern only Jews, so many did not think it was that bad. Nothing had been learnt from history — it begins with us Jews, but goes on with others.

Frank tells us of several decrees that have been announced, and that the penalty is death if they are not obeyed. He says the Germans mean it seriously, so it is probably best to obey their orders.

Frank is also able to tell us that the people living in the big apartment building in Aleja Kosciuszki and had been hounded out of it, had not been allowed to return. The Gestapo has now turned it into their premises; people are arrested and taken there — to the Gestapo headquarters. Many of them never come back and no one knows what happened to them. Those who do come back are often broken men; in that building, they beat and torture people. One man jumped out of a third floor window. It is best to be careful, for there are informers — often caretakers are forced to be informers, others report people voluntarily — and then there are Volksdeutscher, Poles of German origin.

On September 16th, only two weeks ago, Frank tells us, the Gestapo had summoned some well-known Jews to them, several from the previous Zydowska Gmina, the Jewish Congregation. Before they leave home, they say farewell to their families. On arrival at the big building in Aleja Kosciuszki, they are received with: Die Hunde sind da - the dogs are here. There they are met by three Gestapo officers and are under arrest for several hours, though without being hurt. Then they meet the same Gestapo men and are ordered to form a Judenrat - a Council of Elders. Frank does not know what this Judenrat is supposed to do, apart from that it is to administer us. The Council's chairman is Leon Kopinski; his nephew Wladek is in the same class as I am and sits in the desk behind me.

Leon Kopinski was to select the other members of the Council and some officials. Pinkus and Frank are agreed that those selected are all known and good people: Berliner, Rothbart, Rotstein, Kohlenbrenner with his assistant Abraszka Wilhelm, the lawyers Pohorille and Gitler, the well-known ex-athlete - Bernard Kurland - and the rector of the Jewish gymnasium - Anisfelt. I wonder who told the Gestapo which were suitable people to organize—e a Judenrat. They clearly knew this and much else, perhaps even before they came to Czestochowa.

It was probably not quite as peaceful in Czestochowa as it had seemed when we had arrived an hour or two earlier.

I have always been a slow thinker; I need time to understand and draw conclusions. Not until later that evening did I begin to understand the significance of what the German private Werhmacht soldier near Piotrków had said to us earlier that day. Just that — a perfectly ordinary private German soldier, not a party member, saying what he said to us, shows that Adolf Hitler has the German people on his side even in their attitude to us Jews. They agree with his plan for our future — it is an important task for them, to solve the Jewish question once and for all.

The Maple Tree Behind the Barbed Wire

The Calm before the Storm

A few weeks go by. We adapt and try to live as normal a life as possible during a war; during an occupation by a power not particularly friendly disposed to us Jews. We have no choice.

There is new money — for those who go shopping. There is food to be bought, though most of it in the shops is rationed. There is more to be bought on what is called the black market. Our new authorities are aware that it exists but choose not to interfere. On the black market, prices and quantities are not regulated and almost everything is available for sale — butter, bread, sugar, eggs, vegetables, shoes, razor blades, cloth — but they are all much more expensive.

Polish agriculture largely consists of peasants with small patches of land which they cultivate with the help of their wives and sometimes their children, but with no employees. Women in kerchiefs come into town pulling carts of their goods, which are quickly snapped up. Servants of the German occupying forces and even wives and friends of Germans can be seen shopping for food on the black market, although the Germans have much better access to food that the residents. During war and food rationing, Polish small farmers do better that other sections of the population. They have become the wartime aristocracy to whom everyone appeals, their importance growing with the increasing shortage of food. The shortage of food in Czestochowa is getting worse, though people don't seem to be starving, anyhow not yet. Gold, precious stones and foreign currencies also exist on the black market, as well as many other things to buy.

There are special shops for second-hand clothes and shoes, and tablecloths, linen, furs and hides are also traded. A good tablecloth can pass from middleman to middleman — several people may make a living from it for a while. People buy sites and even properties, which for the moment are not worth much. Apartments don't bring in rents or income, but they can be expected to regain their value after the war. They say arms can be bought on the black market, too, but that trade is truly black — jet-black.

Pinkus opens his workshop again. Several but not all his old employees return. There are customers wanting suits, trousers or overcoats — some of them new customers. I now have more time to be in Pinkus' workshop.

Our ordinary schools are closed, both the Jewish and the Axera gymnasiums. Instead, secret courses are started up, organized by Professor Mering. He was the history teacher at the Jewish gymnasium — a rather dry and dull teacher. His wife, Professor Meringowa, a teacher of Polish language, tries to appear strict, but is uninteresting and faint-hearted, and then Professor Brandes, an excellent teacher and pedagogue who taught mathematics. These three

The Maple Tree Behind the Barbed Wire

are now teaching us in all previous subjects — except Hebrew, Jewish history, Bible and religious studies, which are not included in the curriculum we are trying to follow. The idea is that these previously important subjects would not be demanded by any authority we hope sometime after the war is to approve our secret schooling — actually they were not required before the war, either for the school certificate or final school-leaving exams.

In wartime, we have to be content with what was most necessary, our values now being revised. Much of what had been considered necessary in school, at home, during the holidays and in our free time, is now regarded as superfluous and fairly easy to dispense with. As long as you have food, you do not have to freeze, you have a bed to sleep in and, perhaps most of all; you have hopes for the future.

Schaffer, our kind and friendly geography teacher, the charismatic Lauer - our Hebrew teacher who was also our class teacher and excellent at keeping us in order, the "little" Hirschfeldt, the algebra and geometry teacher, the "great" Hirschfeldt - the rabbi who was said to eat ham and taught religion and Bible studies, the red-haired Ginsburg who taught Latin, the stately Leopold Pfeferberg who taught gym and enchanted all the girls when he came to school in his Sub-Lieutenant's uniform although he was actually in the Reserve - all these people and many others in our fine old Jewish gymnasium are no longer with us. The teaching goes on in smaller groups, at the home of one of the teachers, and lasts at the most for four hours a day. We have old school books, new curricula and are given marks at the end of term.

As good as all of Class IIB at our old school often continue to meet, though not all at once. Social life is lively and pleasant. We fall in love, are happy, unhappy and disappointed, as young people usually are in their mid-teens. We kiss, some even hug when they think no one's looking — things are much as usual. We meet in private homes and not as before on the promenade stretch beneath Pazderski's clock on the left-hand side of Second Aleja. We are too young to be taken for forced labour and so relatively safe — so far.

We belong in the Generalguvernement, what is left of Poland after the Germans had annexed huge areas in the west and the Soviet Union annexations in the east. Hans Franck is the Governor-General. He lives in Wawel - a mediaeval fortress full of valuable objects, hand-made tapestries and carpets, beautiful and valuable pictures and furniture, one of the fine old traditional palaces of Polish kings from the days when Kraków was the capital of Poland. Warsaw is in ruins, and so Kraków, a historic place full of the proud memories of the Polish people, is the city of residence of the Governor-General.

Governor-General Hans Franck is a mediocre lawyer. His main merit is that he has been Hitler's lawyer and whenever necessary, he defended Hitler and his closest party friends when the German courts were still free. They no longer have any need for lawyers, for they are now the legislators and dictate the judgements of the German courts, are judges themselves in the occupied territories and carry out their sentences immediately — on the spot, whenever they like. In 1924, Adolf Hitler wrote that if he comes to power he will abolish democracy — and he does, too, including the free courts, an important part of a democracy. And defense lawyers? They probably still exist but have no really important function in Hitler's Germany.

The majority of the characteristic bi-lingual manifestos posted on the walls of buildings are now signed by the Stadthauptmann. He is a German, usually a lawyer with a doctorate title, is often a party member and replaces the democratically elected civilian mayor. But one of these public notices is signed by the Governor-General himself, the lawyer Hans Franck. On it, he hammers in that it is we — the Jews - who have wanted this war, that the war is our doing. We are parasites and have no right to stay in his Generalguvernement, which is Deutscher Lebensraum - German living space — whatever that may mean. What shall we do if we may not stay in Hans Franck's province? We have nowhere else to go, and also, according to another manifesto signed by Herr Stadthauptmann, we may not leave Czestochowa. Jews in general may not travel without special permission. Some must have had this permission, otherwise it would not be mentioned in the decree, but I don't know of a single Jew who has had permission to travel outside Czestochowa.

All that is left of the Polish administration are the blue-clad order police, and the fire service with their red vehicles and gold-colored helmets. But a lot of new uniforms have appeared on the streets. We soon learn to recognize the uniforms and ranks of these new people in power. This can be useful, as we are totally dependent on their whims.

Seen most of all are the German order police in green. Those that have been posted to Czestochowa to keep order in our town are a section of the regular order police in Leipzig; here they are called "the Greens - Di grine". Wartime Leipzig has to manage with rather fewer order police. In Czestochowa, there is also the Gestapo - which I realize is supposed to mean the German state secret police. They have tailored steel-grey uniforms and badges of rank on their black collars — though they are usually in civilian clothes, for they are supposed to be secret. There are semi-civilian Germans in the party's dark brown uniforms, red armbands with swastikas on them and the party badge on their chests. We see the Wermacht in the dark grey-green uniform of the infantry, the air force grey-blue uniforms, and the terrifying tall powerful soldiers of the SS troops, all in black with their gleaming polished jackboots and silver skulls on their black caps — they seem to be highest in rank and like the Gestapo have their badges of rank on their collars.

The Maple Tree Behind the Barbed Wire

A number of Germans in civilian clothes have just the red-white-and-black party badge, NSDAP - the German National Socialist Workers Party. A number of the uniformed Germans, and some civilians, also have the menacing SS-badge of the storm troopers on their chests.

It is clear that the Germans love uniforms and glossy steel-shod jackboots even when they are in civilian clothes, as they proudly wear their badges on their chests or their lapels to show where they come in the hierarchy, in the state and party apparatus. Quite a number are party members, but only a few have the SS badge, the two silver flashes of lightning against a black background.

When they meet, most Germans greet each other by raising their right arm and saying Heil Hitler - then shaking hands. Those with a party badge do that, but many of those who wear neither party nor SS badge also use the Heil Hitler greeting.

All these uniformed men are Reichdeutscher, state Germans, the real Germans. It has turned out that a number of people we knew and thought were Poles are really Volksdeutscher, of the German people, but not German citizens. Many of these Volksdeutscher move freely among the Germans, on German police premises, even in the much-feared Gestapo building. Some wear the NSDAP badge and were previously party members, but had kept it secret. The Volksdeutscher are feared. You never know which among the Poles they are, perhaps they are someone you have known a long time. It is said that there are even friendly disposed Volksdeutscher who are said to help — usually for payment — but they are few, so it is best to be careful. I have not yet heard of any Reichdeutscher who in any way in any context has been helpful to a Jew.

The Jewish council — the Judenrat - has organized itself. Leon Kopinski, chairman of the council, is called by the Germans the Elder of the Jews although he is not at all old. Kopinski had to select the ten members of the actual council and organise something resembling a government with fifteen departments and fifteen departmental heads. All these departments are called Amt. They are finance, labour, social, education, industry, post, housing, just as in an ordinary government, though in miniature. Everyone in the Judenrat and all heads of departments are well known and generally esteemed people and it is agreed that Leon Kopinski has made a good choice, he and his assistants have the confidence of the Jewish people and also live up to it. Bernard Kurland is appointed head of the important Arbeitsamt, the labour department. The rector of our Jewish gymnasium, the well-known mathematician Anisfeld, becomes head of the school committee — though no Jewish schools exist to administer, officially.

The Judenrat registers us all — children, adults and the old, distributes ration cards and arranges public kitchens for those who cannot afford to buy the food with their coupons. They are all given a piece of black bread and quite nourishing hot soup for their coupons, and also if people have no coupons, but then they are exhorted to get themselves registered to acquire food coupons for the next time.

All adult Jews must have work and what is called Arbeitspass. Those who at German razzias turn out to lack work-passes risk being sent away to forced labour and many of them disappear. It is the Judenrat which distributes jobs and passes, and nearly all adults have such passes. If you haven't been able to find work yourself, then the Jewish official finds an occupation that is then given on the pass. It seems to work well — so far.

Nearly all of us are registered — that is German thoroughness and orderliness. Without registration — no ration cards, no food, no Arbeitspass protecting you at razzias. Cleverly planned and logically carried out to catch us in a trap, but none of us understand that, not yet.

People are arrested — usually men, but sometimes women — for no given reason and they disappear without anyone knowing where. Groups of young Jews are taken out at unexpected razzias on the streets or from their homes in quarters that are suddenly barricaded off, and they are sent to forced labour, no one knows where. At some razzias, even an Arbeitspass is not valid.

The Germans clear the streets of beggars and handicapped people. It is said that they are killed with an injection at one of the town hospitals, by a German doctor or nurse — but this is perhaps just a rumor. Anyway, they suddenly disappear and no longer exist.

I feel sorry for the backward and always smiling girl dwarf in her not always clean, but pretty red frilly dresses, who goes round on her misshapen legs on the Jewish side of Second Aleja and is given coins by passers-by. Her name is Rywka and we called her Mesygene Rywka - Potty Rywka. She couldn't speak, but could smile and shyly hold out her little hand. Suddenly she wasn't there. We miss her. She was a friendly patch of color whom everyone liked. No one would dream of doing her any harm, although a few years ago there was a rumor that she had been raped. Did they also kill this harmless dwarf? If so, why? She disturbed no one.

At the beginning of November 1939, the green German order police van drives into the big rear courtyard of our apartment block. Three policemen get out, come up the stairs and knock on our door. They are polite and wish to speak to "Herr Schneidermeister Pinkus Einhorn", and ask if they may come into the living room — then do so before Pinkus has time to say they may. One is an officer - Oberleutnant - the other two subordinates, ordinary policemen, but the officer has an SS badge. He introduces himself - Oberleutnant Überscheer - without holding out his hand — you don't shake hands with a Jew. Überscheer tells Pinkus that they have orders from Berlin to requisition seven

The Maple Tree Behind the Barbed Wire

paintings in our home — we are to be given a receipt. He takes out a list, shows it to Pinkus and asks with a sharp edge to his voice whether the listed paintings are still there in the apartment. Pinkus looks at the list and says — yes, that's right, they are here. Oberleutnant Überscheer relaxes and asks to look at the pictures.

They are our finest pictures. But Pinkus shows no emotion, just goes round pointing out to Überscheer the paintings on the list and explaining who the painters are and what the pictures represent. Oberleutnant Überscheer listens, but does not seem particularly interested. He gives orders to the two policemen with him. The pictures on his list are taken down, two old French ones, a couple of our best Polish ones, one by a Russian artist and a drawing by Chagall which Pinkus acquired many years ago.

With some help, Pinkus had written a letter to Marc Chagall, telling Chagall that he himself was an artist, though as a tailor, but he would like to have something by Chagall and was willing to pay whatever it cost. He asked if Chagall would like to have a suit made for him. Chagall did not, but Pinkus was allowed to buy an original drawing, and now they are taking it. They leave behind other paintings by Jewish artists or with Jewish motifs, except a large oil painting by Menkes of a praying Jew, a modern painting with an unusual dark red background, Pinkus' favorite.

The Oberleutnant leaves a receipt for the seven confiscated paintings, though the receipt does not say which they are. A receipt in advance signed with an illegible name, not even the usual stamp on it with the great eagle above the swastika in the circle. The two policemen go down and back up the stairs several times before they have all the listed paintings stowed in their van in the courtyard — there is no lift in our apartment house. A driver is sitting in the van, another non-commissioned officer in the German order police. They salute politely and leave. It seems to me that they are impressed that Berlin wants to have the Jew Einhorn's paintings. Pinkus looks at the receipt — he can read neither German or Polish, only Yiddish - then hands it over to Sarah and asks her to keep it, for you never know.

Sarah and I think Pinkus is miserable, and we don't know how to console him. Nearly all the money he has saved from tailoring has gone on his paintings. He has not bought land or property, nor has he saved money in the bank. Twice, when he had bought a particularly fine painting, the whole living room had to be repapered so that the background would suit the new picture. But Pinkus says he is not miserable, and I can see he means it. He says: "Jurek" — he is serious then, as otherwise he just says Josele - "there are different periods in a person's life and different things can be important on different occasions. Now it is important to survive. It is sad, but they can have our pictures as long as we may stay alive, have food to eat and beds to sleep in. When the war is over I can start again, buy new pictures. That receipt is not worth much." He goes back to his real life — his workshop. He meant what he said, he really is not miserable — an amazing man, my father.

Our local newspaper - Glos Czestochowy - is coming out again, apparently the same paper, the same emblem, the same layout, the same title and the same typeface. Despite this, we find it difficult to recognize it. Not so much because it is so much thinner than before, only four spreads, eight pages — but because of the content. Everything the occupying powers do, according to the newspaper, is good; everything is for the best of the people. France and England are our enemies. So naive, do they really imagine anyone will believe it? But if it is repeated often enough, perhaps some will, how would I know? There are few advertisement in the paper, new decrees published instead, looking just like the posters on the walls outside, though smaller.

One new decree concerns Jews only. We are forbidden to possess more than a hundred zloty — which is not much — any other money is to be deposited in a bank. The same applies to all specified types of valuables and jewelry. These are to be handed in at a given assembly point — otherwise the penalty is death. Despite this, many break that particular rule. People know that they are going to need those valuables to buy food and other necessities for survival. People know that even worse times are to come — before they perhaps get better. We go on hoping, but no longer know what for.

With the aid of a small pointed pair of scissors, Sarah eases the precious stones out of rings and bracelets Pinkus has given her or she has bought herself. She hands the gold in at one of the two-stated assembly places — they just throw it into big boxes. No one asks who has handed it in, nor are any receipts given. Sarah sews the precious stones into a corset — she shows me which one. "Remember this corset, Jurek," she says. "We'll always have this with us so that we have something to live off when worse times come, and then when the war is over." She is clever, Sarah. Whichever way you squeeze the places she points out in the seams, you can't feel the precious stones sewn in. But nor are her stones all that big. We could not afford large precious stones for Sarah as well as paintings. Also, Sarah was never fond of showy jewelry, so she encouraged Pinkus to buy paintings.

Jews are no longer allowed to own shops or factories. The new administration appoints its own "good men" - Treuhänder - who are to take over Jewish businesses. The owner may not take anything out of the business — otherwise a sentence of death. There is no question of compensation. Almost a third of the population of the town, now over 35,000, are Jews. The Jews have contributed to the development of the town, built up several industries, developed many smaller and

The Maple Tree Behind the Barbed Wire

larger shops, so there are a great many Treuhänder to many businesses. But the decree does not apply to craftsmen and their workshops, which are not to be taken over, so Pinkus can carry on with his workshop. In many of the businesses taken over, the new Treuhänder want the previous Jewish owner to stay. He is often a clever professional who has developed his business, working twelve or more hours a day, in the smaller businesses often with the help of his wife, perhaps even the older children. Without the previous Jewish owner, the Treuhhänder can scarcely run the business.

In the larger factories, the regime's Treuhand is a Reichsdeutscher, in the smaller ones usually a Volksdeutscher, and a particularly deserving Volkdeutscher may well be the Treuhand for several businesses. Very few of these Treuhänder of smaller and middle-sized businesses are specialists in whatever is being produced in the business they have taken over. Some, however, are previous employees in the same firm. The Treuhand in Horowicz' large factory manufacturing leather goods, for instance, is the previous bookkeeper, who turns out to be a Volksdeutscher. But the Reichsdeutscher who come from Germany and take over the big factories are often specialists with experience of management, and there are several larger businesses of that kind which the Jews of the town have developed. The largest is Gnaszyn clothing factory with Director Zygman, and the Cegelnia brickworks with Director Helman, both providing employment for several hundred Polish and Jewish workers. I know Zygman and Helman. Pinkus makes clothes for them, and Helman's son Tomek was in the same class as I was at the Zofja Wygórska Folwasinska elementary school.

On December 25th - Christmas Day, 1939 - another Jewish pogrom breaks out, clearly planned and ordered by the new powers, but it is Poles who fight, lash out and burn. This pogrom is well organized, swift, purposeful and effective--it lasts only a few hours. Our lovely synagogue, built up by many donations and collections among the Jews of Czestochowa, is burnt to the ground — with everything in it, even our old holy scriptures, which we have always cared for so reverently. We stay at home, frightened. But no one harms us.

After a few days, I go out to look at the synagogue. I have gone to it for all our major festivals, usually with Sarah, sometimes Pinkus with us. That was what it was like the year before, when I was thirteen and to celebrate my Bar Mitzvah - the traditional maturity celebration for Jewish boys. I had to stand on the lower of the two prayer places on the podium, and I read from the Holy Scriptures, sang out of tune and was taken into the congregation.

Now I look at the burnt remains of the synagogue, nothing but bare smoke-streaked walls left of it. But you can still see how beautiful it

The Maple Tree Behind the Barbed Wire

had been, at least if you had seen it before. The handsome portal borne on four pillars, the three sets of steps up, where everyone meets at the entrance to the synagogue, the windows vaulted at the top, with their lovely painted glass — all the windows are now smashed. Why have they burnt down our lovely synagogue?

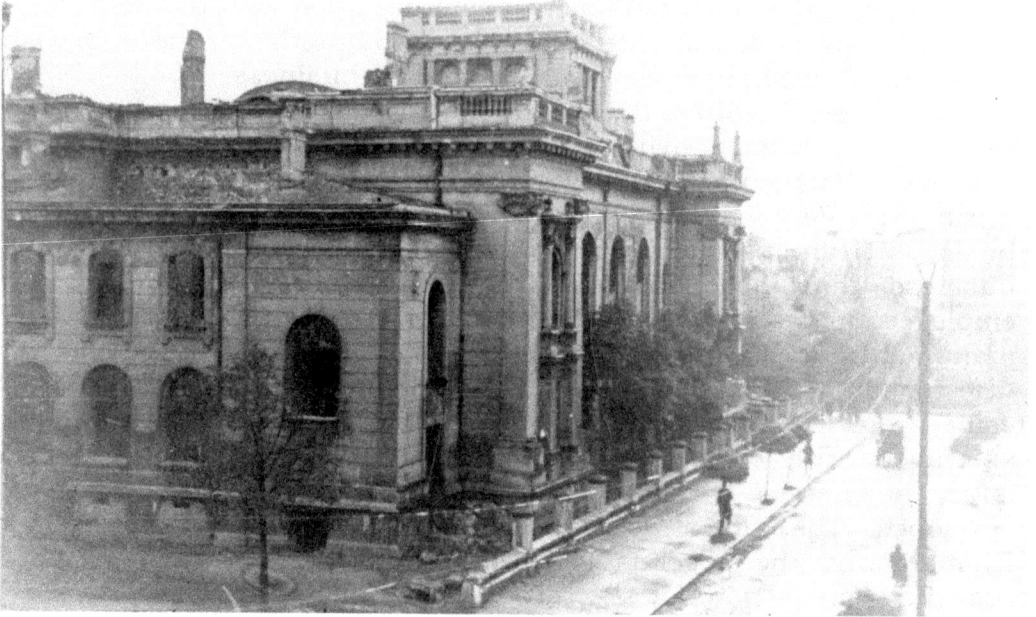

During the 1939 Christmas Day Jewish pogrom, our beautiful synagogue was burnt to the ground, leaving nothing but its smoke-damaged walls. This was where only the year before I had had my Bar Mitzvah and had been taken into our congregation

Jews may not go to the cinema, the theatre or to concerts — that is strictly forbidden. I like going to the cinema, and so does Sarah.

One day Sarah manages it — black pleated skirt, white silk blouse, a little black jacket with small white appliqué and interwoven silver threads. I am wearing a white shirt and a tie. Sarah says we are to go out, but she does not say where, not until we get to the Odeon. We have been to this cinema many times before, as it is the nearest to where we live.

The cashier is the fat heavily made-up pani Kogutowa. In Pinkus' workshop, they like to joke about her, rather coarse jokes. I remember when Berek asked who would want to hold Mrs. Kogutowa if she needed to pee. I guess he meant hold her like a little child who is to wee in the grass.

The first performance starts at five o'clock. We arrive a few minutes past five and everyone has already gone in and sat down. Sarah knows

The Maple Tree Behind the Barbed Wire

Mrs. Kogutowa, goes up to the ticket-office and says she wants two tickets. Mrs. Kogutowa takes the money — the exact sum — and hands over two tickets without looking at us. We go into the already dark cinema, sit down in our seats in the back row, near the exit.

The films is called "Bel Ami" and has just begun. It is a German film, as most are, with Polish sub-titles. A sob story from the turn of the century with grandly dressed untroubled lovely people, balls, singing, elegant homes and much love. They had a few problems, mostly misunderstandings and complications, nothing serious that seems threatening, all ends well and Sarah weeps. Before the lights go on, Sarah takes my hand and says we must go. I realize we have to do that at once, so do not resist although I won't be able to see the last scenes of the film. We come out on to the street before the others. It is dusk and we hurry home — soon a curfew begins for Jews.

This is the loveliest and most gripping film I have ever seen. At night, before I fall asleep, I think about those lovely well-dressed people, always smiling, with nothing but trivial problems which are easy to solve. Everyone in the film is kind and it is difficult to recognize them in the Germans we see. It was nice to see that film in the middle of the misery around us — ration cards, curfews, forced labour, looming poverty, unmotivated arrests, torture and death penalties for infringments which in normal times seem banal. Before I fall asleep, I like to think of something pleasant. I suppose everyone does, and then I think about the film "Bel Ami".

But that Sarah dared — it is so unlike her to take any unnecessary risks — to go to the cinema? I am grateful to Sarah for taking me with her and so that in all the misery I am reminded that there is another world, in the future, too, perhaps even for us Jews. On that day I experience a side of my mother I had had no idea was there — that she could be so light-hearted, so girlish. We become closer to each other as a result of this common secret, and I understand even better why Pinkus once fell in love, wanted to marry and have a family with Sarah. But that she dared! Perhaps she had spoken to Mrs. Kogutowa beforehand?

My mother and I were never to mention this visit to the cinema, not even when we met after the war. I have not asked and have only the faintest idea why she did it.

When in the spring of 1947 I arrive in Uppsala to read medicine, "Bel Ami" is being shown at the Fyris cinema, in the same building as I am living in - Järnbrogatan 10B. I go and see the film again, but I should not have done so. It is a sickly soap opera with people and events that never occur in any normal life. But by then I am again living an almost normal life and going to the cinema is no longer a risky business, and Sarah is no longer with me.

The Maple Tree Behind the Barbed Wire

A few days after Sarah and I had been to the cinema, at home I see a young, self-confident man in a middling brown trench coat, boots, breeches and a jaunty Tyrolean hat with a feather stuck in one side. He looks like a Volksdeutscher, and is said to have papers to say so, but he is actually called Wróblewski and is a Jew with false papers. Wróblewski has lunch with us. In spite of rationing, Sarah manages to arrange a good lunch and I am allowed to join in. Wróblewski comes from Warsaw and tells us that Maurycy, Magda and Rutka are having a bad time, that they are starving. Pinkus says he wants them to come to us, that what we have is enough for them as well, and Sarah agrees. But can they make their way to Czestochowa? I am sent out of the room and they go on talking.

Wróblewski leaves the same afternoon and comes back two weeks later with Maurycy and Rutka, but not Magda. She did not want to come with them, but would perhaps come later. I realize she has left Maurycy and is now living with another man.

There are quite a lot of people in our apartment now. Apart from the workshop and the four of us - Pinkus, Sarah, Roman and me — there are Karola, Rózia, Maurycy, Rutka and sometimes other temporary guests. All the same, it doesn't seem overcrowded — it is wartime, even more live in many Jewish homes, and Sarah has always been hospitable.

A new decree is announced. All Jews are to wear armbands to distinguish us from the rest of the population — a white armband with the blue Star of David on it is to be worn on the right upper arm. If a Jew is found on the street without it — death penalty. We are given a week to arrange it, and trade in armbands begins. There are armbands in various sorts of cloth and in hard glossy cellophane. Those who cannot afford armbands are given one made of waxed paper at the Judenrat. We are careful always to wear our armbands, even little children, and at our home there are reserve armbands in a bowl in the big cupboard in the living room. Now we are labelled — everyone can see which are Jews.

One day a German soldier is standing in our living room, a private in the grey-green uniform of the Wehrmacht. He has come from Lódz, where Sarah's parents live. Before the war, Lódz was in Poland and the country's next largest town — now Lódz is in Germany, in das Reich, and is called Litzmanstadt. The soldier is telling us that Sarah's old parents are having a bad time, especially now it is winter. In Lódz, a Jewish ghetto is to be formed, so things will be even worse for them, and also it will be impossible for them to travel.

I have to leave the room, but they are talking in loud voices and I can hear Sarah crying. She and Pinkus appeal to the German soldier — can he help Sarah's parents get to Czestochowa? He says that is difficult, but he does not say no. I wonder — would it be possible to get

The Maple Tree Behind the Barbed Wire

Szyja and his beard, his pajes, yarmulka, his black kaftan, and Szprynca with her wig to Czestochowa? But a German soldier can arrange it. Has Szyja still got his beard, for that matter, and does he still wear his Chassid clothes?

Pinkus asks if the soldier can take money to them with him. Yes, he can do that, but as the Generalguvernement money is no use in Litzmanstadt, we would have to find other money. In an hour or two, Sarah and Pinkus have acquired some "other money" — that is not difficult these days as long as you have something sufficiently valuable to give in exchange. Most sought after are old Czarist Russian gold coins. If you are caught, you can say you collect coins, and many people believe that helps.

I know the German soldier has taken with him the "other money" but I don't know what sort, how much, or what Pinkus and Sarah gave in exchange for those coins. The soldier leaves. We never see or hear from him again.

That is the last time we hear from Szyja and Szprynca, whether they were even still alive when the soldier came to see us. We shall never find out what happened to them.

This friendly man who is a German soldier was presumably previously a Pole - he spoke faultless Polish. He ought to be a Volksdeutscher, but he lives in Litzmanstadt, so he becomes a Reichdeutscher and is conscripted into the German army. What are they doing — the Germans - with all the people they have in their power? They segregate us into some kind of hierarchy in which the Reichsdeutscher are at the top of the scale, the finest in the world, and we Jews, the scum of the earth, are at the bottom. Reichsdeutschers are to rule over the others, and they do, too, as Adolf Hitler had promised before they elected him to the highest office in the realm — he promised them that it was to be like that for a thousand years.

The workshop is going reasonably well. There are still gentlemen who want tailor-made suits from Einhorn the tailor. There is no shortage of cloth, but there is a shortage of good cloth, the kind Pinkus has, and there is beginning to be a shortage of sewing thread and buttons, even in our workshop.

Even Germans start coming to Pinkus, at first only the odd one, but then more and more. Some bring cloth with them, others want to buy. Pinkus sells to all who ask - when it comes to Germans he has no choice. Certain Germans pay, others don't and pretend they have forgotten. No one reminds a German - Volkdeutscher or Reichsdeutscher - when he or she forgets to pay. Nearly all of them behave well. People do when they meet Pinkus. Many Germans also behave well when they are not on duty, when they are not given orders to do something else and when they are not annoyed. Some of the Germans who come to the fitting room are polite, addressing Pinkus as "Herr Schneidermeister". Pinkus pays the workers in his workshop regardless of whether the customer pays him or not — just like in the old days.

All younger men risk being taken out and sent to forced labour, and some of them disappear. Sarah goes to the Judenrat and says my Arbeitspass is wrong - I was born in 1926 and not in 1925. I am fourteen not fifteen. The Judenrat functions well and I am given a new pass showing what Sarah wants. Sarah explains to me that I am really fifteen, but nonetheless it is best it does not say so, in case they start taking out even fifteen year-olds for forced labour.

On those dark red double-folded pieces of cardboard — our Arbeitspass - it says in large letters that the holder is a Jew, that he or she has a position or regular work. The security they provided when we were tempted into being registered was soon to prove to be false, yet another example of the methodical and purposeful efforts by the Germans to get us on to their lists, know how many we were, where we were, and if necessary find out if we were to stray.

So 1940 goes by. When I think back, it is a fairly calm, almost idyllic time during the war compared with what was to come later.

The Jewish population is impoverished, but adapts. There is no coffee, at best ersatz chicory, only herbal tea, and no ordinary tea. There is a shortage of sugar, and lemons and other imported fruit do not exist at all. There is a shortage of apples, pears, plums, and onions have become a great delicacy. Several people who before the war suffered from stomach ulcers, gallstones and other ailments of prosperity say they are healthier. My school is closed, but I do my courses with Professor Mering and am given my marks. Many people are hungry, but no one dies of hunger thanks to the Judenrat's soup kitchens, which still function. It is said no suicides occur — everyone is prepared to fight for survival. We wear our Jewish armbands, but we are allowed to move fairly freely, if only within the boundaries of the city. The workshop continues, almost as usual, though fewer people work there now and there are different customers. Heniek Epstein continues to receive customers when Pinkus is busy in the workshop; Karola seems still to be in love with Heniek Epstein, or thinks she is.

I am fifteen, although my pass says I am only fourteen, and I am in love with Stusia Najmark, and she is in love with me. Sometimes Stusia sits on my lap and I hold her and like doing it, but am not particularly excited.

My brother Roman is growing fast and starts getting wavy, slightly reddish hair. When we are alone, he likes to tease me, calling me names he knows I dislike, Zulta kaczka - yellow duck, or flejtuch — dirty pig. Sometimes he takes my things and I get sad and angry. The parents see only that I am angry, but not what had happened before. My explanations do not help; no one listens to them. I am big brother

The Maple Tree Behind the Barbed Wire

and should know better — he is so small, Sarah says. I don't think he is small at all, he is nine and rather troublesome.

Actually, I admire my younger brother Roman. I am a rather submissive child and Roman on the other hand dares to protest and does what he likes within fairly wide limits. It has been like that as long as I can remember.

We know that France has fallen and is occupied by the Germans, and our hopes that the war would not last long are crushed. We realize the Germans are powerful and the war will be long. But none of us hesitates. They must lose. I do not know a single Jew who believes otherwise.

At the same time, we know that only England is left. But England is powerful and they say the whole of the British Empire will help. We have heard that in London there is a Polish government, that the prime minister is called Sikorski, that there is a Polish army and a Polish air force in England, that soldiers from Canada, South Africa, Australia. New Zealand, India and other parts of the great British Empire are gathering in England. Rumors go round about America coming into the war, perhaps quite soon. Churchill, Sikorski and Roosevelt are legendary, longed-for people in Poland, not least among us Jews. We talk about what it will be like when they come to Poland. Sikorski will not be coming on a white horse, but in a military plane or perhaps a tank. He is a real soldier, not like those who fled to Romania in September 1939. Before I fall asleep, I fantasize at night on which uniforms the American soldiers really have. I have heard they are coffee-brown, but can't remember who told me. When things are difficult, the imagination is a good refuge from reality, just like all good but unfortunately untrue rumors.

In reality, it is not going to be American, British or Canadian, but quite different soldiers who come to rescue us - the very few Jews who are to survive in Czestochowa.

CHAPTER III

PREPARATIONS

The Large Ghetto

It is April 1941. We have had a severe winter and the days are longer now, it is not cold and it often rains.

On April 9th, 1941, the latest decree from Dr Wendel, our Stadthauptmann, is posted all over the streets of Czestochowa. In future, Jews may live only in a few given streets. The area stretches from ulica Nadrzeczna by the river Warta in the east to ulica Wilsona in the north, from ulica Strazacka in the south to ulica Kawia in the west-- a rather small area in the older southeast part of the city. Most of the streets are in the poorer parts of the town, with often badly maintained old buildings and poor sanitary conditions. However, in the western part of the area are one of two better-maintained streets such as Katedralna and Third Aleja. Worst of all is the area south of Stary Rynek - the Old Market Square - the Jewish quarter.

Everyone calls the area a ghetto, the Germans, too, although the word is not mentioned in the decree that is to regulate this comprehensive moving process. Most inhabitants of the area where the ghetto is being established are Jews. But most of Czestochowa's Jews live outside it — so our ghetto is probably going to be fairly crowded.

Jews who live outside the ghetto are systematically moved, according to a detailed and publicized plan that has been drawn up in advance. The few non-Jews living in the ghetto area are to be moved out. They are the first to be allowed to choose among what were previously Jewish apartments; after the Reichsdeutscher and Volksdeutscher have requisitioned the apartments they want to have. Although the Germans are allowed to choose first, the choice of apartments is nevertheless great, as the majority of the city's 35,000 Jews live outside the ghetto and now have to move and leave their apartments. A real migration starts — there is some hurry as the moving of the Jewish population has to take place within the course of three weeks.

It is not forbidden for Jews to take what they want with them, but for practical reasons they cannot take everything they have. Only a smaller part of their belongings will fit into the space allocated by the Judenrat's housing committee: usually one room per family, shared kitchen and shared toilet. A great many people have to be crammed into a small area.

The Maple Tree Behind the Barbed Wire

The Polish population has already had an opportunity to plunder Jewish properties — in connection with the pogroms in December 1939 and later when the Jews had to hand over their shops and businesses. The moving of the Jews to the ghetto, however, now gives them their best opportunity hitherto. There is a shortage of housing, good furniture, porcelain, fine pictures, carpets, tablecloths, towels and linen. When everything that cannot find space in the new and very limited housing of the Jews has to be sold or left behind in connection with the move, the Polish population then receives the rich crumbs from the Germans' laden table of years of Jewish toil and savings, often the labors of several generations — for Jews have lived in Czestochowa for a couple of hundred years.

It was going to be crowded in the ghetto when all the Jews in the town had moved in, but that is not all. Similar cleansing of Jews is going on in other towns and villages, but no ghettos are being established there, and instead the Jews are evacuated to the ghetto in Czestochowa. They are moved from communities near to our town, and also from such more distant places as the towns of Piotrków, Klobucko, Przyrów, Krzepice, Mstów, Jedrzejów, Zarki and Wloszczowa. In contrast to the resident population of Jews in Czestochowa, they are given only a few hours to pack and they may take with them only what can be fitted into the vehicles the Germans transport them in to Czestochowa's future ghetto. Many arrive destitute. In a week or two, Czestochowa's already overfull ghetto is filled with almost 20,000 more Jews and when all this moving is to come to an end is not known.

There is unrest in Pinkus' workshop, which lies outside the future ghetto. A week has gone by of the three weeks within which we have to move, and we still have no news from the Judenrat housing committee. Pinkus is feeling stressed. Will he be able to go on with his tailoring? He talks to his employees. They all stop work and gather round the cutting table, but only the older men speak. Together they try to estimate how much they can get done before we have to close down. When shall we start refusing new orders and new customers?

Three more days go by with no news. Pinkus looks worried when he tells his customers that we won't be able to finish that suit, I am sorry but I cannot promise, perhaps you had better go to someone who knows he can go on. Pinkus gives several names and addresses and says he doesn't know what is going to happen to his workshop, nor does he know whether there will even be any Einhorn tailoring firm.

One of his customers is a tall, distinguished dark-haired German, austere but always courteous, who had introduced himself as Herr Lohart. Pinkus has made a grey sports suit for him. He had brought his own cloth and thread with him, even buttons — everything. Lohart is pleased with his suit, comes back and wants Pinkus to make a pair of riding breeches for him; he has cloth with him, and I happen to be in the fitting room. Pinkus informs him of the situation — as usual unhappy and worried. He cannot do it, however much he would like to. Herr Lohart looks at Pinkus and says calmly: "I know, but you'll have time to make my breeches. For that matter, you can go on accepting new orders, but only from German customers." He notices that Pinkus looks puzzled and adds: "It's already arranged. We usually think of everything," he says quietly and thoughtfully, as if to himself, smiling inwardly. It is the first time I have seen anything like a smile on this austere German's face. Pinkus looks as if about to ask a question, for of course he wants to know more, but then he realizes the conversation is over, and he seems rather doubtful. Pinkus measures Lohart for the breeches and Lohart leaves. Pinkus turns thoughtfully back to the workshop, saying nothing, and we really don't know anything more, and nor do we even know who Herr Lohart is, except he is a German in civilian clothes.

Later that afternoon that same day, Herr Kohlenbrenner, head of the Judenrat housing committee comes. We do not know him. He sits down in the workshop and tells us we have been allocated space for the workshop and living quarters in Aleja 14 - "the dom Majtlisa". Larger apartment houses in Czestochowa are often named after whoever built them and had been the first owner. Aleja 14 was built by a dentist called Majtlis and his two brothers — one a lawyer. Kohlenbrenner is trying to answer all our questions.

Yes, there will be room for both living quarters and workshop. No, he doesn't know how many rooms we shall be given, as they haven't yet divided up the rooms in the building. Yes, he has been told to inform several others who are to live in the same building, different kinds of craftsmen, fifteen in all. Yes, like all other Jews in Czestochowa, we can take with us all the equipment we have now in the workshop and which we think we shall need in future, indicating sewing machines, pressing irons and cutting tables.

Sarah is with us and was the first to ask questions — now everyone is asking them. Kohlenbrenner is in a hurry, but goes on answering. No, he doesn't know any more. Yes, the Magistrat told them about this the day before, or perhaps it was two days ago, but there has been so much to do, they haven't been able to inform us earlier, as so many are to be housed. No, he really does not know anything more, no, he doesn't know who Herr Lohart is, has never hear the name before, he adds when Pinkus finally quietly asks.

Lively talk breaks out the moment Kohlenbrenner has left, everyone talking at once — speculating on what we have just heard. But Pinkus interrupts and getting up, says "back to work". We know what we know and there is no point in speculating. We'll see. Pinkus enjoys his work and is clearly to be allowed to go on with it. He has said to me before that work is the best tranquilizer, so we go on working, as usual.

The Maple Tree Behind the Barbed Wire

After a while, Sarah comes back into the workshop, as she wants to talk to Pinkus. Do you mean now? Yes, now, she has to arrange certain things. Pinkus always leaves the workshop when Sarah asks him to, which she doesn't often do. He goes out to Sarah waiting in our living room and I go with him.

Sarah says she wants to place some valuables outside the ghetto, the best of our remaining pictures, a couple of small rugs she had bought in Warsaw, our table silver and a few pieces of Rosenthal porcelain she points out and of which she always takes great care — they are in the locked glass-fronted cupboard. Pinkus thinks for a moment. Sarah and I look at him. I see Sarah is tense and impatient. She will no doubt persist in this matter, and even Pinkus notices. Yes, he says — best to do that perhaps, and it is not prohibited.

They discuss whom they will turn to. Sarah wants to talk to Mrs. Plowecka. That's good, Pinkus thinks, they are fine people and instill confidence — if you can have confidence in anyone these days. Mrs. Plowecka's husband is a public notary and was the Social Democrat's PPS delegate at the town hall.

Pinkus selects which pictures are to be placed with Mrs. Plowecka and which we are going to take with us into the ghetto, then he goes back to the workshop. That is more important to him than the question of which of our valuables are to be left with other people and with whom. That is for Sarah to arrange. Pinkus makes clothes and is good at it, Sarah arranges everything else, and she's good at that.

Sarah now undertakes the entire procedure without discussing any more details with Pinkus. What we have reverently collected over many years is now dispersed and kept by other people, whom we know only rather superficially. We are forced to forego more and more of what was part of our home and life we thought to be of importance, because we live in occupied country and we are Jews.

No one talks about why we and other Jews want to leave our things with strangers and for what purpose. We probably just hope other times will come, better times, when we can have them back. But we don't say so, for among the Jews in Czestochowa, there is less and less talk about better times and hopes of better times have faded. News of German victories keeps appearing. No one dares hope that the Germans' attitude to us Jews can be changed, but we nevertheless act as if better times would come. I think people always do that in hopeless situations — right up until they give up and then they die. We have, after all, not given up.

Karola has at last abandoned dreams of Heniek Epstein, and has married. Her husband, Antek, is a decent, safe and good-humored man, liked by everyone and touchingly considerate to his Karola. You can see on them that they are in love with each other and despite everything happening all round us it is clear that Karola is at last happy — a successful ghetto marriage. You can be happy even in

The Maple Tree Behind the Barbed Wire

difficult external circumstances.

The head of the German order police, Captain Degenhardt, tells Leon Kopinski that the Judenrat must ensure that a Jewish police force is established in the ghetto. Degenhardt talks about how many policemen he wants to have, and how the police are to be organized. The Jewish police are to be in civilian clothes, wear special police caps and armbands, as well as the blue and white armband all Jews have to wear. Degenhardt leaves it to the Judenrat to select their policemen, but he says nothing about what the police are to do. The Judenrat commission Dr Anisfelt, chairman of their education committee, once the rector of the Jewish gymnasium, to appoint and organise the Jewish police force. This is a good decision, as are almost all the decisions made by the Judenrat in its three-year history. Anisfelt's farsighted choice of Jewish police is to put its stamp on conditions in the ghetto to come.

Rector Anisfelt was a well-known mathematician and teacher, an excellent head of our school, a wise and farsighted man, interested in his pupils and good with people. When assigned to organise the police, Anisfelt sets up a working party. Apart from Anisfelt himself, it includes two of the most trusted teachers, one from the Jewish gymnasium and one from the Axera gymnasium, and consulting with them, he chooses the candidates. The working party, sometimes with Kopinski and Kurland, interview the candidates. I don't know what questions they ask or what criteria they have for their choice — but they succeed. The Jewish policemen in Czestochowa become friends of the ghetto inhabitants. They turn out to come up to expectations and do not allow themselves to become demoralized — whatever happens. So neither have we, the inhabitants of the ghetto, become demoralized. But they were all to be sacrificed; not one of those fine boys, several of them some of my older school friends, are to survive, except the two who fairly soon resigned, took off their police caps and saved themselves, one of them over on the Aryan side.

The Jewish police have three officers. After the first chief of police, an elderly schoolmaster, was dismissed by Degenhardt, Parasol becomes the chief. He had been a non-commissioned officer in the Polish army and has two stars on his cap. An ex-officer in the Polish army - Auerbach - and a lawyer become his closest assistants, each with one star on their caps. Otherwise the Jewish police have no badges of rank.

The great majority of Jews obey the decree; move and go to live in the overcrowded ghetto, though a few take the risk and stay outside. They acquire false papers — according to them they are not Jews. Others talk of doing that, but few dare.

After nearly three months, on the morning of August 23rd, 1941, without warning the Jewish ghetto is hermetically sealed off from the rest of Czestochowa, from the rest of the Generalguvernement, from

The Maple Tree Behind the Barbed Wire

the rest of the world. According to the housing committee's calculations we are up to 48,000 registered Jews in a small area and it is very crowded. In reality we are more, though no one knows for sure just how many, but the number 56,000 is mentioned. We who live at Aleja 14 are not quite so cramped.

Aleja is the most fashionable street in town. Along it are apartment houses on each side and three stretches of promenades separated by two right-angled through-roads. On the widest promenade, in the middle, small patches of grass are regularly placed out, on each patch of grass a tree. The street is really called Aleja Najswietszej Marii Panny - Holy Mother Avenue, abbreviated to NMP, and in everyday speech just called Aleja. Everyone knows what is meant by Aleja. Streets in Czestochowa may be called either ulica, or if they are wider, aleja. But it is only the pride of the town that is simply called Aleja. All the others are called, for instance, Aleja Wolnosci, where we lived before, or Aleja Kosciuszki, where the Gestapo have their house of terror.

Aleja leads from Nowy Rynek to the monastery, which from its hill dominates the entire central part of the town. Aleja is divided by a railway bridge into First and Second Aleja and by a large grassed area in front of the Magistrat - the town hall — in Second and Third Aleja. All buildings along First Aleja are older but well maintained, at most four stories high. The trees along First Aleja are the oldest and the most beautiful great leafy trees.

Aleja 14 is at the end of First Aleja, before the railway bridge and on the corner of ulica Wilsona, which constitutes the west boundary of the ghetto. It is an old handsome white-plastered three-story corner house with two small attic apartments in the roof. On the outside it is decorated with small columns that frame the low windows in the attics. Above the actual corner the building has a round roof cupola. This is the boundary building to the ghetto. We live on the second floor. From the protruding bay window of our living room, in one direction we can see the whole of First Aleja, in the other a large part of Second Aleja, and in the distance the monastery on the hill.

When I wake in the morning of August 23rd, 1941, and look out, standing in the exit from the ghetto are a blue-clad Polish policeman and a Jewish policeman in his round navy-blue cap with its broad dark red stripe. A barbed-wire fence has been put up, shutting off the whole of the wide Aleja. If necessary, the police can open a gate in the barbed wire fence for passing vehicles, but vehicles seldom pass in or out of the ghetto. There is a narrow opening in the fence for pedestrians. The Polish and the Jewish policemen are always on duty there and no one may go in or out without being checked. There are several notices by the entrance. On the Aryan side it says: "Owing to the risk of infection, entrance is strictly forbidden." On the Jewish side

The Maple Tree Behind the Barbed Wire

it says: "Jews who leave the ghetto without permission will be shot. Non-Jews who enter the ghetto will receive a prison sentence." The Germans are very swift to show that they mean to take the death penalty seriously.

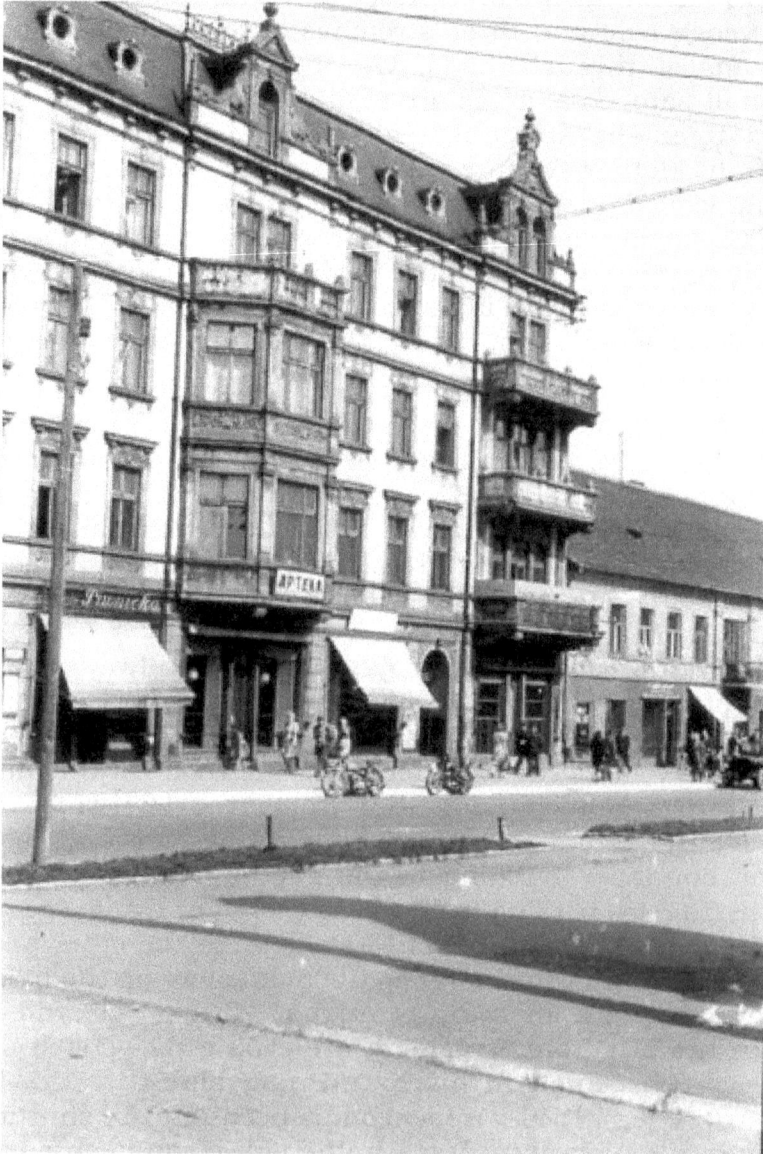

House of Craftsmen - Aleja 14 - is the boundary building to the Czestochowa ghetto. We live on the second floor. From our living room bay window we can see the whole of First Aleja and a large part of Second Aleja - which lies outside the ghetto. The main entrance to the building is on the Aryan side, a smaller entrance on the ghetto side.

The Maple Tree Behind the Barbed Wire

From the window in our apartment we can see the Polish policeman checking the documents of the few people passing. I also see that there is always a uniformed German policeman nearby. The Germans never talk to the Polish or the Jewish policemen, only to the green-clad German who appears when needed. They hold strictly to order of rank — it is inconceivable that a Jew or even a Polish policeman would check a German - one of the Herrenvolk.

The main entrance to our building in Aleja 14 is on the Aryan side; the customers come and go through that. But the building also has a smaller entrance on the ghetto side, and if you are stopped at this side entrance it is always by a Jewish policeman. It is relatively easy to get a temporary pass to Aleja 14. The Judenrat issues them, but it has happened that the Jewish policeman has let in a Jew without a pass of that kind. Once inside the building, through an appropriate apartment, you can pass to the exit on the Aryan side. That can be done through our apartment. It seems easy, you just walk out. But nonetheless, you have to be careful — if you are a Jew - the German police are almost always somewhere in the vicinity.

The day after the ghetto was closed off and the barbed wire put up, August 24th, 1941, Senior Constable Handtke stops a man coming out of Aleja 14 on the Aryan side. Handtke speaks to him for a brief moment and the man shows his papers. Handtke takes the man to the right, to Wilson Street, and shoots him. We hear two shots.

He shot the young man on the spot, without any previous investigation, without asking anything, without trial, but not fatally. This all happens at around four in the afternoon. It is raining slightly. The man is left lying in the street; from our window we can sometimes see him moving, turning over on his side and clutching his stomach, but he is so far away we can't hear him. No one may go near to help the young man, and he is left lying there all night. In the morning he is no longer moving. Not until then are two stretcher-bearers from the ghetto summoned to fetch him. He dies alone in the night, in the rain, on the hard stones of Wilson Street; he was a Jew.

I don't know what Handtke said to him, or what he replied. I don't know what papers he showed Handtke, or what his errand was. But I heard Handtke shoot him with two pistol shots, both in the stomach, so that he would not die quickly.

Everyone in the ghetto recognizes the green-clad German order police from Leipzig. They are our contact people with the outer world and uninhibited lords over our lives. Inside the ghetto we know several of their names - Schott, Oppel, Schmidt, Rohn, Kinnel, Klufaz, Opitz, Tsopot, Handtke, Überscheer, Schimmel, Hiller, Unkelbach, and then their chief, Captain Degenhardt. Most of these policemen have ghetto names, too. Handtke, who is thin, pale and very fair, with bleached eyebrows, always has a thick white scarf round his neck under his uniform coat and is called "der Weisse Kopf" - white head. He is trigger-happy--- an ordinary German order policeman who must have been trained to prevent illegal acts and to protect people. He has a corporal's badge on his shoulder straps — no SS or party badge

Sometimes Handtke comes to the ghetto even when he is not on duty. Then he talks to his German police colleague at the entrance. I can see them laughing, then he goes a little way into the ghetto, takes out his pistol and shoots one or two Jews.

I once see him shooting first a fine-looking man, then a relatively well-dressed woman walking along Third Aleja with a small, quite longhaired grayish-white dog on a short lead.

Perhaps Handtke shoots them because he thinks it inappropriate that two Jews take a walk with a little dog, although this is not forbidden, or perhaps he thinks they seem to be enjoying themselves. Perhaps he was just bored at his garrison. He pats the dog but does not bother with what happens to the couple he has shot, turns slowly round and walks calmly out of the ghetto. At the exit he exchanges a few words with his police colleague — neither of them shows any interest in the shot Jewish couple.

The little dog, clearly confused, is left standing on the street, spins round for a moment and then runs, clearly frightened, into our house, Aleja 14. Sarah goes down and picks up the little dog, which is trembling as Sarah clutches him to her; she cries as she tries to comfort the dog. It stays with us as long as we live at Aleja 14.

"Der Weisse Kopf" Handtke makes several excursions of this kind into the ghetto — they are always crowned with success. He shoots one or two Jews he has selected quite at random. Handtke is trigger-happy and is allowed unhindered to give outlet to his desires. No one in the ghetto would even think of complaining; he has the right to do this for he is German, a policeman, and we are Jews.

In Czestochowa, there is another German policeman from Leipzig called in the ghetto Itcie - a Jewish nickname. He has never shot a Jew. Itcie often patrols with Schmidt. Schmidt has no ghetto name and is called Schmidt even by the Jews. Schmidt is considered quite good-natured, but not as good-natured as Itcie, and he has been seen shooting two Jews. Of all the German police from Leipzig only Icie has never been seen to have shot a single Jew, and then Captain Degenhardt. Degenhardt has not shot a single Jew. Despite this, he is really the most dangerous of them all, and he was to turn out to be even more dangerous than we could possibly have imagined in our worst nightmares.

Another of the German police officers, fat Lieutenant Tsopot, seems quite good-natured. He often comes to the Judenrat premises in the ghetto, and then expects to be served scrambled eggs with as many eggs as possible cooked in butter. He can eat many eggs and is angry if he is not offered scrambled eggs. Although there is a great shortage

The Maple Tree Behind the Barbed Wire

of eggs and butter in the ghetto, Tsopot knows he will always get his scrambled eggs, cooked in butter. Tsopot has been seen leading razzias and he has even been seen shooting a woman, but not the child she had with her. Nevertheless, he is reckoned to be one of the good-natured ones because he does not often shoot, he seems friendly and likes talking to Jews. The thin Oppel is also trigger-happy; he has probably, for no reason, shot as many Jews as Handtke has. Oppel does not do it so often, but he takes several Jews at a time. He is also an ordinary German order police from Leipzig - not SS, not even a party member.

Groups of Jews are taken out for forced labour in places outside the ghetto. Early in the morning they are to go to a given place, their names are called out and they are counted by Jewish policemen — sometimes there is a German policeman present as well. Forced labour groups are then taken under close guard out through the main entrance of the ghetto, early every morning, not to return until late in the evening. They have to work hard, but they are also our breathing space. Some of them meet Polish workers at their place of employment and hear some news. They can take things out of the ghetto, either their own things or things someone else asks them to smuggle out and sell, then when they come back they have with them the food they have got in exchange. Otherwise no Jew goes out and no Jew comes into the ghetto, only the Germans can come and go and even they do so rarely — except the German order police from Leipzig who move freely across the boundaries of the ghetto. Sometimes a German from the forced labour place has some errand at the Judenrat and sometimes a Gestapo man passes — on some special errand. It is always an ill omen when the Gestapo man comes, always bad news. Otherwise the Judenrat administers the ghetto with their police and officials on various committees.

But there is one other breathing space in the wall of barbed wire, police and prohibitions surrounding us, and that is Aleja 14, the house of craftsmen.

At Aleja 14, fifteen craftsmen live with their families, all of them experts, the best there are among the Jews of Czestochowa. There are two shoemakers, one who is very good at boots — his name is Dorfsgang - and the other who is good at ordinary shoes - Szydlowski. Mrs. Parasol is known for her hand-sewn underclothes and pajamas — she is married to the head of the Jewish police. One is a carpenter, three make clothes for ladies — best known is Katz, who lives on the first floor, below us. There is also a hat-maker, a corset-maker - Frau Sarah Frank - so Herr Frank is still living in the same building as Pinkus. Two are military tailors, their names Baum and Grin, and one is a gentleman's tailor - Pinkus Einhorn, my father — with him live Sarah, Roman and I.

The Maple Tree Behind the Barbed Wire

When there is unrest in the ghetto, some of the employees and some of the family stay overnight in our Aleja 14 as they find it safer. In the ghetto, the building is called Das Wajses Hojs - the white house — or Czternastka, number fourteen. The building becomes increasingly important in communications with the Aryan side.

More and more Jews understand that the reality is more threatening than we imagined, as we realize how methodically the Germans are setting about encircling us. First comes registration — to be able to get an Arbeitspass which we think is to give some security. Then the blue and white armbands — to mark us out, still harmless as long as we wear them. Then they herd us into limited housing areas, crowded but possible to live with. Then they close the gates and screen us off from the world outside. All this appears to have been thought through and well planned — we begin to see the pattern.

Frank, Pinkus and Katz are talking about what will come next while I am there listening. Frank says nothing much more can happen — they can't shoot us all — we are 50,000 Jews in our ghetto, out of three million Jews in Poland. Katz is upset that Frank can even make such a suggestion — the world would not allow it. Pinkus agrees but says at the same time that reality can surpass a nightmare, if it brings with it events we can't even imagine.

More and more we realize we are in a trap and imagine the worst, but we have no alternative. We have nowhere to go — it is just as dangerous outside. Few would help us and we can understand that, for the penalty of hiding a Jew is death. Several of those who have nevertheless tried to get out in order to save themselves on the other side, come back frightened and subdued, many don't even manage to get back to the ghetto although they want to. Outside the ghetto are professional informers — szmalcowniki - Poles who have specialized in recognizing Jews. They stand at the exit from the ghetto or outside Jewish forced labour places or just walk the streets. When they recognize a Jew they follow him and find his hiding-place if he has one. They get everything they can out of the Jew and then report him. The Germans compensate the szmalcownik with two kilos of sugar for every hiding-place they uncover. He does not tell the Germans that he has already got out of the Jew everything he possesses.

Those who go out to workplaces outside the ghetto have seen small boys spending their time informing on Jews. They run after lone Jews or a Jewish family shouting Zyd, Zyd in Polish, or Jude, Jude so that the Germans shall also understand — until the Jew is stopped and arrested, or let go if it turns out the boys have got it wrong. But they are usually right.

I think, how terrible it must be for a lone Jew to be out on the street. A boy, perhaps twelve years old, looks at you, follows you, and starts shouting that you are a Jew. He is soon joined by other boys shouting until a German, or more often a Polish policeman in blue stops him

The Maple Tree Behind the Barbed Wire

and orders him to show his papers, which aren't in order. A German may kill him at some nearby secluded spot or in the middle of the street — it is up to him. A Polish policeman takes him to a police station. Why do these boys do this? They don't even get anything for their trouble; to show how clever they are? Or is it pure thoughtlessness, the need for something to do for those with nothing to do, or is it perhaps hatred? Don't they think about the price we have to pay, how we must feel when they start following us? The lone quarry's paralyzing terror, the terror of helplessness, the terror of rapidly approaching death. These boys know what happens to those they point out; a Jew they discover is usually killed the same day. Do they hate us so?

I am aware that the security the ghetto provides is false, but not at any price do I want to leave this false security. At least I don't have to be alone here — whatever happens I am at least allowed to keep my own identity, Jurek Einhorn, sixteen, son of Pinkus and Sarah, a Jew. I also have an unrealistic faith in that my strong father will manage things one way or another. This provides me with security in an insecure existence, gives authorization to my thoughts on days after the war, what the moment of liberation will look like, what we shall do then — when it is all over. A healthy person cannot constantly feel insecure, constantly be afraid. I think a Jew on "the other side" is constantly afraid, as he has no right to be there. Here in the ghetto, at least I have the right to exist, as long as it lasts. Why didn't we appreciate freedom and security when we did have it? Just imagine — moving about freely, walking and traveling wherever you like. What a privilege it must be to choose, to be allowed to walk in a street, any street, anywhere.

But there are Jews regularly going in and out of the ghetto for other purposes. Some do so at night or in the early morning by trying to climb over the barbed wire surrounding the ghetto. They risk being shot and left hanging on the wire — until they die — or being arrested by a merciless Polish blue policeman, or being discovered by a szmalcownik waiting for his victim on the other side of the barbed wire. Others use Aleja 14 as a transit place.

One of all the rumors circulating is that at a camp outside the town of Chelmno, they gas to death Jews from the ghetto in Lódz. The Germans use car and tractor fumes, killing several thousand every day. Could this be true? How hideous it must be to be shut in a room with many others, then fumes being pumped in and slowly suffocating all those inside. People dying all round you, you wait for yourself to begin to lose consciousness — it is no use holding your breath, for how long can you do that? A teenager with a reasonable imagination has time to think of a great deal before he manages to push the idea away from him, into his subconscious.

The Maple Tree Behind the Barbed Wire

Not many in the ghetto believe the rumor, but some do. A consequence of that is that the underground ghetto movement, which is spoken of rather patronizingly, is strengthened, becoming more visible and well organized. Not until we move into Aleja 14 do I understand how extensive that movement has become.

They call themselves Zydowska Organizacja Bojowa, the Jewish Struggle Organization, abbreviated to ZOB - in ordinary ghetto language they are called partisans. They are said to be three hundred and have their headquarters in a building in ulica Nadrzeczna number 66 in the south part of the ghetto. ZOB is said to have branches in several Jewish ghettos in Poland, contacts with Polish resistance movements and through those with London and the Jewish organizations in other countries. Those in Czestochowa call themselves Group 66 and use Aleja 14 largely as a transit place for their couriers — those who dare go in and out of the ghetto.

Those I see passing through our apartment are only a few years older than I am — boys and girls — mature, purposeful, self-confident and brave. They often stay overnight with one of the craftsmen, but we who live here never tell anyone when or with whom. We trust each other but it is best not to talk. You never know when one of us may be arrested and taken to the Gestapo in Aleja Kosciuszki or what might happen to the arrested person. There are methods to make even the bravest talk.

The couriers tell us things that have happened and are happening though never anything that touches on their own activities, their contacts and organization. What they tell us we then discuss with each other, so we who live in Aleja 14 are fairly soon informed — for good or evil. These ZOB couriers often know much more than the Poles the Jews meet at their workplaces. What the ZOB couriers tell us is rarely encouraging and never hopeful — their stories are true.

A great many rumors circulate when reading newspapers and listening to the radio are prohibited. It is human in our situation not to believe the worst rumors; you want to believe it when the news is good, preferably when it is about distant foreign countries, or the Allied troops. But these good rumors are few. The Allies are inaudible and invisible, and most of the news of the war is about the successes of the German army.

Those who stay overnight in our apartment change their clothes, their hairstyles or dye their hair. They all have false papers. Some of them are school friends, older than me, only one from my old class; class IIB at the Jewish gymnasium - Janusz Stawski.

Janusz and I talk nearly all night, not so much about what is happening now, but about the old days, about our school, what we know about our school friends, teachers, the caretaker, and towards morning we talk about our dreams and hopes, about what we are

The Maple Tree Behind the Barbed Wire

going to do after the war. We never talked much when we were at school, but that night we came very close to each other.

This is the last time I see Janusz Stawski, my serious, calm and confident classmate. He hasn't dyed his dark hair but has acquired a mustache. Janusz Stawski is sixteen and is not to survive the war. He never returns from this assignment — no one knows what happened to Janusz Stawski, an unusually young ZOB courier.

Some of the people passing through Aleja 14 are those wanting to escape and are trying to establish themselves on the Aryan side as non-Jews, and those who have been on the other side but have been forced to return. We meet Jews who have been recognized and who have managed to escape from their szmalcownik at the last moment when their hiding place has been revealed — "burnt". Jews pass through after having stayed on the other side, but have had to return to the ghetto when their money has run out and they can no longer pay the host who has hidden them. In the long run, it is impossible to survive on the Aryan side in Poland, they say. Pinkus and Sarah usually know in advance when someone is coming from the ghetto on the way out, but not when anyone wants to come back.

One afternoon a girl with a guitar in a large shabby case comes to our place. She wants to get out of the ghetto. She is slightly older than I am, perhaps seventeen or eighteen, with a round face and a warm serious smile. Her name is Hanka and Sarah calls her Haneczka. Hanka is an open inquisitive person and likes talking about her, but not about what contacts she has on the other side, whom she is to meet, where she is going when she leaves Aleja 14.

The adults in the building meet in small groups in the evenings. We young people also meet in groups and in different apartments. This evening several come to ours, Genia Frank, Pola Grin and a few others. Hanka takes out her guitar — it is clear it is very important to her — sits on a backless stool, props the guitar against her right thigh, leans forward, looks at the strings, plucks lightly to tune the guitar, then starts playing a melancholy German pre-war tune — "Zwei Gitarren am Meer", - two guitars by the sea. She gets going, no longer looking at the strings. She raises her head, looking at us without seeing, concentrated, serious — she is a very pretty girl. You have to like Hanka when she is playing, but also otherwise. I like her very much and am at once entranced.

When the others have all gone, Hanka talks to Sarah about having to make her hair lighter. She goes into the bathroom and stays there a long time, then comes out with a pink towel wound round her head. She is to sleep in the same room as Rózia, with the towel round her head — you have to do that when you dye your hair. The dye has to work all night.

The Maple Tree Behind the Barbed Wire

When Hanka wakes up early the next morning, her hair is lighter but has acquired a greenish tinge, is part pale green. It is difficult to get hold of good hair dyes in wartime, especially in the ghetto. Hanka must have got some particularly bad dye or she applied it in the wrong way. It is hard on her lovely dark reddish-blond hair and Sarah and Rózia say she can't go out like that, as the color is so unnatural. But Hanka has decided — she is going. Hanka cuts her hair short and Rózia gives her a floral shawl that has a little green, Hanka covers her hair with the shawl, ties it under her chin — then leaves. We watch from the window, as, guitar in its big case in her right hand, she walks steadily out of the entrance door and crosses the railway bridge over to Second Aleja. I stay by the window on my own, watching until she disappears between the trees in the centre of Second Aleja.

I still remember and occasionally think about pretty and purposeful Hanka. Where was she going, did she manage, if so where is she? I don't know, just as I don't know what happened to most of those who passed through Aleja 14 and I happened to meet. I remember some of them better, some I hardly remember at all, but I remember Hanka although I don't remember her surname. Every time I hear "Zwei Gitarren am Meer" I remember her. Sometimes I want to hear the tune in order to think about this fascinating girl.

If the war had not interrupted the natural history of her life, Hanka would have become a person appreciated by everyone, would have easily found a good husband, had a family, been a good mother. And perhaps she has, somewhere in some country here on earth — if she is alive. I like to think so, although I know that very few of the Jews who set off and tried to survive the war "on the other side" managed it. Hanka will remain in my memory as long as I live, perhaps my memory of her all that exists.

It is June 1941 and already very hot. Another rumor starts - Germany is at war with the Soviet Union. The German supreme command has blacked out what is happening at the front, three days have gone by and no news has come. Rumors abound and arouse wild hopes. In the enclosed ghetto we long to be able to hope the war will soon be over. They cannot possibly cope on two fronts - Britain in the West and the great Soviet Union in the East.

But our joy is short-lived and our disappointment great. The German army is succeeding even against the Soviet Union. At Aleja 14, someone has found a copy of the local paper - Glos Czestochowy. It has big black headlines - Victory in the East. The text repeats victorious bulletins from Das Oberkommando der Wehrmacht. In a pincer movement, the victorious German army has surrounded and wiped out the Russian army in the North, and reached within two days the Baltic countries — the Lithuanian capital fell on June 24th. In a few days, the German armored units have reached Smolensk and the

The Maple Tree Behind the Barbed Wire

Russian army in the South is encircled in a gigantic pincer. Pinkus and Frank agree that they are exaggerating, that some of this is propaganda, but some of it must be true and that is bad enough.

During the following lovely summer weeks of 1941, the news reaches us from various sources confirming these victorious German bulletins. In a short time, the Germans had reached the Volga and the Caucuses, were now nearing Leningrad and Moscow and still advancing. How would this end? Are they invincible despite the fact they are so evil?

This brief period of positive expectations turns into dejection inside the ghetto. But we rapidly recover, everyday life in ghetto goes on, new rumors are put about, refuted, confirmed or remain hanging in the air — rumors which keep us busy, influence us, fulfill a function and are forgotten if not confirmed.

It is the beginning of 1941, an unusually cold beginning to another long winter. The stream of bi-lingual decrees in thick black frames no longer reach the ghetto. Orders from the authorities reach the inhabitants of the ghetto through our Judenrat and its less dramatic, often handwritten notices. The latest is that everyone is to hand in any furs they have, the death penalty to anyone failing to do so. There are two collecting points, the northern one, nearest us in Nowy Rynek - the New Square. As usual, there are lots of questions. Pinkus asks an official from the Judenrat if the decree applies to just fur clothes, or also to fur hats and untreated fur goods — he has a few like that left in store for customers wanting a fur collar on their overcoats. The official says he thinks they have to be handed in, but he is not sure. Sarah takes out the lovely fur coat Pinkus had given her when Roman was born in 1931 - the one she regretted not having with her in Warsaw during the siege. Sarah has always looked after it well. She looks so good in it and now she has to hand in. She takes the fur collars off her winter coat and Rózia's. They have to hand in the collars, but they intend to keep their warm overcoats.

Pinkus and one of his assistants take all the furs with them when they go to collecting point in Nowy Rynek. They also take Pinkus' handsome grey overcoat, fur-lined and with a carefully selected Persian lamb collar. He hands in the whole coat. They also take with them the bits of fur Pinkus has in store. Pinkus says to me that it's not worth risking one's life for a fur.

Within forty-eight hours, our Judenrat hands over to the Germans a goods wagon filled with furs collected from over 50,000 people.

When they had moved from their homes to the ghetto, many Jews had chosen to take their furs with them so as not to freeze in winter, and now they were being made to hand them over, so had no warm clothes for the winter. What are the Germans going to do with our furs? Perhaps things are so bad at the Russian front they need the furs for their soldiers?

It is January 1942, a very cold and hard winter that has only just begun. More and more people queue up at the Judenrat's soup kitchen, fewer and fewer try to leave the ghetto through our building. It is more difficult to survive "on the other side" when it is so bitterly cold. Frightening rumors are circulating about what has happened to Jewish hiding places that have been found and to the Jews found there.

But in the forests outside Czestochowa, there is said to be a group of Jewish partisans who have joined the smaller of the two Polish resistance movements. The Soviet-supported socialist people's army - Gwardia Ludowa (GL) The larger, London-supported nationalist Armia Krajowa - the army of the country — does not accept Jews. It is rumored that they murder Jews they find in the forest or in any of the villages they visit.

Gutka Baum

Nowadays, the young people living at Aleja 14 mostly meet at Genia Frank's. The Franks live on the ground floor, their windows facing the courtyard. Among those who have been coming recently to our evening meetings is the Baums' son, Moniek Baum.

Moniek is younger than I am and was in a class below me at the Jewish gymnasium. He is quite tall; a cheerful youth with straight brown hair, dark brown eyes and an open smile, which makes everyone smile back. He finds it easy to laugh and is the youngest in the group.

Moniek has a sister - Gutka - the leading beauty at the Jewish gymnasium. Gutka had to re-sit a year and is only one class below me. I have heard her playing the piano at school — she plays very well, with empathy and sensitivity. I have also seen Gutka on several occasions at school, in the street or recently in the stairway of the building, but she is and always has been inaccessible to me and I have never spoken to her. Gutka Baum is not there when we meet, we never see her and she always stays at home. The Baums live on the same stairway as we do, in the apartment above ours. Sometimes piano music can be heard from their apartment, and it must be that invisible Gutka.

Occasionally we meet somewhere else besides at Genia Frank's, but Moniek, who comes every day now, has never on any occasion suggested that we should meet at his place, nor do the adults ever meet at the Baums'. The old military tailor Baum is a pleasant, open, talkative and friendly man. His wife is quite sturdy, her dark hair scraped back and worn in a knot at the nape of her neck, and she is

The Maple Tree Behind the Barbed Wire

not so friendly. They never invite anyone home, nor do any of them go out in the evenings, except the son - Maniek.

One evening Gutka comes with her brother to the Franks' place. Maybe she is curious and wants to see all of us who meet here and have a nice time, as Moniek has told her. This is the first time I have seen her at close quarters. Gutka is even lovelier than I remembered, a dark beauty, her head held high; smooth skin, red lips, strong black eyebrows and a deep melodious voice. She has long, thick, almost black hair, long thick plaits which she often lets hang down her back, but sometimes brings them forward and even then they come almost down to her waist. She fastens her long plaits up with a broad slide, so it looks as if she is wearing a crown, and you feel like touching the thick plaits, but you don't. A serious beauty with a natural innate dignity, she is a wonderfully beautiful young lady.

Gutka also comes the next evening; perhaps she arranges it or it just happens that she and I find ourselves sitting slightly apart from the others on a sofa in a dark corner. We talk — about all sorts of things. From the very first, it is no superficial conversation to pass the time. We talk about Gutka and her mother, Gutka's dreams of the future and the kind of piano she wants to have. Gutka comes the next meeting, and the next. After only a couple of meetings we are suddenly sitting there in the dark, holding hands. Gutka has a soft warm hand, full of life, her fingers long — she holds my hand and lets me hold hers.

She and I now sit every evening in the darkness on the same sofa, talking and cuddling. The others pretend they neither see nor hear, Moniek, too. What does this proud, beautiful, mature and serious Gutka see in me at all? I wait for her to come every evening, and when she comes, I am happy. If she does not come one evening, I miss her. Then I talk mostly to Moniek.

This is no game — it is serious, a perhaps rather immature young man's genuine love, a love that shapes, changes me, and is to be part of me for ever. They are the kind of feelings that make a boy soon to be seventeen mature, a love in which desire exists but does not dominate. We loll on the wide sofa, talk and hold each other, I caress Gutka gently and cautiously and it is clear she likes it. I don't try to go any further and she appreciates that.

Gutka increasingly talks about her dreams, the future, how she is going to marry, and one evening the conversation acquires a deeply serious undertone. I realize that Gutka would be pleased if I could say more about what she means to me. She wants me to talk about my own plans for the future, whether I also want to marry, perhaps not now but some time in the future, perhaps even marry her. I realize that is what she wants to hear, but I don't say all that. I have no education, no profession, no means of supporting a family; it would be irresponsible of me to talk about marrying, even if that meant some time in the future. From the very first meeting I have realized that this is serious and not a game, nor is it for her, and I am afraid of hurting her. So I don't say what I think she wants to hear.

We go on seeing each other every day, talking, cuddling, kissing each other in the dark, but Gutka does not take up her plans for the future again. I wish she would imply a future together again, but I have neither reason nor any right to take up the subject myself. I have nothing to add, nothing concrete.

It is the end of April 1942. Southwest Poland, where Czestochowa lies, has a marked inland climate with hot summers and cold winters. The past winter has been unusually severe and long, only now beginning to let go of Czestochowa's tormented Jewish ghetto. The inhabitants of the ghetto have less and less to sell to each other or to people on the other side, poverty is on the increase and more people are undernourished.

The ghetto is being decimated, the number of inhabitants falling, but slowly. Some are taken by the Germans for questioning, for forced labour or for no reason at all, and disappear. Some are shot, usually by one of the German green police. Fewer and fewer try to escape from the ghetto, fewer and fewer have the money needed for any chance of surviving on the other side. The GL guerilla is said to accept Jews - but only strong young men, preferably with their own firearms and previous experience of military service. The AK does not accept Jews. There are SSZ units in the forest, the right-wing guerillas who kill any Jew they get hold of.

Many young people get married younger than they did before the war. Several boys and girls who were at school together now marry, but as yet no one from our class IIB. Very few children are born in the ghetto, for people are definitely advised against having children in these uncertain times. The few children born all the same are everyone's favorites.

By the middle of May 1942, Gutka has stopped coming to the our meetings at Aleja 14, nor does Gutka's younger brother Moniek come as often. But one evening, a week or two later, Gutka comes, as usual with Moniek. She is even warmer, tenderer, more loving that evening than on any previous occasion. She is serious, cuddles up in my arms on the sofa and starts crying — quietly. I don't ask why, and Gutka says nothing, just lies softly against me and I hold her gently. She whispers quietly into my ear, so quietly that I only partly grasp what she is saying. It is about feelings, about that I am to know that she likes me, and I whisper back that I know.

I am happy, but my delight is clouded by the seriousness of what is happening, though I am not really clear about what is happening, nor do I ask, just keep holding my lovely, beloved Gutka. I can see I

The Maple Tree Behind the Barbed Wire

cannot influence what is happening, but what I do not see is that it is the last, or the next but last time we are to meet. We stay longer than usual that evening, then part reluctantly and go back to our own homes.

After that evening, Gutka no longer comes to our meetings. As before, she does not appear at all, does not leave their home in the evenings. Moniek still comes, and he says their mother is ill so Gutka cannot come as she has to look after her mother, that their mother demands it. We all know that Mrs. Baum is a determined strong-willed woman, and also that she is ill.

But only a week later, everyone in Aleja 14 knows that Gutka has married Mietek Sojka. We find out that old Sojka, a widower, has been living in secret with the Baums with his son, Mietek, ever since the day we moved into the building, which was probably why no one was allowed to go to their place.

She wanted to marry, my lovely proud Gutka, wanted the security, to have a family or at least plan to have one. But Sojka, fat and several years older, that superior and rich Sojka?

I am in despair at not being allowed to be with her, hold her, gently stroke her hair. I love her just as warmly as before, and I long for her. Sarah sees what is happening and it is obvious she is suffering with me. I lie on my bed, gazing at the ceiling for hour after hour, and I eat practically nothing. Sarah has known all the time that I have been meeting Gutka. You know that kind of thing when you live in the same building, but Sarah did not know I was so deeply in love, or that her young son could experience such strong emotions. She behaves towards me in a different way from before, with another understanding. She is wonderful in my first crisis in life, my mother Sarah, for I am going through a crisis.

In the end I tell Sarah. I have to talk to someone and there are not many to choose from. I don't tell her what had gone on between Gutka and me, for she understands that anyhow, but I tell her about what I had felt like, and what I feel now. I tell her much Gutka liked to talk to me about getting married, now or in the future. Sarah looks at me with her great sorrowful brown eyes and says practically nothing, does not even try to comfort me. She perhaps thinks I ought to have said more to Gutka about how strongly I feel for her, but Sarah doesn't say so aloud, she is wise, cleverer and more sensitive than I had realized before, perhaps thinks like that because she finds it hard to see me suffering. Sarah is there, and I see that she feels helpless, but it helps me that she is there. It requires a war and long-lasting exclusion in a single building for a still immature and yet quite grown son to confide in his own mother on such matters. Perhaps more sons ought to try to do that.

Worst of all, but also wonderful, is when I hear Gutka playing the piano in the apartment above. Then I again lie listening on my bed, saying to myself that she is playing for me — can she do that when she is married to Sojka? Girls like Gutka are faithful, even in their thoughts.

After a while, Moniek tells me what had happened, once only, that when their mother was admitted to the ghetto hospital and was having a blood transfusion before an operation, she made Gutka promise she would marry Mietek Sojka - to ensure her future. I do not know if I am to believe this, but I do believe it when Moniek tells me that several months ago, Sojka had already asked his parents and then Gutka if she would marry him, and I understand him - Mietek - you have to be in love with Gutka when you are close to her. I sincerely hope she will be happy.

Gutka and I are to meet only one more time.

A year later, when the extermination of the Jews of Czestochowa has largely been carried out and those of us who are still left live in the Small Ghetto, Gutka comes to see me. We walk down the worn uneven stone stairs, stand in the narrow porch entrance to the earth-covered courtyard. She takes my hand, holds it for a moment, and squeezes it lightly with her warm sensitive long fingers. It is very dark, I feel her warm cheek against my cheek, and again am allowed to hold my hand on her long thick plait down her back. We just stand there for a moment, saying nothing, for there is nothing to say. She mumbles — 'bye, and goes. As I stand in the courtyard of the house in the Small Ghetto and watch her go, I still feel strongly for her, but my profound despair and melancholy have gone. I am no longer thinking about what things would have been like if ...

What happened is probably for the best, anyhow. As I stand there alone in the dark in the narrow cobbled street, I think she had probably done the right thing, beautiful Gutka with her long plaits. We had our evenings together and I am grateful to have experienced being with her for almost six months. I am sure she loves her Mietek, and he is also able to give her everything she so warmly desired. It is natural for her to want to say goodbye, perhaps also to her other acquaintances before what was to happen, among them all, even me.

The very next day I hear that Gutka and Mietek Sojka, the morning after Gutka and I had met, have left the ghetto to join Sojka's father, who had a hiding place on the Aryan side. They were caught, spotted on the road near their hiding place and both of them, though not old Sojka, were shot after a brief interrogation at the police station.

Beautiful Gutka and rich Mietek. Poor Gutka, who was to prepare for the future, who sought security. In our world, the world of the Jews, there is no security, only poverty, hunger, threats and death, but also a desperate attempt to build families, to keep a hold on a tiny ray of hope and a strong will to survive, despite everything. To plan for the future, for the time after this and not just live for the moment, that is an expression of a kind of defiance of the fate awaiting us.

Moniek Baum, the youngest in the family and the one who did not plan for the future, is the only one of the Baum family to survive. We are to meet again many years later, when my wife Nina and I visit him at his home near Tel Aviv.

Moniek Baum stayed for a long time in Czestochowa after the war, longer than any other survivor from the Jewish and Axera gymnasiums. He is one of the last of the Jews to emigrate from our town, where so many Jews had once lived. Moniek is a civil engineer and has made a life for himself in Israel with his wife and his two sons. When we meet at his home in Herzlia, we talk for a long time about our roots, about Czestochowa after the war, what he had lived through and I know so little about. Neither of us say anything about our time in Aleja 14.

I had hoped we would talk about Gutka; I wanted Nina to hear about Gutka from Moniek as well. I try to steer the conversation towards those days and events, but I see that is painful. Moniek Baum will never get over what happened, although he seems just as lively and open as he was during that long winter of 1941 and the brief spring of 1942, when we met so often. I realize he does not want to talk about his family and what actually happened at their home in Aleja 14.

At the time Gutka Baum and Mietek were murdered in 1943 for being outside the ghetto, the Soviets had already broken the backbone of the German army. The German front was retreating in increasing disorder, the fortunes of war had turned, and the war in principle lost, their murder utterly meaningless.

Old Sojka was to survive the war. When taken in for questioning, he managed to persuade the German police that they should phone the Treuhand who had taken over his business — a Reichsdeutscher. The latter says he needs Sojka, and it is urgent. Sojka is sent to prison and from there is allowed to help his Treuhand. There must be several Jews who survived the war in German prisons, but I have never heard of any other apart from the lonely old Sojka. I know Jews who have survived on the Aryan side, but I know none, have never even heard of a single Jew caught on the Aryan side and despite that survived — except old Sojka.

The Maple Tree Behind the Barbed Wire

The Last Days

In mid-July, 1942, it is warm, the previous long and unusually severe winter not forgotten but already distant. The majestic great trees lining the central promenade in Holy Mother Avenue - Aleja - provide pleasant shade. From the windows of our house in Aleja 14 we can see people outside the ghetto walking in the sunlight, mothers in floral summer dresses pushing their children in prams. We see no prams in the ghetto.

German, Polish and Jewish police guard the main entrance to the ghetto. Fewer and fewer are taken to forced labour. With approaching summer, there is more food to be bought on the black market, but less money in the ghetto to pay for it. Germans continue to come to the Craftsmen's House, among them two tall serious men in civilian clothes. They say little, behave strictly correctly, and bring cloth, thread and buttons — everything with them. Pinkus makes a pair of trousers for each of them. Trousers also have to be fitted before they are finished, including the length of them. We already know I am not going to be a tailor, so I mostly help in the fitting room, and I am usually there.

Pinkus kneels, as tailors always do when they are deciding on the length of trousers, and he does so in front of one of the Germans. Pinkus turns up one trouser leg, looks into the mirror and says: "Is that the right length?" The German looks, turns his head slightly to see better and agrees. "Ja, danke" — thank you, that's good. Pinkus stays crouched down, one knee on the floor and takes pins from a green velvet pincushion on his left lower arm and pins the trousers at the right length and marks the width of the turn-up — as usual, he is very thorough. The German trying on the trousers says to Pinkus in a calm conversational tone: "Sagen Sie mir bitte, Herr Schneidermeister, was meinen die Juden, wie geht's für Deutschland im Krieg? - Tell me, Herr Tailor, how do the Jews think the war will go for Germany? I stiffen, thinking the whole room must be able to hear how loudly my heart is beating - I can feel it in my chest, even in my throat.

Pinkus pretends he has not heard the question, but looks in the mirror, then up at the German and asks if the length is all right, and the German nods. But the other man standing to one side and waiting for his turn, says in a sharper voice but still formally correct: "Herr Scheidermeister, haben Sie nicht gehört?" Didn't you hear? My colleague asked you a question", then he adds in a sharper tone: "Do not wish to answer?"

I hold my breath and feel sick. Is this how our end will come? I am very frightened.

Pinkus gets slowly up and looks at the other German - the one who has demanded an answer of him, and says: "Nicht nur die Juden

The Maple Tree Behind the Barbed Wire

wissen" - not just the Jews, but everyone knows "das Deutschland Schillers und Goethes nie verloren gehen will" - Schiller's and Goethe's Germany will never be lost. Just as calmly, in a conversational tone Pinkus goes on, saying he has finished, that the customer can put on his ordinary trousers. The two Germans exchange looks. The one who had told Pinkus he must answer looks questioningly at the one who had asked the question — he shrugs slightly and it is all over, the other German tries on his trousers. One of them says they will send a messenger to fetch the trousers — when will they be ready? Then they leave. Epstein is not in the fitting room at the time, so I go with them to the door, then from the window see the green-clad German policeman at the ghetto exit click his heels and salute smartly as they leave the building.

When I go back, Pinkus is clearing up after his customers' visit - I can see his hands are trembling but otherwise not a muscle moves to show that we were in great and immediate danger. We know that a German can do what he likes with a Jew, whenever he wants to and with any Jew. We have also learnt that the most dangerous Germans, the ones who decide everything in the background, are always polite and that both those Germans are dangerous — both were wearing the badge of the much feared SS, the two silver flashes of lightning.

The driver who fetches the trousers two days later is a uniformed non-commissioned officer with rank badges on his black collar and an SD badge on the narrow band far down on the left-hand sleeve of his tailored steel-grey uniform, Sicherheitsdienst - a Gestapo uniform.

I have always admired my father, but never so much as on this occasion — he was able to cope with that kind of situation as well. Pinkus never brings that event up with me, nor do I with him. We tell Sarah nothing, nor the men in the workshop, but I go on wondering about his clever answer. A few hours later, I wonder what Pinkus would have said if he had had to answer the next obvious question, what will happen to Hitler's Germany? But they do not ask the question. Perhaps they will think about it later — just as I do.

At the end of August 1942, another rumor appears: Jews are being deported en masse from the Warsaw ghetto. They are being sent away, tens of thousands every day, in cattle wagons. Wladka - one of ZOB's couriers — is on her way from Warsaw to our ghetto. She is a self-confident, sturdily built, dark-haired girl in a hurry and she stays with us only to change her clothes. She confirms that what we have heard really is true. Wladka has seen it, from the Aryan side. As we listen to her, it is the first time I hear the expressions "Aktion" and "Selektion" in the terrible sense that those words have come to mean for us Jews during this war.

Sarah says to Pinkus that we have to do something, at least one of us must be saved; she says Roman ought to get out on to the other side, the Aryan side. They have clearly talked about this before, there

The Maple Tree Behind the Barbed Wire

are detailed plans, but Pinkus is hesitant. Sarah does not let Pinkus go back to the workshop — we must not put it off any longer, we must decide now, it may be too late next week. Pinkus has just heard what the courier had said and is anguished, so he half-heartedly agrees. OK, we'll do it. Sarah is relieved; things seem better when you are not totally passive and you do something about a situation, which seems hopeless. Sarah is and has always been a person of action.

Two days later — just after lunch, at the end of the week - Sarah comes into the workshop and says quietly to Pinkus: "Aren't you coming to say goodbye to your child?" Pinkus puts down his big tailor's scissors he uses for cutting out a suit and goes out with Sarah. I go, too.

In the living room is a woman, a well-dressed woman in her early middle years, perhaps forty. She is speaking kindly to Roman, who is standing in front of her, dressed and pale. With a friendly smile, the strange woman is looking straight at my brother, but he looks away, my little brother, eleven now, with whom I have squabbled so much because he took my things. He looks lost as he stands there in front of this kindly but totally strange woman. Roman's little suitcase with his things already packed in it is on the floor.

Sarah talks to the woman about the remaining details, how payment is to be made in the future, while Pinkus looks on. The woman smiles at him. Sarah says: "Aren't you going to say goodbye to Roman?" But instead Pinkus goes over to the woman and says: "We are so pleased to be able to meet you at last." He asks about the estate she owns together with her husband, wanting to know how many work there and how she was going to arrange things for Roman. Then he goes even closer, takes her hand and says in his very broken Polish: "We are grateful you are going to look after and try to save our little son, because you want to do this in these difficult times when we do not know what will happen to us tomorrow. But I would like to ask you to do us yet one more service." He goes over to the window, points at Cukiernia Blaszczynskiiego - the big tea-rooms on the other side the street, on the Aryan side — and says: "Would you go down to the tearooms, take with you the advance payment my wife has given you for my son's keep for six months, and have a cup of tea and a pastry. If you want to look after and try to save my son, then come back and take him with you. To make it easier when you leave the house together, take his suitcase with you, leave it at the tearooms and fetch it on the way home. It is safer to go out of this building without a case."

Sarah flushes, is upset. "How can you? How can you suspect the lady wants to help us?"

Pinkus looks at the woman and says: "I don't suspect you of anything. I am entrusting you with the most precious thing I have, our son. But I, an old father, would be eternally grateful to you if you

The Maple Tree Behind the Barbed Wire

would do as I ask you, then I will feel even more assured." The woman is not at all upset. "I understand, Herr Einhorn," she says. "We have mutual friends, but you do not know me personally. You know very little about me or our estate. I shall do as you ask." She takes Roman's case and says to Sarah that she will leave the case at the tearooms and will soon be back. We watch her crossing the street with Roman's little case in her hand, then going in through the glass door to the big tearooms. She does not come back. We were never to meet that friendly woman again, or see Roman's case ever again, or the advance payment.

Pinkus and Sarah stand by the window for a while, waiting. Then without a word, Pinkus goes back to the workshop. Roman seems relieved; without anyone saying anything to him, he takes off his outdoor clothes and starts doing something else.

As usual, Pinkus makes no comment on the matter and does not reproach anyone. But the question of one of us being separated from the others, sending Roman over to the other side, is not brought up again, not for several months, and several months is a long time in wartime.

When I think back on this time in the ghetto, it certainly does not appear to have been any kind of idyll. But I can think back to most of what happened during that period, perhaps not with yearning and nostalgia, but anyhow without any feeling of anguish. That was the only period of youth and maturing I was to experience, and it does actually seem to have been a relatively secure time compared with what was to come — and come very soon.

The Maple Tree Behind the Barbed Wire

Prelininaries and Silence

In recent weeks, a fateful atmosphere has descended on the Czestochowa Jewish ghetto, for a great many reasons each week becoming worse.

Few still want to believe that thousands of Jews are being gassed to death every day in furniture vans adapted for the purpose and special chambers, but the rumor persists and causes anxiety. Many people maintain that the rumors are outbursts by prophets of doom spreading terror, or they are sick fantasies — those who pass on these rumors are called groilmacher — scaremongers. Some say the rumors must be false, that they are absurd, that they are deliberately spread by the newly formed Labour Council, which has its premises in a building in First Aleja. The Labour Council, which assembles increasing numbers of known people in the ghetto, largely intellectuals and radical left-wing sympathizers, alternately want to co-operate with and act against the ghetto's Judenrat, but most of all the council issues propaganda for a strike among those selected for forced labour. Unrest is increasing, nourished by new rumors of increasing hunger and distress.

In May 1942, many of activists on the council and nearly all their leaders were arrested in a well-planned razzia by the German police. They are all sent to a concentration camp said to be called Auschwitz, near the town of Oswiecim, not far from Krakow, and the rest go underground. Then no more is heard about the Labour Council, but despite this, the rumors of mass murders of Jews persist.

In mid-June, 1942, Captain Degenhardt issues an order for an Appell - a roll call — of Jews at three o'clock. The appell applies to all Jews between fifteen and fifty — men and women — who live in a part of the ghetto designated by him, plus the entire Judenrat, their officials and the Jewish police. The staff of the cottage hospital inside the part of ghetto concerned is exempted.

A few hours before the stated time, a migration again occurs, this time within the ghetto. Children are left at home with older relatives or neighbors who do not have to appear, or are taken to areas untouched by the order. But adults pour in, filling Stary and Nowy Rynek - the Old and the New Market Square - and part of First Aleja. The Judenrat, their employees and the Jewish police are lined up nearest to the entrance to the ghetto — for the first time I see how many they are.

At exactly three o'clock, Captain Degenhardt arrives in the ghetto with his entourage of green-clad German order police and one or two Germans in civilian clothes. Degenhardt speaks in friendly terms to members of the Judenrat. Some of them, among them Leon Kopinski, go with him to the New Market Square, where he inspects the lines,

The Maple Tree Behind the Barbed Wire

here and there commenting on something to those with him. Halfway through the inspection of the ranks of Jews, Captain Degenhardt declares himself satisfied, turns on his heel and goes back to the entrance, Oberleutnant Überscheer orders the Appell to disperse and the German police leave the ghetto. We can make nothing of it, an apparently utterly meaningless whim of the German police. Many people want to know what Degenhardt and his police had said and they discuss it later, others talk about Captain Degenhardt's friendly manner.

Captain Degenhardt behaves, and is also to do so in future, formally correctly, is sometimes almost friendly. No Jew in Czestochowa has ever seen or is ever to see him angry or agitated, hear him raise his voice, hit or shoot a Jew. Captain Degenhardt is the perfect organizer of mass murder — cold, efficient, listening in a friendly way, understanding opinions produced by Jews. Like so many others during this period in the history of Germany, as an order policeman from Leipzig he is only doing his duty — he himself has never killed of even struck a Jew. No one can accuse him of that.

Three months were to go by before we realize that this was one of the final preparations for a well thought-out Aktion, a dress rehearsal that was carried out in the minutest detail all over the Generalguvernement, then all over German-occupied Europe, well-planned mass extermination of us Jews, all Jews and gypsies — children, adults and old people.

Certain changes of plan had to be made. Experience has shown that it becomes far too expensive and time-consuming to shoot and bury us, we are too many. Faced with such a comprehensive project, lessons had to be learnt from industrial planning to develop a more efficient, more purposeful and cheaper technology for producing the mass-death of healthy people. The latest gains in technology had to be taken on board — the integration of chemistry, medicine, construction and insulation, to build a functioning communications network and training people — victims and the murderers — to carry out the necessary tests for the production line to run smoothly once it has been started up. Another important lead in the planning is to replace expensive ammunition and the old-fashioned mass poisoning with carbon monoxide, which also requires the combustion of valuable fuel, with more efficient poisons.

This is a monumental project. But those needed for it do appear — scientists, inventors, chemists, architects, German industry, and the executioners who are to carry out the actual deeds. The majority involved know, the rest must have some idea what the aim is, all except the victims. And when even we understand, by then only a few left, we anyhow attempt hopeless resistance.

Innumerable German doctors, scientists and psychologists make themselves available. Everything is scientifically, or pseudo-scientifically explained, for better or worse, but explained — superior races and inferior races, Aryan race, nice and tidily motivated, and also — no one wants these Jews, no one wants to accept them; we Germans are doing mankind a service.

It is to be wondered just where these many thousands of German order police, lawyers and doctors who collaborate in this received their basic training — has their training not been about preserving and protecting lives, administering justice, not judging anyone unheard, thinking critically? But it is true that no one wanted us, although up to 1939 and even for a time after that the German authorities agreed to Jewish emigration, a form of solution to the Jewish problem. No one wanted to accept these Jews. That is used against us and in Germany is a good argument for mass murder being the only solution.

Germany is at war, but we unarmed Jews are the main enemy, and all of us — men, women and children — must be exterminated. And those needed to collaborate, not just the Gestapo, the SS and party members — parts of the Polish population also collaborate, not only passively but also actively, by informing on those who attempt to save themselves by fleeing.

It is not possible to excuse, but it is possible to try to explain the collaboration of the Germans - fear, threats, order, mass-psychosis — we human beings find it difficult to stick to an opinion which deviates from the general view. But I cannot explain, cannot understand — however much I try — why the leaders of nations all over the world consciously chose to keep secret what was happening.

Several Jews, Germans and Poles risked their lives to inform you. Why did you choose to say nothing? The chairman of the Warsaw Judenrat - Czerniakow - understood and committed suicide. That information reached you abroad. The Jewish member of the Polish government in exile in London - Samuel Zygelbojn - committed suicide in 1943, leaving behind him a letter containing convincing documentation. Can anyone make a greater sacrifice, show greater heroism and despair than to commit suicide in safe London to draw the attention of the world to our plight? Several senior German embassy officials, a few individual German officers and Polish couriers risk their lives to pass on what they know and inform, all in vein. You all knew - Roosevelt and Churchill and Stalin, every single Head of State, the Polish government in exile and the Swedish in Stockholm - but you chose to suppress the information that reached you through great personal sacrifices by heroic people. I still cannot understand why you did not offer us the little help you were able to by informing the world that you knew. Was it so as not to worry your own population? In that case, it is a paltry explanation.

It is unreasonable to blame it all on Captain Degenhardt and his like, nor is it enough to condemn just them, to describe and take

The Maple Tree Behind the Barbed Wire

offense at what they did. They were given orders, perhaps feeling themselves threatened if they did not carry out the orders; they could be sent to the front. We human beings are weak, our free will, and our ability to think freely and without bias is limited — even if we are reluctant to admit it.

But you, who lived in free countries, you were not threatened, you were not exposed to massive propaganda for ten years, were not exposed to the same mass hysteria as the Germans were. And yet you said nothing.

I am sorry, but when after fifty years I manage to think about what happened and try to analyze it, I cannot get away from that you — several of the leading heroes of the second world war — through your incomprehensible silence, you must be regarded as passive contributors to genocide. For fifty years you were also my noble heroes. We who were shut in and many who risked their lives to inform were naive when we believed something would happen if you were told. But nothing happened, on the contrary. You silenced the information of which there is evidence that you received from various independent and unanimous sources. Formally, your hands are clean, the majority of you have justifiably been honored in the history books for your contributions during the war. But had you or have you — if you are alive — clear consciences? It was not you who condemned us to death, but through your criminal silence you condemned us to die in silence, denying us the compassion of the world surrounding us, in an isolation that feels a very, very great burden.

In addition to that, no one will ever know whether the murdering would not have continued, or continued in the same way as actually happened, if the world had known, if opinions had been aroused through the free press that nonetheless existed in your countries. And I cannot get away from what is for me the painful insight that it was you, the heroes of the Second World War, who took this little chance away from us.

Others who were not victims can perhaps understand better, are perhaps more suited to explain than I am. I and my few fellow brothers and sisters, we who were saved when you won the war, we are not the most suited to make such analyses. We find it difficult to grasp your reasons and to explain your deafening silence — perhaps others can. I cannot, although I try.

CHAPTER IV

HOLOCAUST

First day of Extermination

Rosh Hashanah, the Jewish New Year, and Yom Kippur, the Day of Reconciliation, fall during the autumn in September or October. They are our foremost religious festivals. Many non-orthodox Jews also go to the synagogue, perhaps to keep up a several thousand year tradition, perhaps to pray "for safety's sake", or perhaps to join in on the fellowship when we greet each other, wish each other a Happy New year and sing together the cheerful songs as a conclusion to the service, the songs we remember from our childhood. Yom Kippur is a day of fasting, when without being disturbed by everyday problems we are to honor our departed, be reconciled with what has happened over the past year and with each other; this is to be a day of undisturbed meditation leading to reconciliation. The day of fasting is to start and end in a meal together.

But the evening before Yom Kippur in 1942, the evening of September 21st, the atmosphere in the ghetto is low-spirited and this evening cannot be lightened by either our presence together at the solemn meal or the evening service.

We have got used to the schools being closed, that our businesses and shops have been taken over without any compensation, that we are overcrowded, are shut in a ghetto and kept away from the world outside, that we suffer from poverty and a shortage of food, for we have learnt to live with all that. Our only remaining aim is to survive — everything else is subordinated, and that aim takes up our entire thoughts. So it is harder to live with the new rumors now circulating - Di Szwarce - "The Black Ones" — have come to Czestochowa.

Rumors about the Black Ones precede their arrival. In various ways, we have heard that these heavily armed soldiers in dark-brown uniforms and black forage caps usually arrive when the Germans are preparing for bloody Aktions against the Jews, that they are called Einsatzkommando, but by the Jews the Black Ones or the Ukrainians, which turns out to be only partly true.

The Jews at the East Station selected for forced labour have already been sent back to the ghetto at two o'clock in the afternoon. They have seen the Black Ones marching and heard them singing melancholy Ukrainian songs — they sing very well, rhythmically with a choir leader. But for us in the ghetto it is ominous news that they are here.

The Maple Tree Behind the Barbed Wire

Before the Jewish forced laborers are sent back to the ghetto, they also manage to see that on a railway siding from the East Station is an unusually long goods train with what they say are up to a hundred closed goods wagons the German order police have begun to inspect.

At about four that afternoon, another group of Jewish forced laborers who have returned to the ghetto confirm that they have seen that the Black Ones have been quartered in the closed school in Pilsudski Street and that the troop consists of two units, one of Ukrainians and the other with men from the Baltic countries. Some tell us a German Vorarbeiter at their workplace has said: "The bloody game starts tonight." All this is second-hand information, but it quickly spreads in the fear-filled ghetto.

The Jewish Council petition to be allowed to meet the new Stadthauptmann, who like the Governor-General in Krakow is a lawyer and is called Dr Frank. They are allowed to meet him that evening. Dr Frank assures them that there will be no Umsiedlung - expulsion — of the Jews of Czestochowa. It is rumored that the delegation had 100,000 zloty with them, collected from the inhabitants of the ghetto to be used in the event of a catastrophic situation, and that they handed over the money as a "donation" to the new Stadthauptmann, but no one in the Judenrat will confirm this.

Soon after nine that evening, Captain Degenhardt uses his special telephone line to the Jewish police. He sounds upset - Herr Stadthauptmann has informed him about the meeting with the Jewish council. Anyone spreading malicious rumours about evacuating Jews from Czestochowa must be punished. At the same time he confirms Herr Stadthauptmann's assurances that nothing is going to happen, and he demands that the Judenrat at once take measures to calm the inhabitants of the ghetto.

The ghetto jungle telegraph is effective and despite the religious holiday these contradictory rumours quickly circulate. People are worried; they very much want to be calmed but many find it hard to believe these new German assurances.

Those who have already gone to bed find that the night shift has been sent back to the ghetto from their forced labour and just after midnight they have seen the ghetto being surrounded by heavily armed troops in the characteristic uniforms and forage caps of the Black Ones. The Jewish police coming on duty at midnight at the exits of the ghetto are sent back by the German police; the Black Ones replacing them are from the Baltic countries - Lithuanians, Latvians and Estonians.

At one in the morning, we who are awake hear single shots in the distance and we realize something awful is happening. We try, each in his own way, to control our sense of anguish and helplessness. I go to bed with an adventure book by Karl May and fall asleep by forcing myself to think about the hero of the book, Old Shatterhand.

The Maple Tree Behind the Barbed Wire

At three in the morning, all the streetlights in the ghetto go on. Captain Degenhardt again uses his telephone and orders the Jewish police to be at an Appell in the rear courtyard of Metalurgia - the metal factory in ulica Krótka - Short Street. They are to be there in an hour, at four in the morning.

I am half-asleep in bed when I hear all this from others who are wide-awake and talking loudly in agitated voices. I would rather not wake up to this terrifying reality but can no longer sleep, so stay in bed trying to read, fleeing from the world into Karl May's book, which is safe, because it does not touch on my threatened existence. I do not want to take part in what is happening, and I can't do anything anyhow.

Early in the morning, work at Pinkus' workshop starts as usual. We find out that at one in the morning the Black Ones had fired on a group of Jews trying to make their way out of the ghetto under the cover of darkness - all were shot dead. That must have been when we had heard the first shots. Someone tells us that at the Appell at four in the morning, Degenhard had informed the Jewish police that after all there might be a Umseidlung - forced evacuation - of Jews from the Czestochowa ghetto. Everyone living in Kawia, Koszarowa, Garibaldi, Wilsona and Warszwaska streets, in two hours at the latest at six o'clock in the morning, is to be in front of Metalurgia in ulica Krótka 13. It is important that they bring with them the red Arbeitspass issued by the Judenrat, for the purpose of the Appell is to check them.

Several of the men working in the workshop have stayed overnight with us, the next youngest - Chaimek - says this can't be right, for only six hours earlier Captain Degenhardt had phoned to say nothing was going to happen. Even I, now out of bed and hauling on a pair of trousers, realise it would be pointless to remind Captain Degenhardt of the fact. Lie is being piled upon lie.

The Jews living in the streets indicated by Captain Degenhardt put on their best clothes and make up small parcels of whatever valuables they have left. Some choose to take prayer books, teflim and tales that are to be used at prayer, others take family photographs or the remnants of money and valuables they have saved for even worse times.

Between our house and ulica Krótka is just one block. We can hear crying coming from mothers with no Arbeitspass and small children frightened by their parents' helpless anxiety. In Pinkus' workshop they discuss what is going to happen to those too old to have a Judenrat work pass.

Before six in the morning, Jewish workers leaving for the day shift are assembled near the exit from the ghetto - no one has told them not to be there. There they are met by the Black Ones, who shout at them

The Maple Tree Behind the Barbed Wire

in a language they don't understand, except the constantly repeated German word - Zurück, zurück. Some of the Black Ones are impatient, raise their rifles and fire straight into the group of confused workers. Their own guards prevent the Jewish workers from leaving the place, and panic breaks out. The German order police look on, at first letting the Black Ones have their own way, then ordering them to stop shooting and taking the remainder of the forced labourers, the ones not shot, away to the general assembly place in front of Metalurgia.

I can see a group of the Black Ones being let into the ghetto. With two German policemen, they go round the injured Jewish workers and shoot the wounded ones - even the slightly injured who have managed to get up and are trying to join the group about to leave.

That is what I see, as do others who work in apartments at Aleja 14 with windows facing First Aleja. The German police kill methodically and efficiency, without unnecessarily tormenting their victims and without any show of emotion. The Black Ones - whom the ghetto inhabitants still call Ukrainians although they know that just as many of them are from the Baltic states - keep jabbing at the wounded with the hard toes of their boots and letting those who have managed to get up take a few steps before they fire - an unnecessarily cruel cat-and-mouse game with those who are anyhow about to die.

Today, fifty-six years later, safely surrounded by wife, children and grandchildren, whenever I try to remember I find it hard to write about what happened on September 22nd, 1942, and over the following three weeks. It is not the same as my memories of the siege of Warsaw, the Large Ghetto and prison camp.

Imprinted deeply in me, I have razor-sharp and detailed images of what I saw during that first day of the extermination of the Jews of the Czestochowa ghetto. But these images are sterile - they are released from the memories of the feelings I had as I watched, saw and understood. These tremendously detailed and clear memories have become part of me and will remain alive as long as I live. It feels as if I had been an outside observer and not one of those involved, one of those directly touched by the process of extermination. I remember perfectly clearly what I saw, but not what I was thinking. I don't even remember whether I was frightened. I don't remember my emotions.

But the memory of those emotions must exist somewhere deep inside me. For when I try to describe what happened and repeat all the details, then severe anguish rises in me, a sense of panic, as if I were in state of acute danger, an increase of adrenalin and signal-substances which today, over half a century later still send my whole body into a state of stress. This stress and anguish rise from somewhere in the depths of my being and do not let go. It is possible I might be able to force my emotions on those days of extermination up

The Maple Tree Behind the Barbed Wire

to the surface of my consciousness, but it is too much to demand and is perhaps unnecessary. Perhaps you, the reader, can nonetheless imagine what I and others with me felt as we looked on, saw what was happening and waited for our turn, which we knew was to come. But it is possible that at the time, September, 1942, I did not feel the same anguish as to do today. I was perhaps anaesthetised, screened off by what is today a familiar defence mechanism - denial, denial of reality - this is happening, but it can't apply to me. This merciful mechanism no longer functions. Today, I realise that the danger did apply to me, and I am frightened.

I have a strong aversion to having to remember, analyse and describe what happened during those three weeks fifty-six years ago. I would rather not - but I must not allow that, for then this book and the account of everything else I have done in my life will be meaningless. In addition, I have promised not to forget, and I hope that you, who happen to be reading these lines, will not forget, either. For those crammed together in the Czestochowa ghetto deserve to be remembered and the eye witnesses left who remember and can bring themselves to tell it, are few. The fact that you and I remember may perhaps prevent any other poor wretches having to live through similarly cruel, methodical, at the same time unnecessary and incomprehensible violence. For the memory of what happened to us in Czestochowa ghetto is a protection, however fragile, that makes a repetition more difficult against us Jews or any other group of people.

But I hope that you, the reader of this book, will be indulgent over that I express myself briefly. During the coming three weeks I am also anaesthetised from what I have seen and understood on September 22nd, 1942. The crystal clear, connected images concern the first and last day - when I myself am forced to be part of it - the rest I experience as very clear but disconnected sequences in a nightmare. And in that nightmare is a skeleton in uniform with a pistol instead of a scythe in its bony hand.

At the agreed time, at six in the morning on September 22nd, a long queue winds its way from the head at the entrance to the Metalurgia factory in ulica Krótka 13 round the neighbouring streets. It is an endless queue of men and women, the healthy and those who try to hide that they are sick, the old trying to look like the young, all dressed in their best, almost all with parcels in their hands or with a rucksack on their backs, except a number of young women instead carrying or holding by the hand one or several children they are trying to calm - often in vain - everyone knows Captain Degenhardt detests crying children. The majority in the queue have the dirty red folded piece of cardboard clutched in their hands - their security - the much desired Arbeitspass they have been ordered to bring with them to show. That is why they have been summoned to the Appell, just to show their Arbeitspass.

The Maple Tree Behind the Barbed Wire

A few metres in front of the Metalurgia entrance is Captain Degenhardt himself. Everyone is to pass by him. He doesn't even glance at the passes held out to him. Disappointed and confused, the Jews filing past look into Captain Degenhardt's face for an explanation during the brief moment he looks at them as they pass with their pathetic red pieces of cardboard in their hands.

Degenhardt stands there surrounded by his henchmen, feet apart, and a short dully-gleaming swagger stick in his hand. With it, he points first to the left - that Jew is taken into the Metalurgia courtyard - then to the right - he has to go to the larger group, the group standing just outside the entrance to Metalurgia, surrounded by the Black Ones. The green-clad German policemen directing the whole performance make sure the queue moves quickly, that everyone goes to wherever Captain Degenhardt points and quickly deals hard-handedly, decisively and efficiently with anyone who tries to say something to him. At his side are some Jewish police, mostly passive spectators. They have to deal with all the questions from the rapidly growing group outside the Metalurgia entrance - questions they cannot answer.

All women carrying children or holding hands with children are shown to the right, all men holding such women by the hand are shown to the right, all older people, all who do not look very healthy, all those weeping, all those who look frightened, all those appealing to Captain Degenhardt, and many others are shown to the right, with only a few going to the left to be taken into the rear courtyard of Metalurgia.

It all goes very swiftly; Captain Degenhardt does not find it difficult to decide. Despite several interruptions because of reports handed to him, in four hours he manages to sort out about eight thousand people and decide their fates - over seven thousand to the right, 340 to the left - into the Metalurgia courtyard. The rest are killed on the spot. What judge has ever managed to work so quickly? He is good at his job, Captain Degenhardt from the Leipzig police.

When he has finished, in good time before lunch, the Black Ones take over. They get those Degenhardt has sorted out into a long column, five people wide, and start driving them, first towards the ghetto exit, then along the streets of Czestochowa, through Pilsudski Street, towards Mirowskie-Zawodzie, the East Station and the new railway line to Kielce.

No one alive today whom I know saw what happened during that march, but some Jewish policemen ordered to go with them, later when I was also there listening, told us how bestially cruel it had been. Not one of those Jewish policemen is alive today, but several of us heard what they had to say, how the Black Ones beat, maltreated, kicked with their heavy boots and constantly insulted the seven thousand people they knew had been condemned to a suffocating death, either during the long journey in closed wagons or directly after they arrived at their end station. Was it not enough that they were to die? How to explain this meaningless and brutal cruelty on the way to the slaughter? The German police accompanying them through the town streets remained passive.

As we live on the border of the ghetto, in Aleja 14, I am present and hear when three profoundly shaken Jewish policemen return from the East Station and tell us about the unusually long train, at least seventy large cattle wagons with only a few ventilation holes and no windows. They tell us about the strong smell of disinfectant sticking in their noses when the wagon is opened - they say it smells of chlorine. They tell of the brutal loading up, the yelling and threats and blows, shoving and pushing the exhausted, thirsty, browbeaten and often already apathetic Jews, one more, one more, into each wagon, so tightly that people barely have room to stand, sit or lie. Then the door of the chlorine-stinking wagon is closed and bolted on the outside, about a hundred people crowded into each cattle wagon. Animals are transported in better conditions. The three policemen neither want to nor are able to stop talking. They talk about those shot lying in pools of blood at the station, how people were shot whenever they dawdled, hesitated or refused to go up the wooden ramp into their wagon. They tell us how one of the Black Ones took a little child by its small feet and smashed the child's downy head against the hard side of the wagon when a mother appealed to him, then shoved the weeping woman into the already overfull cattle wagon.

In the afternoon several hours later, Julek comes to Aleja 14. He is a Jewish policeman and has been ordered to go with a group of German police into the already emptied part of the ghetto. He tells us of the end of one of the prides of Czestochowa Jews - the strong, always friendly gentleman boxer, Hans Zylberberg, twenty-four and district boxing champion for three years running, called Hans by everyone, even by the local press, an unusual first name in Poland. Hans Zylberberg has refused to leave his apartment. When the German police inspecting the evacuated buildings come to his apartment, Hans hurls himself at them, shouting at them in a commanding voice and pointing at the door - out of here, this is my apartment. He quickly knocks down two of the intruders and injures a third before the first bullet hits him. He has nothing but his bare fists with which to defend himself. His last words before the fatal shot hits him are defiant: "I refuse to leave my apartment - my apartment", then he remains silent on a rug, lying in his own blood but still in his own apartment. Hans Zylberberg chose his way, not believing the German assurances that this was about a transfer to another labour camp. He escapes any further degradation, the cruel transport in packed cattle wagons and the efficient German death chambers.

The Maple Tree Behind the Barbed Wire

When the "Selektion" - as we are to call these individual events in the major Aktion - is completed in good time before eleven o'clock, the fair-haired German policeman, Senior Constable Schimmel, selects out fifty or so men from those Captain Degenhardt has directed into the Metalurgia factory courtyard. With several Black Ones to help him, he lines them up in three rows and they are ordered to take our dead away on carts that have been driven up and to bury them in a mass grave in the Jewish cemetery.

Captain Degenhardt and his assistants have done a good day's work. It is not easy in only a few hours to hunt 8,000 people out of their homes, sort them all out into the 340 allowed to live a little longer and the 7,000 who are to be sent away - have time to pack in the 7,000 into a goods train of only slightly over 70 cattle wagons and kill sufficiently many of us on the spot to make an example and inculcate terror to get us to obey. But on the other hand, the entire Aktion is extremely well prepared. Everything is planned in advance after the decision on the Endlösung - the final solution of the Jewish question - has been taken by the highest administrators in the country on January 20th, 1942, at a conference in a luxury villa by the beautiful Lake Wannsee outside Berlin, where they have discussed various methods of exterminating six million defenceless people, all in accordance with the clearly pronounced intentions of their democratically elected and appointed leaders.

The details important for success in these plans - choice of places, means of transport and the most suitable poisons - could be worked out later, described and practically prepared within a wide circle of knowledgeable and in their own field experienced representatives of various sectors of the well-organised German society - representatives from medical and chemical research, the chemical industry, the transport services, the administration, the police service and the construction industry, even psychologists brought in to instruct which lies should be served up to us. Everything is planned with the starting point in Chancellor Adolf Hitler's public speeches and declarations on the Endlösung of the Jewish problem - from the Wannsee conference in January 1942 and the expansion of the railway network to cope with the comprehensive transportation of human beings, to the construction of Treblinka's gas chambers, the choice of poison - the effective cyanide gas so carefully tested several times - and the conclusion in specially built crematoria for the mass-cremation of human corpses. In a modern, highly industrialised society, with the aid of all these experts, a detailed thought-through and thoroughly well-timed network has been built up, a network that demands great resources and covers a large part of Europe.

This all-embracing process includes several elements still not described. Who had the brilliant idea of Jewish Arbeitpass which were

The Maple Tree Behind the Barbed Wire

uniformly introduced into all the ghettos all over the Generalguvernement and lulled us into a false sense of security? Who thought up all the elements in the technique applied in all ghettos with the help of the Judenrat, the Jewish police with identical uniform caps, with the same lies and the co-operation of the local administration to lull us into a false sense of security? In Czestochowa it was Stadthauptmann Frank; I wonder whether he ever thought it unpleasant to lie to us.

It all ended with a uniformly organize—d collection of all the last possessions of the murdered people. Everything that remained in the impoverished Jewish ghettos and everything usable left behind by those sent to various extermination camps is uniformly taken in hand — gold teeth, and women's lovely hair cut off soon after they were killed.

This was the first time in the long history of mankind that industrial slaughter of six million human beings was carried out — the majority within one single year — and in which everything we possessed was efficiently taken care of, even parts of our bodies which might be of use to German society.

Captain Degenhardt and his retinue of German police from Leipzig and the Black Ones - the ones we see and I am writing about — are important, but nevertheless only small cogs in a large machine with one of Germany's largest industrial complexes at the top - IG Farbenindustri, the producer of the efficient poison. But we see only these small cogs receiving orders and carrying out their craft. Many of them who collaborated on various levels are still not yet identified, will never be identified, others deny their collaboration - some in good faith. People like forgetting what they want to forget.

September 22nd, 1942, the day before our Yom Kippur, is a sunny, for the time of year unusually warm day. Late in the afternoon, out of our window I see people outside the ghetto walking in the sun — young and older, men, women and children, some holding hands — as if nothing had happened. Towards evening, at about half past five, I see that Senior Constable Schimmel with his forcibly selected Jews has got as far as ulica Wilsona. Some of them weeping, I see them loading our dead from the day's Selektion. I don't see, but I know, that for the 7,000 who find themselves inside those overfull, closed cattle wagons, the lovely sun and the unusually late autumn warmth is yet another severe trial.

I would prefer to forget that day, but I cannot and must not. Trying to express what I myself saw or heard from several unanimous and reliable eyewitnesses, has entailed a greater strain than I could have even imagined when I began to write this book. At the same time, it feels liberating to have done so, my anguish when I think of the first day of the Extermination still there, but now easier to deal with.

The Maple Tree Behind the Barbed Wire

Last Day of Extermination

It is early morning on October 4th, 1942, the day of the last of the deportations of Jews from Czestochowa and the last day of the great Extermination Aktion. In principle, this Aktion was carried out according to the same pattern as before. Captain Degenhardt is responsible for the Selektion, and with his short swagger stick decides who is to live and who is to die. The Black Ones take over at the ghetto boundary, heading the grim marches through the streets to the long goods train, which then crammed full with its human cargo leaves the Kielve siding from the East Station every third day. Some practical arrangements have been slightly changed owing to experience the Germans have hitherto acquired, and have also been adapted to the buildings in different parts of the ghetto.

In contrast to the previously cleared parts of Czestochowa with their numerous small old buildings, today's Selektion concerns the big multi-occupied buildings situated on the west boundary of the ghetto; First Aleja lies in that area. Instead of driving 8,000 Jews out and lining them up in a long queue in front of Metalurgia, those of us standing in the bay window see the group, the indefatigable Captain Degenhardt in the lead, carry out the Aktion inside the large courtyards of one building after another. With the usual yells, threats and the occasional shot, they drive out all the occupants and do their Selektion in the courtyard - the people are divided into two groups, which we see are either taken to the ghetto boundary where the Black Ones take over, or are driven into the Metalurgia area.

We can't see what is happening in the rear courtyards of individual buildings, but we do see the Aktion slowly coming to Aleja 14, the last building on the boundary of the ghetto.

I go on taking refuge in my adventure stories, this time Janusz Meisner's book, an exciting world of brave aviators, a world in black and white, in which the good have their problems, but I know they will finally win and survive. But that is not my reality. In my reality, the good do not seem to win. I try, but find I cannot screen myself off from what I have seen and heard from numerous and unanimous eyewitnesses over the last thirteen days.

Last week, three members of ZOB, the Jewish resistance movement - among them Rywka Glans, who has stayed overnight with us before — with the help of the Jewish police have managed to make their way into Aleja 14, now cut off from the rest of the ghetto — they want to find out whether they can get out of the ghetto this way. That turns out to be impossible, but that evening they tell us that during the two days after the first Aktion, September 23rd and 24th, the cleared area was searched by German patrols with specially trained police dogs going round looking for Jews who have tried to hide in cellars, attics or

The Maple Tree Behind the Barbed Wire

ingeniously constructed "bunkers". Rywka tells us that the Jews the Germans find are kicked, maltreated, threatened and urged to inform on other Jews who have hidden and managed to escape the Aktion. In ulica Kawia they had found a big room hidden behind an ingenious construction of walls, a room containing several families with small children. I hear them talking about the method often used by the Black Ones, holding up small children by their feet and in the presence of the parents smashing their soft skulls against a wall. Several of the Jews found hiding in the bunker have taken their own lives to avoid being interrogated, to escape torture and the risk of giving way and informing on other hidden Jews. Every searched part of the ghetto has then been barricaded off and supplies of water, electricity and gas also cut off.

On the morning of September 28th, the day for the third Aktion, the German police drive round in green police cars announcing through loudspeakers that the Jews taken away on the two previous transports have arrived at their labour camp and are well, that the Jews at today's assembly point for the next transport will be given half a kilo of bread, some jam and hot soup. This is a "successful" ploy to ease the carrying out of the third Aktion. Many Jews tormented by hunger in the barricaded part of the ghetto turn up at the given assembly point. Some perhaps believe the German assurances, others are certainly aware that they cannot escape their fate — so they might as well enjoy hot soup, bread and jam for one more time.

This time the Germans keep their word, but only when it comes to the food. The promised bread, a dab of jam and the soup is handed out to those who come voluntarily for the third transport from the ghetto to the Extermination camp in Treblinka. Others, who have resisted the temptation and do not come voluntarily, are driven out of their apartments in the usual way and forced to join the transport all the same.

Over the next two days the large area that has been the target of the third Aktion is thoroughly searched - Nadrzeczna, Garncarska, Targowa, Prosta and Stary Rynek. The fourth Aktion could start.

ZOB couriers are - in a way unfathomable to me — very well informed. They tell us that the large group of those crowded together in the Metalurgia courtyard — over 1500 - has been sent away to new forced labour workplaces — to Pelcery, the large previously French-owned factory for the manufacture of woolen goods, to the Czestochowianka factory, to Huta Raków and to the stone quarry in the village of Bur.

I hear about Hasag for the first time, a German firm - Hans Schneider Fabriken A.G. - which is to take over Pelcery. The workplace is called Hasag-Pelcery and becomes the largest camp for those Jews allowed to stay in Czestochowa - Rywka tells us that the Jewish workers are dismantling the factory machines, which are then sent

The Maple Tree Behind the Barbed Wire

back to Germany. Nothing was ready when they got there. They have to work for more than twelve hours a day, sleep on stone floors with no mattresses and they have only three toilets between them. If they need to go to toilet at night, they have to lie stretched out face down and announce their need to the guard. They are given a slice of black bread per day, black chicory coffee in the morning and hot but watery soup in the evening. ZOB has heard that the man in charge of the kitchen, a French Volkdeutscher called José, sells on the black market most of the food intended for the Jewish forced laborers at Hasag-Pelcery.

Between two Aktions three Germans in civilian clothes and a group of Black Ones visit another of these camps. They force one of the Jews to take off all his clothes, then beat him black and blue until he is bloody, just to frighten the others. Then all Jews are ordered to hand over within five minutes any gold or precious stones they have, wedding rings as well — anyone later found with gold will be shot.

At Hasag-Raków, one of the tasks of the Jewish forced labour force is to unload the railway goods wagons arriving daily with loads of coal and coke for the plant's great blast furnaces. Nothing is known about those taken to the stone quarry in Bur.

ZOB also knows that in the first Selektions, Degenhardt has sent too many away, leaving behind too few, and nowadays more are being taken out to the group allowed to stay behind.

The three couriers stay for two nights with us and then return to the ghetto when they realise they are unable to get out on to the other side through Aleja 14.

It is nearly eleven o'clock in the morning of October 4th, 1942, when we go through what other Jews in our ghetto have previously gone through. I hear yells and the tramp of boots as the German policemen run up and down the stairs, banging on doors and shouting Raus, Raus, Schnell, Schnell, leaving all the doors open. They no longer say anything about our Arbeitspass; even the Germans have realized that they are no longer any use as conveyers of false security. Instead they shout that everyone is go to the courtyard immediately. Before I leave our apartment, I see the Black Ones are waiting outside the ghetto, quite close to our building.

We go down and try to keep together - Pinkus, Sarah, Roman and I, the people who work in Father's workshop and those who stay overnight in our apartment.

Captain Degenhardt is in the middle of the courtyard, talking to some officers in his retinue, which includes a couple of German civilians I have never seen before. The police who have been round the building assemble in small groups after having reported to the officers with Captain Degenhardt. Some have individual Jews with them who had been unable to get to the assembly point in time, or had perhaps tried to hide, but we hear no shots.

The Maple Tree Behind the Barbed Wire

There is now a large crowd in the courtyard, among them many familiar faces, our neighbors from our building, but also quite a number I cannot remember ever seeing before. There are several we have made friends with during the eighteen months we have lived here and have met every day. We could not be more than three hundred people. There are also a lot of green-clad German police, blue-clad Polish police, and a few Jewish policemen standing to one side, everyone except the victims and the Jewish policemen looking relaxed. We are lined up three deep in a large semi-circle.

Once Degenhardt has received reports from all the police sent out, he signs to them to start from the left, quite near where I am standing. Degenhardt is surrounded by German police as he starts the Selektion.

With his now famous short officer's swagger stick, which I see for the first time at close quarters, he makes his choice. I see him glance quickly, though to me with a penetrating look, at each of us as he passes. His grey-green eyes are watchful, his gaze sharp — he is quite short, seems vigorous and relaxed, a self-confident man who has accumulated considerable experience of what he now has to do, a man who knows he has great power.

He divides us into two groups — a larger one who have to stay in the semi-circle and another smaller who are assembled inside the circle, to the left directly opposite me. Those taken out to the smaller group outside the semi-circle are guarded by an older blue-clad Polish policeman who looks good-natured and rather bored.

It all goes very rapidly. Pinkus is in the second row, his left hand, almost white, resting lightly on Roman's right shoulder. Sarah and I are on his right, I in front of Sarah. Sarah has powdered her face and put on a little lipstick, but no rouge on her cheeks — she has no need to. I can feel her holding hard on to me with her left hand. She is looking straight ahead, trying to seem relaxed, which she is not - I can feel that in her hand which is almost clutching me. Degenhardt approaches, walks past Pinkus, Sarah and me, and I think he looks a trifle longer, perhaps slightly inquisitively at Pinkus, who with his impressive stature and lion's mane of grey hair is the eldest of the Jews in the courtyard; Pinkus looks him straight in the eye. I recognize two of the German police in the retinue. They have been to Pinkus' and he has made clothes for them, but at this moment not a flicker of recognition is to be seen in their faces. The rest of the retinue and the two German civilians are standing a little way away, talking to each other. They don't seem particularly interested in what is happening in this Selektion of Jews in Aleja 14. They are waiting for Degenhardt to finish. Degenhardt passes without taking out any of the four of us.

We don't know what is going to happen to those of us left in the semi-circle, or to the even smaller group taken out — mostly younger

The Maple Tree Behind the Barbed Wire

men and women standing less than ten meters away from Sarah and me, guarded by the older Polish policeman Degenhardt usually has with him at his Aktions.

Once Degenhardt has passed us, Sarah asks the Polish policeman if I may go over to the group taken out by Degenhardt. I don't know why she asks, or whether I want to join the group opposite — there are several people I know in it now. The policeman shrugs his shoulders and Sarah whispers in my ear: "One of us must be saved", then pushes me out of the semi-circle. I take the few steps across to the group in the middle. Once there I wonder whether it is right.

They are mostly younger Jews in the group; it is also smaller and in the Selektions hitherto, the larger group — children and older people — has been sent away, while the smaller group — of younger Jews - has been allowed to stay. I am rather confused and would prefer to run away from what is happening around me, but no longer can. It is strange, but at this moment I think about what Pinkus said to me a long time ago when I was to start school — we mature late, the men in our family. I am fairly immature for my age and find it difficult to make vital decisions. But suddenly, as I stand there in the courtyard of Aleja 14 beneath an almost clear sky, my thoughts and the consequences of what is happening clarify.

I look round the courtyard, at the people left in the three rows in the semi-circle — many of them known to me, among them Sarah - my mother, Pinkus - my father, and Roman, on to whom Pinkus is still holding hard. Pinkus is looking straight ahead, giving me no guidance, perhaps not even wanting to. And Sarah, despite all the hardships my still markedly beautiful mother is looking at me, her great dark-brown eyes filled with sorrow. Then I look at the group round Degenhardt slowly making its way over to the rest of the semi-circle, their backs to me now, and finally the older Polish policeman guarding us — he is also watching Degenhardt rather absently, for what is happening is clearly an everyday event to him. I now think with crystal clarity and realise that I have to decide, not Pinkus, nor Sarah.

What insanity is this — am I voluntarily to separate myself from Pinkus, Sarah and Roman? Am I to choose to be alone? I want us to be together whatever happens, my father, mother and brother and I to be together regardless of whether we are sent away or we stay. I do not ask, but say to the policeman that I am going back to my place in the semi-circle — he shrugs - I clearly can do as I like. No one in our group reacts, perhaps even notices what is happening — they are all staring at Degenhardt's back. I take the few steps and go back to my original place. Sarah looks at me with her sorrowful eyes as I whisper briefly, decisively and slightly reproachfully: "We are to be together." She clutches me by the arm again, mumbling something I don't catch, and when I turn towards her I see she has tears in her lovely big eyes. I don't think many have noticed what has happened - Pinkus' and

Sarah's elder son going back and forth.

For a brief moment, I don't know how many seconds, I had my fate, my life and death, in my own hands - I had to decide for myself and there I was. I am where I want to be, with my family and nowhere else — as long as I am allowed to be. The Polish policeman has not stopped me going across, nor from coming back when I want to — he has let a Jew choose, which is very unusual these days.

Two Polish policemen who had continued the search of the building come out into the courtyard with four Jews they have found at the last minute, two women and two men. Degenhardt indicates they are to join the smaller group.

With that the Selektion has been completed, swiftly, smoothly, neatly and in an orderly manner, with no noise except the barking of the police dogs and the usual shouts - Raus, Raus, Schnell, Schnell - as they drove people down into the courtyard; no one had to be killed on the spot.

The smaller group is taken away under escort by Polish and German police, and at the ghetto boundary handed over to the Black Ones already waiting there, guarding the growing group of Jews to be taken to the long train and its at present empty cattle wagons at the East Station. Captain Degenhardt, chatting calmly with his retinue, strolls away through the main entrance and heads for Second Aleja - in the rear the older Polish policeman who had let me choose. They are to have lunch, in good time before twelve o'clock. No one turns round. I cannot remember any one of them showing any emotion. The two Jewish policemen hitherto standing quite passively to one side now tell us we can all go back to our apartments and we will be told more later.

I had done the right thing, even when it came to survival. But soon, already the same day, I am to be separated from the rest of my family, and in the future, for the rest of our lives we are to be together for only short periods, against our will, for we want to be together, but the actions of various people and authorities are not to allow it.

We feel no joy, only sorrow as we return to our workshop. The relief of being allowed to stay is short-lived and we feel more vulnerable than ever. We are aware that in these times of insecurity, the relative security of the Craftsmen's House has gone. We don't know what is going to happen next, but we know things will never be as they were before the Aktion reached us. Those who rule over our destinies are sure to have plans for our future — and that can only be worse.

I still bear within me an unrealistic faith in my strong father, but common sense tells me that there is little he can do. My safe father is one of the victims like everyone else, and my beloved mother's advice may not always be the best. I am also dimly aware that by pinning

The Maple Tree Behind the Barbed Wire

unrealistic hopes on my father and taking refuge in the unreal world of adventure stories, I am trying to escape from the grim reality I am being forced to live in, a reality the content of which has to be experienced to be understood and which you do not want to understand when you do experience it. The bitter truth is that we are being helplessly drawn into a mill which grinds on and on, and which will go on grinding until not one single Jew is left alive in Czestochowa.

It is the middle of the afternoon. The great Aktion to exterminate the Jews of Czestochowa ghetto has been just about completed, the ghetto has to be cleared and that applies to Aleja 14 as well. But in the various workshops there is work ordered by the Germans but not yet completed — half-finished shoes, boots, suits, coats, shirts, dresses, brassieres, corsets. At about two o'clock some German police come and two of them - Schmidt and Hiller - sort those of us who are left into two groups. One group is moved to a temporary workshop owned by a Volksdeutscher - Mrs. Mosiewicz. They are to live there until the unfinished orders have been completed. Pinkus and Sarah are included in that group and Pinkus is allowed to take one of his assistants and Roman with him. None of us has ever heard of this workshop before, or of Mrs. Mosiewicz. The remainder — the majority of us — are to be moved to Metalurgia where other Jews who have been selected to stay in Czestochowa already are. But two of us, I one of them, are taken to a small group who are to clean up in the ghetto. Those not going to Mrs. Mosiewicz are given fifteen minutes to pack and say goodbye.

Sarah is practical — she starts packing. I think she is putting far too much in and weed some of it out, but I take my old school books. We have no food to share between us. Pinkus gives me a big hug and says in Yiddish: "Met uns treffen" — we shall meet again. Roman clutches at me and says: "Where are you going?" "Don't know," I say, patting my little brother on the head. There is no time for long farewells, which is just as well.

Down in the courtyard are several Polish and a few Jewish policemen who are to take us to our new locations. I am taken to a building in Garibaldi Street, a location for those who are to clear up the ghetto. The Jewish policeman with us - a fellow pupil of mine at the Jewish gymnasium, but four years older than I am, called Moniek Kamras - tells me on the way that over half the Jewish police and almost the entire Judenrat have been sent away on the last transport, only Kurland is left. He tells us about the bad conditions for those at Metalurgia.

The Maple Tree Behind the Barbed Wire

There are about twenty Jews already in the house in Garibaldi Street - all young men, and several more are on their way. We are allocated sleeping places — straw mattresses on the floor, a blanket and a pillow with no pillowslip, five or six men to each room. The room contains a table and a couple of chairs. We are given a quite thick slice of moist black bread, a dab of jam with no sugar and soup which has gone cold during transport from Metalurgia.

More Jews are brought to Garibaldi Street, mostly men, all young and in relatively good physical condition. They are allocated their rooms and sleeping places. As darkness falls, we are considerably more than fifty people, all tired and frightened, many having arrived too late for the bread so are hungry — we who have come earlier have no more food left to share with them.

The lights all over the building are turned out and for the first time I am alone, longing for the warmth of our family. We go to bed early, for work starts early the next morning — what kind of work will it be? Exhausted and drained of emotion, before I fall asleep melancholy creeps up on me — there are so few left of our fine lively Jewish community in Czestochowa. My last thought is that I am no longer with my family. What will become of us? How long have we to live? Then I sink into the merciful darkness and emptiness of sleep.

In thirteen days, between September 22nd and October 4th, 1942 - between Yom Kippur, the Day of Reconciliation and Simchas Tora, the Feast of Joy - the Germans have wiped out a Jewish community laboriously built up over two hundred years in Czestochowa. The Aktion has been led by a section of the ordinary police loaned from Leipzig under the command of its Commissioner - Captain Degenhardt.

The Maple Tree Behind the Barbed Wire

End of the Large Ghetto

On October 11th, 1942, a week has gone by since I had been taken to the Garibaldi group cleaning up the cleared large ghetto.

For the first days we are isolated from other Jews still in Czestochowa, but we tell each other what we have seen and been through. The last seven to arrive, five men and two women, were at Metalurgia during the last day of the Aktion. They tell us that the remaining 190 Jewish policemen were summoned to an Appell. Captain Degenhardt himself divided them into two groups, one of 160 who are to join the last transport and carry on as police in the labour camp which — according to Degenhardt - the Czestochowa Jews are being sent to, the other thirty to stay in Czestochowa. The division is said to have been rather random. The entire Judenrat has to go on the same transport, except its chairman - Leon Kopinski - who is shot on the spot owing to his lack of loyalty, and Bernard Kurland, who is still at Metalurgia.

The Rector of our Jewish gymnasium, the gifted mathematician and teacher Anisfelt, is sent on the last transport on October 4th. Before he has to leave, he tells some of those who are staying that he has continuously noted down everything that has happened in the Juderat and in the ghetto written down any verbal information from the German administration and the police, as well he has saved some of the original German communications in the original. He has put all the documents into four watertight containers and buried them deep down in the ground. To date, not yet a single one of Anisfelt's containers has been found, although many people have tried. When they are, I am convinced they will be an important record of the end of the history of the Czestochowa Jews.

A methodical search is being made for Jews hiding in the big ghetto. The search is begun in the cleared area of the ghetto immediately after the latest Aktion and ends the evening before the next Aktion is to start. During the two weeks the Aktions have gone on, the Germans have had the help of the Black Ones, though later they have to do it on their own.

We who are cleaning up may go only into the parts of the ghetto that have already been searched. The Germans use dogs trained to sniff out people in cellars, attics, abandoned derelict buildings, even walled-in bunkers well concealed from to the human eye. Clearly many Jews have tried to save themselves in hiding places such as these. I have seen two bunkers already cleared by the Germans. One of them in ulica Warszawska 6 was very thoroughly planned and well protected, able to hold quite a number of people for a long time. In this bunker, where the whole of the Mitelman family had tried to save themselves, they had stored dried food, tins and other food to last for two years, and it also had access to running water. Not even the dogs had found it. The Mitelmans were betrayed by an acquaintance of the family, a Jewish policeman, who with his wife and two children were taken out to the last transport and promised amnesty if he reported Jews he knew were in hiding. He knew about the Mitelman bunker in ulica Warsawska and informed on them to save his own wife and children. He himself died under torture when he failed to report any more Jewish hiding places, but his wife and children were not sent on the transport. They were let into Metalurgia, though I don't know what happened to them later. The entire Mitelman family, seven people in all, were all shot— on the spot. In their bunker, which was considered "safe", the Germans found and destroyed the memoirs Professor Mitelman had carefully noted down on the events in Czestochowa.

Those who had tried to hide in the ghetto and were not shot on the spot were assembled in a special building and they turned out to be quite a number. Most of them were children and old people — some people considered hiding the only way to survive. They were interrogated, threatened, beaten, tortured and promised amnesty if they reported other Jews in hiding in the ghetto, or on "the other side". They were all sent on the last transport to Treblinka.

It must have been very important to the Germans to find and kill every Jew in Czestochowa; a great deal of work and resources went into making sure no one survived. Specially trained German police, other experts, dogs trained for the purpose, and special equipment were brought into Czestochowa at this time and used to seek out those trying to survive. I am surprised when several months later, I find out that nonetheless, over twenty Jewish boys were successfully hidden and saved.

When we in the Garibaldi group are let into the cleared parts of the ghetto, we are the only people there. To prevent looting of what is left, no others are allowed in, the Germans themselves are to do the looting — our group and myself are their helpers.

The streets, the buildings and their courtyards are ghostly and empty, not a human being audible or visible in the persistently beautiful and mild autumn sun. On two occasions, I see small groups of uniformed Germans, five or six of them, and on one occasion two women in civilian clothes walking round as if they had come on an outing. On one occasion I see two steel-grey Gestapo-uniformed Germans walking round inspecting the empty ghetto.

In Wilson Street numbers 20/22, which both the Germans and we call the Furniture Store - previously the Lewkowicz furniture factory — the Germans assemble Jewish artisans such as carpenters, locksmiths, painters and electricians. Their first task is to equip two buildings in Garibaldi Street for a new purpose — the storage of

The Maple Tree Behind the Barbed Wire

everything of value we find. We who are to clean up the ghetto are then to collect up all men's clothing into one hall, men's underclothes into another, then women's clothes, women's underclothes, better furniture and lamps, sewing-machines and electrical goods, pictures and sculptures, precious metals such as silver and gold, other metal objects — all neatly sorted out into a room each. It amounts to a great deal, for it all comes from over 50,000 people.

I am in a group that Handtke - "der Weisse Kopf" — is in charge of and I am the youngest in it. Under his green uniform coat, Handtke wears a not very regulation white scarf, scarcely noticeable against his white face, bleached light eyebrows and almost white hair. He has hitherto not shown any of his shoot-to-kill-habits, perhaps having satisfied his needs for a while ahead at the Aktions and during the search for hidden Jews. Handtke behaves quite humanly, in an almost friendly way towards us in his group.

We start with the oldest, poorest part of the ghetto, near the River Warta. When its streets are cleared of everything that can be considered of value, Jews from various temporary locations are moved in — those at Metalurgia, Hasag-Pelcery, Hasag-Raków, Czestochowianka, the Furniture Store, and those of us in Garibaldi Street - but not Pinkus, Sarah, Roman and the others in the small group quartered in Mrs. Mosiewicz's workshop. The Germans call the area Das kleine Ghetto, the Little Ghetto. Every morning, we are taken out to our workplaces and every evening brought back after a working shift of at least twelve hours.

Those of us clearing the ghetto are called "fasownikes". Although it is forbidden, some of us put on a smarter garment or take with us something which the next day another Jew takes to his workplace to exchange for food or to sell to Polish workers, the profit then shared between the two who take the risk. This means more food can be got into the small ghetto. The Germans don't notice, or perhaps don't bother when one of us is better dressed, but some are often searched at random. On one such occasion, the Germans find two small silver spoons on a woman. Constable Schimmel, in charge of the strip search, shoots her on the spot and in everyone's presence. Then the rest of the group is let in through the gate to the small ghetto. It is said that some of us "fasownikes" nonetheless dare to take jewelry in particular, which they keep, and some are said to have accumulated a fortune, but I don't think that can be true.

One obstacle in our work is the number of doors that are actually still locked. People forced to leave their homes were urged not to lock their doors behind them, so perhaps these have locked themselves or been locked after the Germans had searched the building. Handtke happens to see me opening a locked door with a kick — in future, he sends me on ahead to open all locked doors.

I have plenty of time, at least an hour, after I have opened the doors and before the group with Handtke arrive, and I can also hear them coming. Meanwhile I go round and look everywhere. Ghostly, empty silent buildings that look as if they were inhabited, as if the owners would soon be coming back. But the owners will not be coming back. They have gone forever. I can see that people have left in a panic, half-eaten plates of food still on the table, food still in a saucepan on the stove. Those who have now gone had perhaps wanted to eat up the food they had saved, but had not had time to do so. I also see they had been in a hurry to change clothes — garments lie thrown on a bed, a chair, or the floor.

Apart from having become good at quickly kicking open locked doors, I have also learnt to find valuables, but don't know what to do with what I find.

One day I find some small glittering stones underneath the waxed paper at the bottom of the middle drawer of a light birch wood bureau — they must be precious stones, for why otherwise should anyone hide them? One large and three smaller cut stones — they look like diamonds. I am frightened and would prefer not to have anything to do with them, but then I think perhaps I ought to take the stones with me. They are easy to hide, perhaps worth a fortune and might turn out useful in exchange for food, or after the war. Yet I don't want to risk my life for a fortune. If I put them back, they will fall into Handtke's hands, and I don't want that, either. I don't want the man I have seen kill Jews to be rewarded like that. But perhaps they are not diamonds, perhaps just worthless bits of glass. That would be relief - I think.

I remember from my physics lessons at school that a diamond is the hardest substance of all, harder than steel. In another drawer in the neat kitchen I find a hammer. Then I put the largest stone on to the steel edge of the stove and try to break it with the hammer — if it is a diamond, then it ought not to break. It is not easy. Several times the stone shoots away, but I manage in the end. After the next blow the stone breaks and nothing is left on the stove but some glittering powder which I sweep up and put into the half-full garbage bag. After a few more attempts, all the stones have been turned into powder, the three smaller ones easier than the first large one. The problem is solved and I am relieved, though at the same time there is a gnawing doubt inside me — perhaps after all they were diamonds I have smashed.

I am perhaps cowardly, I accept that, but at the same time I do not need to risk my life, and Handtke is not to get his hands on any diamonds in apartments I open up. In future, I have the hammer with me whenever I go into another building. If anyone should ask, I can say I need it to break the lock. But no one asks and during the week ahead I find four hidden stones in yet another place, glittering white and green stones — they are all smashed, turned into powder and left in the garbage bag of the cleared apartment.

The Maple Tree Behind the Barbed Wire

I can see why the Germans allowed the small remnant of Jews to stay in Czestochowa. We are not a particularly good work force, nor do they use us particularly efficiently, for it takes a lot healthy Germans to guard us instead of being at the now retreating front — but all the same they are to put us to work. I do, however, often wonder why they let Jews stay in the prison camps of Ravensbrück, Buchenwald, Bergen-Belsen in Germany itself. Perhaps we were needed as a motive for certain deserving Germans to be rewarded with a secure occupation and escape going to the war fronts. Or was it that some high-up person in Berlin saw us as objects of barter, an insurance in the event of things going wrong in the war?

For the fortunes of war have already turned and the war is already lost when the annihilation of the Czestochowa ghetto takes place. By then, eighteen months have gone by since Adolf Hitler's closest confidant - Rudolf Hess - whom he had appointed as his successor — flew to Great Britain to try to negotiate peace. Nine months have gone by since the twenty-six Allied states had signed the Washington declaration in which Germany is designated the main opponent and the Allies have pledged not to sign any separate peace treaty with Germany, to accept nothing but unconditional surrender. Germany's industrial capacity has begun to weaken despite its total conversion to centralized arms production. Germany is suffering from a shortage of troops and materials, while on the other hand the industries of Great Britain and the United States are working at full pitch on arms production. The losses of the German submarine fleet exceed production and at the same time the Allies occupy Iran in order to be able to send war materials to the Soviet Union by land.

Almost ten months have gone by since owing to the cold Hitler himself was forced to break off the huge winter offensive in the Soviet Union. Owing to lack of material and manpower, the summer offensive had to be limited to the southern part of the front and had already ebbed away. A huge concentration of Soviet troops is under way. Under Marshall Vasilevski's command, in a month they are to begin their powerful winter offensive against the overextended German lines along the two thousand kilometer long front.

The skillfully carried out German offensive led by General Rommel in North Africa has been halted. Later in October, Allied troops under the command of General Montgomery are to break through the Axis front at El Alemein. After their early spectacular initial successes, even the Japanese offensive has been halted. Five months have passed since the battle of the Coral Sea at which the Allied fleet stopped the Japanese attack on Port Moresby, four months since the Japanese suffered great losses during their failed attempt to take Midway Island, and also their offensive in the north to the Aleutians has been halted.

The Maple Tree Behind the Barbed Wire

Germany has already lost the war when the order police from Leipzig, with the aid of a great force of experts sent there — among them the Einsatskommando of the Black Ones - on October 4th, 1942, complete the successful, almost total extermination of the great, unarmed, over two hundred year-old Jewish community in Czestochowa. But we do not know that the German fortunes of war have already turned. To us, we still regard the Germans as the predecessors of an invincible evil power.

I know many people wonder how we Jews could fall in with the German decrees and that some despise us for not resisting but allowed them to deport and then gas us to death. Why didn't we resist when we were so numerous, why did we wear Jewish armbands or yellow stars on our chests. Why did we allow ourselves to be crammed together into ghettos, ranged up at assembly points for Selektion, allow ourselves to be driven up ramps on to cattle wagons, believing the lies that we were to be sent to labour camps?

But was it really so strange that we believed them? Was it not more difficult to imagine that one of the leading cultured peoples of Europe in the middle of the twentieth century could send train after train of several thousand people in each to an extermination camp?

Our people grew up in ghettos, with a mentality formed in that ghetto environment. We were forced to live in that environment for fifty generations - for over a thousand years. Almost everywhere in Europe during those thousand years we were alone and isolated, discriminated against by the population outside our little circle.

When Adolf Hitler came into power, our process of liberation was still in its infancy. Herzl, Ben-Gurion and Zabotinski, Zionism, Revisionism and Bunt - the organized resistance of the Jews to oppression in our homelands — were still new phenomena. Our liberation had not had time to develop before nine out of ten of us were to be exterminated, mostly in a single year — while the outside world pretended it knew nothing.

And where would we have gone? Those who managed to escape were forced to creep back into the ghetto, the surrounding people giving us no alternative. People reported us when we tried to escape. With what would we have defended ourselves when granted minimal and the worst sort of the arms which Jews in other countries managed to persuade those in power to parachute in to us.

Our young people were not accepted, and those who managed to escape out of ghetto to join the resistance movement were often murdered. We did not receive even the little help that was quite possible to give us by bombing the only railway line to any of the extermination camps, or bombing a single one of the gas chambers. The historic leaders of the second world war knew, but kept silent on the these mass murders. It was allowed to continue in silence.

The Maple Tree Behind the Barbed Wire

I was there, in Poland, where the majority of Jews lived during the German occupation. I saw it, experienced it, I know what it was like. I have heard from my parents, read about what it was like before and despite all the degradation, I am full of admiration.

I was proud that our people were able to survive the difficult exile with several hundred years of almost unbroken persecution. Proud that sufficient numbers held on so that our religion, our traditions, and with that our people were able to survive, although it was so easy to escape discrimination and persecution. It was easy to escape twenty-five years of military service with constant harassment in the Russian army — as long as you gave up being a Jew, but they chose not to give up. I am proud of the solidarity in my people during the difficult centuries, of their willingness to sacrifice, which meant my people were able to survive, but I am also deeply grateful to all the friends who appeared for different, often good reasons to help us. They were sufficiently many for a dispersed people their identity intact and with no land to be able to survive for over 1900 years.

I feel a profound sadness and am wounded in my soul by what has happened. But at the same time I am proud that we could go through even the Holocaust with our self-esteem intact. I am proud of the solidarity we experienced in both the large and the small ghetto of Czestochowa, then also in the prison camp. I am proud there were no traitors among us, at least, I have not come across one, that in the end we managed to organise weak but nonetheless some resistance. I am proud that a whole division of motorized and armored SS élite troops had to be withdrawn from the eastern front in order to quell the rebellion among our brothers and sisters in the Warsaw ghetto — and proud of the hopeless armed resistance in our and several other smaller ghettos, even in the Treblinka extermination camp.

To be a Jew has in no context meant an advantage to me, though many disadvantages. Yet I am proud to belong to the Jewish people, because the historic misery of our people demonstrates the ability of mankind to survive with their dignity and faith in people intact.

The Maple Tree Behind the Barbed Wire

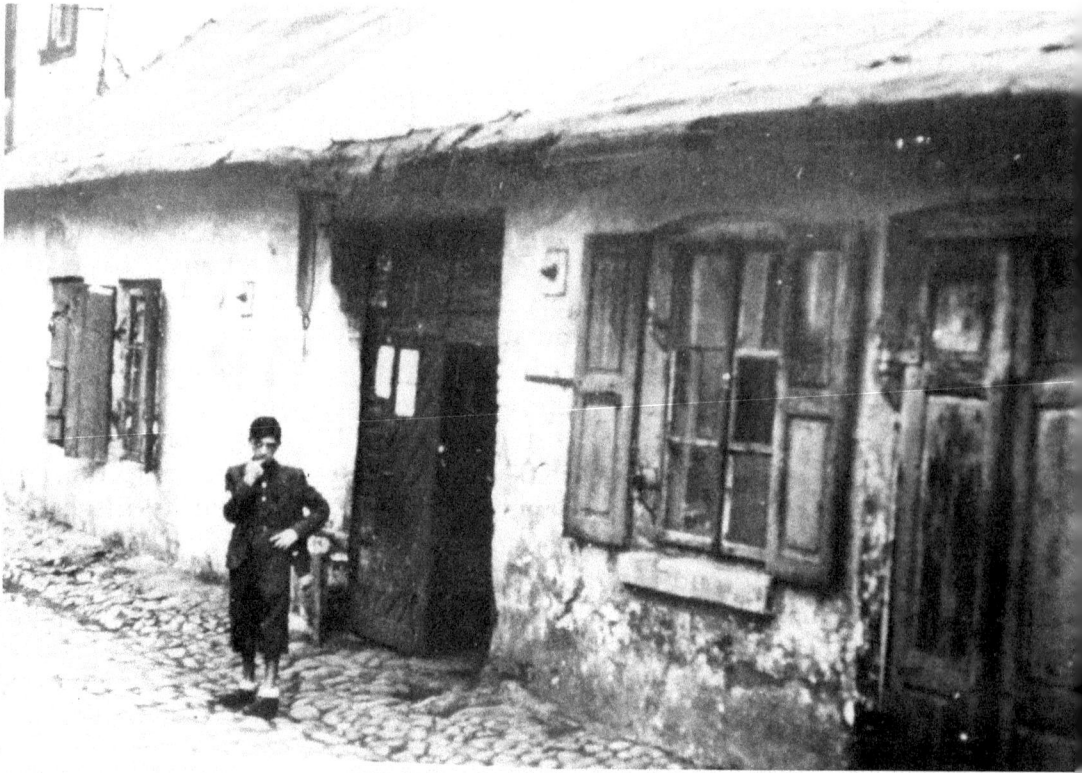

The small ghetto, where the remaining 5,200 Jews of Czestochowa were housed after the Aktion consists of a few short crowded alleys. This is the oldest, poorest and worst maintained part of the town.

The Maple Tree Behind the Barbed Wire

The Small Ghetto

The Small Ghetto, where the remaining Jews of Czestochowa are housed after the Aktion, consists of ulica Kozia and parts of Nadrzeczna, Mostowa and Garncarska Streets, which are really no more than cramped little alleys. This is a small area for the 5,200 people officially registered in the ghetto and is also the oldest, poorest and least well maintained part of the town. All the houses are small, with outside toilets, many with no running water, but they do have electricity. Only one street is asphalted, most surfaces large brown or grey cobblestones, others just trampled dark earth.

This small ghetto is surrounded by a man-high barbed wire fence consisting of coarse barbed wire twisted firmly between large posts. All the houses surrounding it have been evacuated, the shops are empty. The ghetto is constantly guarded by heavily armed soldiers patrolling day and night in the streets beyond the barbed wire - Jaskrowska, Senatorska, Ptasia and the continuation of Mostowa.

Most of those trying to get out of the ghetto have been shot and left hanging on the barbed wire fence. Despite this, it is said that there are several Jews who repeatedly manage to get in and out; they know about places where the wire has been cut or prized open.

I am among the first, Pinkus and Sarah among the last to move into the Small Ghetto from our temporary quarters at our workplaces; we have now been together for a week. We are seven - Rutka, Maurycy and Rózia are living with us in this tiny apartment, though it is no worse or more crowded for us than for anyone else. When Rutka and Maurycy later move, we have more space than many others. In this ghetto, the total number of rooms is 1,200. Apart from the 5,200 registered Jews, there are said to be over 500 unregistered - I cannot understand how and where they managed to escape the Aktion.

We have been given one room and a tiny kitchen on the first floor in a decayed two-story house in ulica Garncarska, quite close to the ghetto exit. To get to our apartment you have to climb the always dark, worn and slippery stone stairs. The old building has two attic apartments and altogether comprises eight small apartments. Three toilets and a cold room with a bath in it is out in the courtyard, from where we also fetch water which has to be pumped by hand from a stand connected to a well nearby.

150

The Maple Tree Behind the Barbed Wire

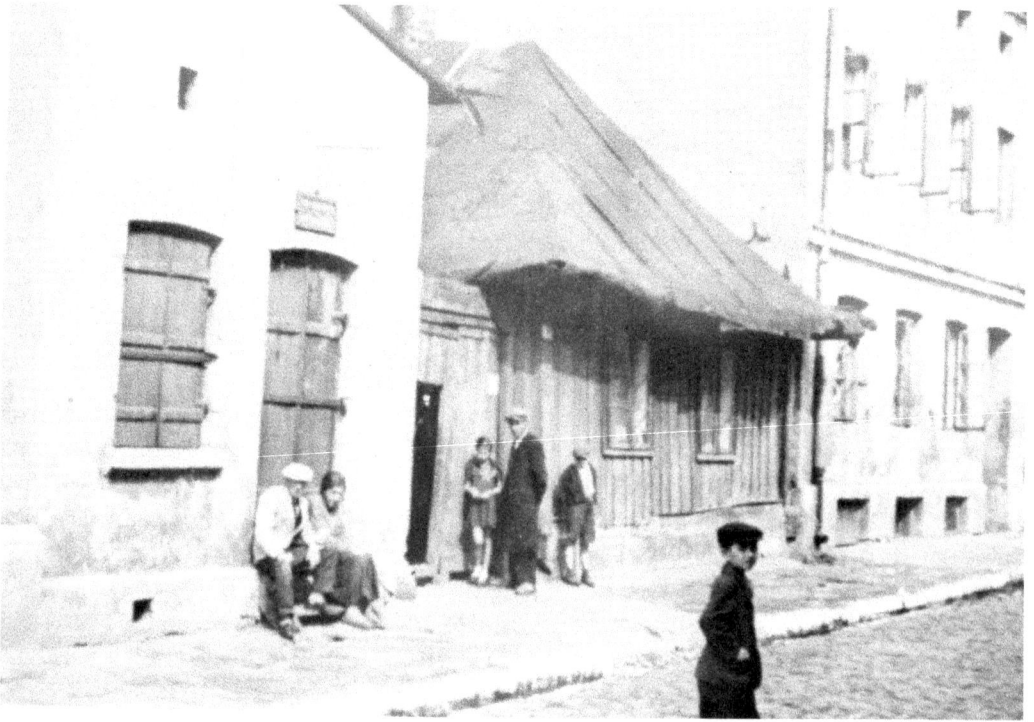

All the houses in the Small Ghetto are small, the toilets outside, many houses with no running water, but they all have electricity. We live in ulica Garncarska, in the house on the extreme right

Sarah has worked miracles with the shabby apartment. The buckled saucepans are always bright and shiny, the heavy black cast-iron pan hanging on a nail in the wall — we seldom have any use for it. She always keeps the apartment clean and tidy, with something pretty on the only table over by the window. She also nearly always has something at home to make the soup go further, or at least give it some taste, the soup, together with a slice of black bread and a portion of chicory coffee dealt out from one of the big pans further down ulica Garncarska in front of the Jewish police station. We have been allocated our apartment because it is to hold seven people, but soon my cousin Rutka is to move, then her father, Pinkus' younger brother Maurycy, also moves out.

Rutka is said to have moved in with a man several years older than she is, a man called Besserglick, who is one of those who manage relatively well in the ghetto. Sarah does not think Rutka's choice is a good one and she tells Rutka so. Rutka does not like that and says so quite calmly to Sarah, then we don't see Rutka for several weeks. Maurycy sometimes comes to see us in the evenings and tells us that Besserglick manages well and so things are all right for them, but Maurycy does not tell us what Besserglick does or what he himself does. Pinkus and I are sad that Rutka does not put in an appearance.

The Maple Tree Behind the Barbed Wire

I think Sarah's interference unnecessary. What Rutka does with her life has nothing to do with us. Sarah is also sad, but does nothing about it.

The only exit from the ghetto is in ulica Garncarska. Outside is an open space called Rynek Warszawski, which we call Ryneczek - Little Square. Every morning, the Germans taking groups of Jews to the various forced labour workplaces come to the square and the Jews are to wait for them behind the fence.

There are no green spaces in the ghetto, the only tree visible is in the square just outside the exit from the ghetto. This gnarled, partly leafless maple beyond the barbed wire is the only greenery visible from our ghetto. We call it the Maple behind Barbed Wire.

Bernard Kurland and his four assistants' Arbeitsamt has fairly modest premises in the corner house between ulica Garncarska and Nadrzeczna, close to the entrance into the ghetto. Almost in the middle of ghetto, in ulica Garncarska, is the Jewish police station, next to it the cottage hospital, which the people working there grandly call the Hospital, but in the ghetto is generally called the Sick Bay. It has two doctors, the senior called Szperling, the other older and called Dr Bresler. There is also another doctor in the ghetto, a young surgeon called Przyrowski.

Everyone likes Dr Bresler. He is friendly and generous with sick-notes, but otherwise not much of a doctor. Bresler is called the AK doctor — he just writes out only two prescriptions — both are powders packed in waxed paper and labelled A for Aspirin or K for Kogutek - which before the war was a non-prescription preparation for headaches.

No one likes Dr Szperling. He refuses to write sick-notes for people who are sick but have no temperature, and those he does pronounce sick, he often brings in to one of his sickrooms although they would rather be at home. He has appointed his wife as nurse, although she has had no training — but she seems to be a good person and is kind to patients and staff.

Several people have heard Szperling criticizing out aloud his colleague Dr Bresler, warning him not to write out so many sick-notes. Bresler is said to have said in his defense that only sick people come to the doctor, not those who are fit, and the sick should be let off work. It is said that Dr Bresler has taken to giving out sick-notes only to those with a temperature, but all the same patients wait before going to the doctor until Szperling is not there.

Dr Bresler is nearly sixty and does not seem to be all that well himself. Dr Szperling is strong and squat, red-haired, red-faced, only just over forty — a superior and unsympathetic man. He was slimmer and more friendly when before the war, six years ago, he examined me and was with me for my appendix operation. What they say about Dr Szperling is certainly exaggerated, but I would nevertheless not want to have him as my doctor.

Although the ghetto is officially a forced labour camp, which means everyone has to have an allotted workplace and everyone has to work, things have become fairly slack at some workplaces. So quite a number of Jews are left in the ghetto during the day and even more in the evenings, despite the fact that some groups work night shifts and go out in the afternoon. Those who are absent from their workplace must have a note from a doctor at the cottage hospital, but some are allocated work inside the ghetto. Some have not been allocated any work at all and some take the risk of staying in the ghetto without a sick-note. Hitherto the Germans have not carried out any razzias in this ghetto. They are not to be seen there and as before, the Jewish police turn a blind eye to what goes on.

Every morning, Pinkus, Sarah and Roman join the group to go to Mrs. Mosiewicz' workshop in the middle of town in Second Aleja 18. Rózia is allocated some obscure task inside the ghetto and comes home earlier than the rest of us, sometimes even staying at home all day.

I am the first to leave my job as "fasownik" the moment an opportunity arises. It is not difficult to change as my job is one of the most sought-after in the ghetto. One afternoon, I speak to my Vorarbeiter - Rotsztajn, and he explains to his German boss that he has to exchange one of his workers, and at the same time manages to arrange with Mrs. Mosiewicz that I have been allotted to her workshop. A week later, I go with Pinkus and Sarah to their workplace and for the first time meet Mrs. Mosiewicz.

She is a rather powerfully built, well dressed, good-natured but efficient woman in her fifties, with grey streaks in her dark brown hair. She is from a German-Silesian family and speaks fluent Polish. Her husband is dead, he, too, a German living in Poland. Mrs. Mosiewicz has built up a small tailoring workshop that does well and flourished during the German occupation. I do not know if she is a Reichdeutscher or a Volkdeutscher, but she mixes with the highest officials of the occupying powers in Czestochowa and at the same time is a clever and honest businesswoman - Pinkus maintains. She has arranged it so that the Jews working in her workshop are not only allowed to finish the work started before the evacuation of Aleja 14, but also that she may receive new orders which we are to carry out.

Mrs. Mosiewicz perhaps arranges this because she is a clever businesswoman, but perhaps also out of consideration for those who work for her — how do I know? Now, at the end of December 1942, Pinkus is fifty-six and one of the oldest in the ghetto. He would be unlikely to have remained if he had not been allocated work that he is

The Maple Tree Behind the Barbed Wire

particularly well qualified for, that he is an unusually good tailor.

We who live shut in this forced labour camp are still hoping for a future — healthy people cannot live without hope. We need a scrap of hope just as much as we need food, drink, and a place to live in face of the approaching winter, which, however, has not been particularly severe. Pinkus takes with him the dark green cloth parcel with the life insurances from the Swiss insurance company, hoping that by redeeming them it will help give us a new start in life — after the war. But no one knows, no one any longer dares prophesy how to make survival possible. They have taken all realistic hopes away from us, and we have nothing left but unrealistic illusions.

We have seen many people shot before our very eyes and we have many a time been betrayed, so only few of us believe the still beautiful Helenka Tennenbaum when she tells us that Captain Degenhardt has told her that everything he has done has been on express orders, but now there will be no more Aktions against the Jews and we who are left are to be allowed to live — not even Helenka herself seems to believe it.

At the same time, when one of the Jews, emaciated and tormented by his memories of hardships, comes back from Treblinka - the Extermination camp for our ghetto, he confirms in detail what we have previously heard. Despite having lost all his illusions, he comes back to the ghetto — he has nowhere else to go.

The fact that we now all know that we can no longer deny the truth has strengthened ZOB - the Jewish resistance movement. They are said to number 300, are well organized and generally accepted as a more powerful authority in the ghetto than the Jewish police, or what is left of this police force and of the Judenrat - that is, Bernard Kurland, who is also said to collaborate with ZOB. The leaders in ZOB all have pseudonyms, the Commandant Mojtek. In the ghetto it is known that ZOB not only have wire-cutters, thick blankets and ladders to get over the barbed wire fence whenever necessary, but they also have firearms and grenades — or what in the ghetto are called grenades — manufactured in their secret workshop in ulica Nadrzeczna 66. ZOB has contacts with "the other side". These contacts extend all the way to the Warsaw ghetto and to AK - the nationalist Armja Krajowa. It is said that AK, in its capacity as a necessary intermediary, help themselves to the arms, ammunition and medicines which are regularly, with the ghetto and ZOB as addressees, parachuted in.

But the insight into what has happened to the rest of the Czestochowa Jews and what must happen to us has also had another effect. Several people make their way over to "the other side", and many throw themselves mindlessly into what is in practice a hopeless situation.

The Maple Tree Behind the Barbed Wire

My first love at the Jewish gymnasium, the precocious and gentle Stusia Neumark, comes to our apartment early one afternoon to say goodbye on a day when I have not gone to work. In my eyes, she is still good-looking, more mature, even softer, even gentler, a lovely young lady. Stusia is profoundly sad. She tells me that both her parents are dead, and that of her whole family, only she and her younger brother are left. She talks openly about when and in what way she is going to get out of the ghetto the next morning, but not where she is going, nor do I ask. We mostly talk about the old days, our remaining school friends, less about the ones who have gone. There is a great tenderness between us, but no hugs or kisses. It seems to be so long ago — in another happy-go-lucky world — when we played and loved each other.

Stusia does not survive the war. I meet her younger brother many years later and even he does not know in what way Stusia Neumark was killed.

At the beginning of January 1943, the winter is still unusually mild in Czestochowa. The gate at the exit from the ghetto, usually open for only a few moments, is wide open early in the morning of January. The groups of Jews at the exit to be transported to their workplaces are instead lined up for Appell, as well as those who come from the night shift. The Jewish police go round the ghetto summoning everyone to Ryneczek immediately. Things begin to become clearer when several German police, otherwise unwilling to pass the gate into the ghetto, come inside to check what is happening and go to the cottage hospital to see if anyone not sick is hiding there. At Ryneczek are a lot of green policemen, many more than those we have known previously, and also other uniformed Germans, but not Captain Degenhardt. It is Oberleutnant Rohn leading the Aktion and next to him is the fat Lieutenant Tsopart.

We stand there for a long time, freezing in our thin clothes; Rohn waits until everyone is lined up for Appell.

At eight o'clock, after we have stood in Ryneczek for almost two hours, a Jewish policeman comes by and says quietly that they are to take 500 of us out to a camp in Radomsko. But nothing happens — we look at the Germans and at the gnarled old maple tree.

It is almost nine o'clock. The pale sun is shining weakly on those of us still standing in the square and on to the ghostly empty area inside the ghetto, when Oberleutnant Rohn with a retinue of green police and Lieutenant Tsopart beside him start walking round inspecting us. In the Degenhardt manner but without Degenhardt's swagger-stick, Rohn points at those he thinks are to be taken out. To what? We are standing four deep in a vast long line and he passes quickly along it. He has picked out up to a hundred Jews, men and women, clearly at random, when I hear that something unusual is happening.

The Maple Tree Behind the Barbed Wire

Oberleutenant Rohn is at the most twenty meters away from us when two young men leave the long line, the one raises a pistol, the other, somewhat younger, is holding a long knife in his right hand, and he cries out, loud and clear, first in German and then in Yiddish: "Myn tur nys hargynyn ynz unbestruft" - you may no longer kill us and go unpunished, you may not! I recognize him — it is Izio Feiner, a school friend, three years older than me, from the Jewish gymnasium. During the last winter before the war, both of us were at the school sports camp with our gymnastics teacher, Leopold Pfefferberg, who taught us to ski - and play cards. I don't recognize the other man with the gun in his hand. For a second it is deathly quiet in the square and for a brief moment these two young Jews have the situation in their hands.

During those seconds, thoughts race through my head as I stand there in Ryneczek, suddenly feeling the cold. At first I am terrified by what is happening, then proud, still frightened, but at the same time exhilarated when I see our two heroes — at last someone is defending us! He is right, Izio - you may not kill us and go unpunished!

But the enchantment and paralysis are shattered when the older Jew with the gun, whom we later find out is Mendele Fiszelewicz, again and again tries to fire, then shakes the gun, which refuses to fire. He has got the pistol from "the other side" and looked after it carefully, but has not been able to try it out in our well-guarded ghetto.

The hitherto so self-confident Oberleutnant Rohn seems to be paralyzed when Mendele Fiszelewicz reverses the pistol and tries to hit him with the butt. Fat Lieutenant Tsopart steps forward to try to stop Mendele, and my school friend Izio Feiner thrusts his knife into Tsopart's right forearm in an attempt to give Mendele a little more time. I just have time to see that he has made a deep cut and hear Tsopart let out a loud yell as he clutches at his bleeding arm.

Suddenly shots ring out, a volley, but not from Mendele Fiszelewiicz' pistol, but from the surrounding Germans shouting and shooting wildly. I can't see how many bullets hit our two young heroes, but it is a great many.

The Germans are shaken but quickly pull themselves together when they realise we have no more firearms, we the hitherto totally defenseless Jews. Nearly all the Germans I can see are now standing there with their pistols drawn, the ones in grey uniforms who had been a little further way before, have come closer and are standing stiffly with their rifles aimed at us. Some start shooting at the Jews in the lines, yelling zurück, zurück — a number of Jews are lying bleeding on the ground, wounded or dead.

Several of the heavily armed Germans whose job is to guard the area round the ghetto come running with their rifles at the ready, and in the distance I hear the sirens of German police cars, which must have been in the vicinity. Oberleutnant Rohn has also recovered, and now only Lieutenant Tsopart is whimpering, clutching his injured arm and threateningly — though I also think with some fear — gazing at the profusely bleeding Izio Feiner lying at his feet, the knife still in his hand. The next moment, Warszawawski Rynek is seething with German uniforms, some Wehrmacht soldiers from the German garrison in their characteristic helmets. In ulica Warsawska, the street leading into the square, I can see an armored car with its machine guns protruding, all this for two young Jews, one with a useless pistol, the other with a hunting knife.

The Aktion is completed, but only 350 Jews are sent to Radomsko where an Extermination Aktion is going on against a Jewish camp and they have to continue on the long train to Treblinka. Over 200 were killed in Ryneczek or were taken away and shot at the Jewish cemetery, which has become our place for executions and mass burials. In all more than had been planned have gone, at least 550 instead of the planned 500. We who are left have to go on standing for several hours in the cold in Ryneczek before we are allowed back into the ghetto. We are given no food that day.

After January 4th, 1943, that to us survivors forever memorable first day of armed resistance among the Jews of Czestochowa, our whole lives in the ghetto change. The relative calm of the last two months is followed by reinforcement of the guards round the ghetto and greater suspicion from the representatives of the German powers; a German no longer dares go alone into the ghetto. The soup handed out becomes even thinner, the black bread the same weight but even moister than before, the previous minute portion of margarine and jam now withdrawn, the guard round the ghetto and of the forced labour groups even stricter.

One of the first victims of this increased guard becomes the hero of my childhood, Maniek Rozen, the boy I met when we moved to Aleja Wolnosci 3-5, the one who showed me that even Jews could defend themselves and fight and who saved me from Zofja Wygórska Folwasinska's school. Maniek lived a fairly hectic life in the ghetto, on several occasions making his way over the barbed wire at night, but he was killed in the end. On the morning of January 12th, we see my once best friend, Maniek Rozen, hanging slackly on the barbed wire fence with his head touching the ground, almost but unfortunately not quite on the other side.

A few days later all of us in the ghetto know the background to the first, apparently clumsily organized armed rebellion.

The leaders of ZOB in the Czestochowa ghetto have decided to make a show of resistance at the next Aktion. ZOB, usually well informed,

The Maple Tree Behind the Barbed Wire

do not know in advance about the January 4th Aktion. That day, several armed members of ZOB have gone out with a group of forced labour workers — they have an assignment outside the ghetto. In the ghetto there is only one pistol left. But Mendele Fiszelewicz, one of the leaders, decides they will nevertheless carry out their collective decision to show resistance with what little they have. He selects Izio Feiner to "cover" for him and hopes to be able to inflict some damage on our tormentors.

I do not know what he had time to think before he died, whether he thought he and Izio Feiner had failed. Those of us left behind are filled with terror over the events in Ryneczek, but also with pride, and in many of us, what has happened raises a will to resist. But with what? Others, perhaps largely the older ones, are critical. Why should Mendele risk our lives; what Mendele and Izio had done was quite meaningless.

To me, Izio Feiner, Mendale Fiszelewicz, the couriers staying overnight with us and all the others in ZOB in Czestochowa are the successors and predecessors of those of our young people — the halucim — who emigrate to Palestine and with great personal sacrifices turn the almost uninhabitable malarial swamp and desert land into a flourishing landscape. Together with the remnants of survivors from German prison camps later to arrive on illegal ships, they are to build Haganah and Palmach, with surplus arms smuggled in to defend the miserable land area which is the lot of the Jewish people as a result of the United Nations resolution, a resolution governed by the guilty conscience of the world.

If the Bible had not already been written, this return of the Jews after nineteen centuries would have been one of its greatest and most remarkable events.

Israel is a small country with a still uncertain future. But to us Jews who have chosen to live in other countries, Israel is a symbol of security. Not to ourselves, for that is unnecessary — but to our grandchildren and their grandchildren. We are bitterly aware that the Holocaust would not have occurred, would not have been possible if Israel had already existed in the 1930s.

Germans are not permitted to have personal servants who are Jewish. But Captain Degenhardt has one, who also spends all day in his temporary private residence in Czestochowa - her name is Helenka Tennenbaum. Helenka is a blond beauty. She is quite tall, taller than Degenhardt, who is quite short for a policeman. Her hair is brushed back into a tight knot at the back of her neck, she has a naturally lovely walk, and green eyes. She is well dressed despite the poor conditions for dressing well in the ghetto, she always looks clean and is naturally polite to everyone. Helenka Tennenbaum is a well brought-up, well-educated girl from what is usually called a "good home" — her family is not wealthy but intellectual and educated.

No one knows how long Helenka Tennenbaum has worked for Captain Degenhardt. Many say he found her at one of the Selektions outside Metalurgia, others that he had already noticed Helenka earlier and ordered her to go to the police station and there said that in future she was to work for him — she is not allowed to leave her job. Helenka Tennenbaum is fetched everyday by Degenhardt's driver, Sergeant Unkelbach. He comes in the captain's official car in the morning at about nine, after all the forced labour groups working outside the ghetto have gone. Unkelbach is polite and obliging, opens the car door for her, but Helenka does not seem to be proud of this treatment, unique for a Jewess. On the contrary, she seems constantly sad, troubled and even tormented.

Helenka does not wish to discuss with anyone what she does at Degenhardt's apartment and no one asks her. It is said that some evenings Unkelbach does not drive her back to the ghetto. Despite this, none of the Jews despises or condemns Helenka Tennenbaum, at least none that I know. It is obvious that she has not chosen this assignment, that her situation is not an enviable one, that she is to be pitied for being marked for life, whatever happens. I feel sorry for the lovely Helenka Tennenbaum, perhaps more for her than for anyone else in the ghetto.

Just before the Small Ghetto is to be exterminated, Unkelbach fetches Helenka later in the day than usual and he is not as polite as usual, nor does he open the car door for her. That same day, Sergeant Unkelbach shoots Helenka Tennenbaum at the usual Czestochowa place of execution, the Jewish cemetery.

Rumours fly round the ghetto. One is that Helena Tennenbaum has been removed because Degenhardt's wife is coming to see him, another that some higher authority has criticized him for having a Jewish servant woman. There are also rumours about what Unkelbach has done with Helenka before he shot her. But all the same, surprisingly little is said in the ghetto about the sad Helenka Tennenbaum - the woman who had to suffer for her beauty.

Several months later, I hear a rumor that Degenhardt really had been in love with the lovely refined Helenka Tennenbaum, that he had been miserable and depressed for a long time after he had given orders for her to be executed.

However, one thing is certain, quite certain. Captain Degenhardt from the Leipzig police would never under any normal circumstances whatsoever have had such a fine person and such a beautiful woman as Helenka Tennenbaum at his private apartment and absolutely never in his bed — if he had not been posted to occupied Poland, been given the responsibility for the Jewish ghetto in Czestochowa and unlimited power over its population.

The Maple Tree Behind the Barbed Wire

Roman, Rózia and Me

After an unusually mild winter, spring has come early and the constant rain has turned the dirt roads and courtyards in the ghetto into a sea of dirty dark-brown mud. Now it is the beginning of June 1943.

One morning, Sarah and Roman stay at home from work. When I get back in the evening Roman is not there. Sarah tells me he is on his way to a hiding place with a Polish family out in the country, near Czestochowa. They are willing to have him and the place seems "safe" - Roman is eleven and far too young to cope at the next Aktion. He has left the ghetto with a group of carpenters, who are to hide him under the tarpaulin of the truck which has been taking them to their workplace in Gnaszyn Górny for the last few weeks, not far from the place where Roman is to be hidden. He has been given a detailed description of how to get to the Polish family's home and they are to meet him on the road.

I am sad, but at the same time see why Sarah tells me all this first afterwards. She knows that I would have opposed the plan. Roman might have become uncertain and that would not have been good for him. I say nothing, for there is nothing to say and my poor tormented mother silently repeats her "one of us must be saved". We know that our situation in the ghetto is hopeless — but we don't talk about it.

I have my textbooks with me from school and the secret courses that ceased when the Extermination Aktions began. I have also acquired books for higher classes. There are plenty of those in the ghetto, for no one wants them. I start reading from where we stopped at Professor Mering's secret courses. Apart from ordinary school textbooks, I have come across books of calculus, booklets of questions in history and geography, examples of subjects for essays, examples of well-written essays, and am hoping all this will make up for the guidance teachers otherwise offer. I sit over my textbooks, often in the evenings, sometimes in the early mornings before going to work and occasionally I take the risk of staying at home without a sick note. Hitherto no one has remarked on this, perhaps because I am working at Mrs. Mosiewicz' workshop.

It is a sunny Friday morning at the end of May 1943, and I am alone at home with Rózia. I have been at my table facing the only window in the apartment since early morning, looking up in textbooks and trying to solve geometry problems, but I am very much aware of Rózia's presence behind my back. I hear her walking round the apartment in her black low-heeled pumps and know she is wearing her gleaming black cotton-satin overall with buttons down the front and that she has no stockings on.

The Maple Tree Behind the Barbed Wire

Rózia is standing behind my back asking me what I'm working on and whether I would like something to drink. She has saved some of the chicory coffee we were given this morning and can heat it up for me — her voice is very soft. I turn round and see that some of the lower buttons are undone and I can see the inside of her plump white thighs, in tempting contrast to the partly open black overall and black shoes. Rózia sees that I am looking greedily at her. Although I am seated she must know, even see what is happening to me. She blushes scarlet, her face becoming almost beautiful. She must have just brushed her dark hair. Rózia sees that I can't stop looking at her thighs, that I am almost devouring her with my eyes. She walks slowly and rather uncertainly across, lightly runs her hand through my long since uncut hair which she has combed so many times, then she takes my face in her two warm hands and mumbles: "What do you want?"

When she comes over towards me I see even more of her body, and never before in my seventeen year-old life have I felt anything like this tremendous excitement.

She has let me stroke her down there before, without saying a word, teaching me what to do, but I have never been allowed to touch or even see any other part of her gleaming, still plump body. I was a very willing instrument to satisfy her strong need, which had no other outlet, but on those occasions she has never shown me any emotion, given any sign of an invitation for me to go further, never touched any other part of my body except my hair. Between us has been a silent agreement that when she — clearly satisfied — has withdrawn, we pretend she has just been combing my hair and nothing else has happened between us.

Quite a number of months have gone by since my Aunt Rózia last combed my hair. For long periods we have lived in different places and the crowded ghetto allows no intimacies in periods when we are living in the same apartment.

But this is something different. I can see, or imagine that she is looking at me in a different way, that in her eyes I am a young man now grown up, less childish, more purposeful owing to external circumstances. And perhaps, as so many others in the ghetto, she decides to get the most out of life before it is too late and I am the only person available.

To me it doesn't matter what it is that is driving this mature woman I have desired for so many years. For the first time she is showing her feelings, she speaks to me, is not silent and morose as on previous occasions of quite one-sided intimacy. This is an open invitation and I neither want to, nor am I able to control myself over what is happening. For a moment I feel as if a window has opened on to a wonderful paradise in the closed hell we live in.

The Maple Tree Behind the Barbed Wire

I don't reply to her question — "What do you want?" — but slowly get up and push my chair to one side. She looks away when, although I am dressed, she clearly sees my erection, but I don't look away — on the contrary, I look at as much as possible, not for one second considering whether what we are going to do is appropriate or forbidden. I lift her lightly off the floor, not even knowing why, and put her down again, then unbutton two of the top buttons of her overall. She is not wearing a bra and for the first time I see her breasts, also white and soft like the rest of her body, quite big and slightly pendulous, the pinkish-brown nipples pointing slightly downwards. I tremble as she lightly pushes me over towards the big bed, her eyes closed, and I guide her there.

I put her down on the bed and she helps me by arranging herself, looking away as I quickly take my clothes off, but pulling me to her when I touch her. I undo the other buttons of her black overall, look hungrily and with admiration at the great white body of a mature woman in front of me. I touch her big breasts and she clearly shows she doesn't want that. I lightly touch her down below, seeing it for the first time open in front of me — she is more moist that I can remember on any other occasion, already before I have touched her. She also trembles when very lightly, I feel the soft insides of her thighs.

She says nothing, squeezes her eyes tight shut when for the first time in my life I pull on a condom I have largely out of vanity saved for several years, then very slowly move into her. She puts her arms round me and kisses me, slightly ashamed, on the throat. Inside her, I can feel a slight resistance that breaks and she cries out as if in pain, but holds hard on to me, letting me stay. I move inside her several times and she moves towards me, breathing quickly and jerkily, and I have a violent orgasm, so longed for so many years and it simply goes on and on. She must feel what is happening to me, for she clings on to me, holding her breath, then lets go. I draw back and see blood on the condom - I must have been her first man. I wipe myself and try to go into her again, but she cries out, again and again when I try. She holds on to me and says quietly: "I want it, I do so want it, but I can't, it hurts so, perhaps in a few days' time". And with great gratitude, I content myself with what has already happened.

We lie on the bed holding on to each other, she does not draw back as before; there is no feeling of shame or regret. I look at her and think she is beautiful although I know she is not. To me her body is the cause of tremendous excitement and a source of endless satisfaction. We want to do what we have done again — in a few days, when Rózia can.

But that is not to happen. Rózia has barely a month to live and we have no further opportunity to be alone together in the crowded ghetto.

The Maple Tree Behind the Barbed Wire

I often think back to that day at the end of May 1943, in the middle of a war in the tormented ghetto, condemned to extermination. As before, it was Rózia who took the initiative. It was good that she had, that we fulfilled it, that we have done it before it was too late. It doesn't matter that she was my aunt, much older than me — we were not living under normal circumstances, we helped ourselves to the delights of life in the midst of great wretchedness, hopeless darkness and meaningless murder.

Many years later I try to say something about this to Sarah, but although I don't tell her much, I realise it was wrong for me to try. Sarah seems crushed and starts apologizing to me and I see she does not understand, cannot understand, so I say no more. Presumably no one can understand. To me it was nothing ugly, but fine, something that perhaps became fine under the circumstances.

I had kissed and fondled many girls, but Rózia was the first woman I had. I was pleased she had time to be with a man, even if that man happened to be her inexperienced nephew. She wanted it, and I am grateful for her giving me what I experienced that day.

I don't think I have become a less good person from what happened between us that day. After what Rózia had previously let me experience, I think the opposite, that it was good, very good for me that she also released me and that I perhaps released her before she was to die in a very cruel way, killed with a heavy hammer by a Meister at Hasag-Pelcery. In a way, Rózia still lives in me; each time I think about that day, I feel excitement.

After an unusually wet spring, June 1943 comes with mild early summer weather.

Everything in the ghetto is in short supply, food, soap, clothes, underclothes, bedclothes, shoes, stockings, and socks. Everything that might be attractive to a purchaser outside the ghetto has already been sold to acquire food. Coffee, tea, sugar and washing powder simply don't exist. But we go on living, our hopes not extinguished despite what our insights tell us and the horrible rumours confirm. We are hungry and frightened, but not demoralized. There is still a solidarity — surprisingly much mutual trust between the inhabitants of the ghetto and what remains of the Judenrat and the Jewish police.

A strange symbiosis has developed between the green German police guarding us and the undernourished Jews in their rags in the ghetto, a symbiosis filled with mutual suspicion. We are aware that thanks to us, despite the war, they have had an opportunity to live a comfortable life and they need us not to be sent away to the front. For us, these policemen are our only source of information on vital matters. We are aware that we cannot rely on this information, but we have no one else to turn to.

The Maple Tree Behind the Barbed Wire

As we go to bed on this June night, almost three weeks have gone by since Roman left the ghetto. All we know is what we have been told by the Jewish carpenters who had helped get him out. They have told us that as far as they could see, he had managed. The two uniformed guards had not seen him crawl out of his hiding place under the tarpaulin of their truck and set off. We know nothing more. We think about Roman and how things are going for him. But no one says anything, for there is nothing to say. On one occasion only, Sarah says, her voice very uncertain: "It is good one of us is on the other side", But she sounds as if she were apologizing. I also hear Pinkus' quiet comment: "Main klaine Avrum Herschele" — my little Avrum Hersch, Roman's Hebrew name. Before I fall asleep, I think about my brother being only eleven. Although we are hungry, we usually sleep soundly after a twelve hour working shift, at least I do.

Early in the morning, when it is still dark and I am half asleep, I hear someone knocking quietly on the front door. Sarah wakes first, opens the door and cries out: "Romek, Romeczek, Romus, jestés w domu" - you are back home! "Co sie stalo" - what's happened? She clutches him to her and both of them are weeping. Roman apologizes between sobs which slowly subside as he tries to explain and tell us — he has a great need to do so. "Sorry, sorry for coming back, but I couldn't." His tears choke him, perhaps mostly from relief at being back. Sarah has let go of him and he is standing there, his arms hanging, and he looks terrible — hair untidy, filthy hands, tears furrowing his dirty face, his dirty ragged clothes in disorder. He has his back to me and I see he has boils on his neck, one cracked with semi-dried pus — how can a boy be so changed in scarcely three weeks?

Roman is still standing by the door, confused and dejected, reproaching himself because he has not been able to live up to expectations he himself has imagined. Neither Sarah nor Pinkus does anything. I have already pulled on my trousers, go over to Roman and hold him — "dobrze ze wróciles" — good that you have come back. "We are pleased — we have been wondering how things have gone for you and we have missed you." He looks at me with some surprise and relief, then starts babbling away incoherently, rapidly, as if afraid someone might interrupt him. He tells us he had sat all day on a chair behind a wardrobe, that at night he had had to sleep in a wide bed with two older girls, and how he had longed for Sarah and Pinkus, how for two nights in a row he had dreamt Sarah had come to him in his sleep and told him he should come back. He tells us how much more difficult it was getting back than going. He just left the house in the country without saying anything to anyone, sleeping in the open the first night in a cornfield. In one street on the long, long journey back to the ghetto, some small boys had approached him and asked him if he was a Jew. He was frightened, but pretended not to hear them, pretending the question had nothing to do with him. He did not get to the boundary of the ghetto until evening, then hid behind the counter in one of the empty shops in the evacuated streets round the ghetto. He had calculated from his wristwatch how often the regular patrol of Germans returned to the same spot — every third or fourth minute. In the end he had fallen asleep behind the counter and early the next morning dared to leave his hiding-place just after the patrol had passed. He had pried apart the barbed wire at a place he had previously seen someone else must have used and made his way into the ghetto. He has deep, still bleeding scratches on his hands and an aching sore on the back of his neck.

He is only eleven, but has been forced to save his own young life on his own. That must have required a strong will, and making the long way back to the ghetto a great achievement.

Roman still has a desperate need to talk, to tell us, to defend himself because he has given up and come back. He is talking to me now, for I am the only one asking questions. Sarah is sitting beside Pinkus on their bed, bewildered, in her pink nightgown, mumbling "sorry — sorry, what have I done?" For once, Pinkus is also at a loss. It is important how Roman is received, and it is not pity he needs. It is getting lighter - I have put on my sandals and say: "Come on down to the washroom and get washed so that you look human. Then we'll go to the sick bay — you must get that sore on your neck fixed. Mamma, will you get some clean clothes out for Roman. We'll be back in a moment." Roman has nothing left of what he had taken with him into hiding on "the other side". Sarah comes back to reality - Roman must have clothes and food.

As I help Roman take off his filthy rags in the washroom I see he has sores and pus-filled boils in several places, his skin is rough, blotchy red and covered with scratches. It is not easy to get the dirt off in our washroom, the water cold and the soap does not lather. The way he looks I don't know how much he should be washed, perhaps it should be done in several stages. I have already thrown away the first dirty water and the water in the bowl after the second washing is not so dirty — that will have to be enough. I also see that Roman is about to be overcome by exhaustion and I leave him in peace. As I dry him with the thin worn towel, I tell him a little about what has happened at home and in the ghetto, mostly just to talk about something apart from his misery.

When we go back across the little courtyard, the ghetto has begun to wake up and the sun has risen just above the horizon. Roman's obvious exhaustion is counteracted by him still being upset, but nonetheless calmer than when he had just arrived. He has cheered up from the washing and his red hair is combed flat. There is a little food on the table - Sarah is amazing at conjuring up something to eat when needed. She has made and put out a thin but hot soup, a piece of

The Maple Tree Behind the Barbed Wire

black bread, despite the fact that nothing had be handed out so early in the morning, a little jam and a hot drink that almost looks like tea. But Roman does not eat much although he must be hungry — he has not eaten for two days. He is finding it increasingly difficult to keep his eyes open and keeps dozing off as he eats. But his joy at being home with us comes through, and is overwhelming, infecting all of us in the room. Sarah helps him to bed before she, Pinkus and Rózia get dressed and go to work. I am to stay at home to be there when my little brother wakes. No one protests when I say — now we all have to stick together, whatever happens — as long as they let us. It was probably superfluous to say so.

It is a cool cloudy June day. In the afternoon Roman and I go to the cottage hospital to get his sores and boils painted with iodine and bandaged; a careful older nurse takes him in hand very professionally. Roman has rapidly recovered after a few hours' sleep, but is still in a wretched state, which can be seen when he has to undress and lie on the hard couch. At the same time, he is childishly delighted at again being able to walk on the cobblestones and trampled earth streets of the ghetto. But neither Roman, I nor the nurse know that the ghetto will no longer exist in ten days' time. We are very soon to be separated again.

When the liquidation of the ghetto starts on June 26th, 1943, Germany has not only lost the war, but is on her knees and the recently acquired Great German Empire has fallen apart. The whole world and the Germans themselves know this.

The Axis army of 250,000 men has already capitulated in North Africa, American troops are pouring into Britain and for six months the United States Air Force and the British Royal Air Force have been participating in increasingly merciless bombing of the German nation — the Americans at night, the RAF in the daytime. The German army no longer has any access to the important protection from the air, for their fighter planes now have to defend their homeland. When the Germans start the liquidation of our ghetto, only two weeks remain before the Allied landings in Sicily and exactly a month before the fall of Mussolini. The turning point has also passed in the war at sea. The Japanese advance on Australia has been halted — it is generally known that at the failed attack on Midway Island not only was a large part of the Japanese air force destroyed but also the core of the Japanese navy — four of Japan's largest aircraft carriers, responsible for so many earlier successes, have been sunk. But most of all - American and British war materials are pouring into the Soviet Union.

The German attack on the Soviet Union has lost all its force. The Germans have not succeeded in achieving any of their aims, neither taking Moscow, nor the oil fields in the Caucuses. The lengthy siege of Leningrad is already over, Rostoff has been re-taken and on February

The Maple Tree Behind the Barbed Wire

2nd, 1943, the German garrison in Stalingrad capitulated - Hitler promoting General Paulus to Field Marshal just before the capitulation was no help. Hitler's insistence on the hopeless defense of what they had managed to take of Stalingrad and the unnecessary loss of the strongest of his army corps, the 8th Army Corps, has devastatingly extended the long German front in the Soviet Union. After the last feeble German offensive's breakthrough in the summer of 1943 - lasting no longer than a week — the increasingly weakened German front is pressed even further back without the Germans having any chance of halting it. The people in the German occupied countries have recovered after the shock of the German invasion and the ruthless terrorization of the civilian population. Almost everywhere, forms of national resistance have arisen, and now they are getting increasingly more comprehensive help via airborne supplies of arms from the Allied powers, now at last equipped for war.

But in the isolated world of the Small Ghetto in Czestochowa, cut off from the outside world, we know nothing about all this when the Germans start the most successful of all their offensives — the offensive against us — scarcely 6,000 undernourished but no longer entirely defenseless ragamuffins.

The Maple Tree Behind the Barbed Wire

Liquidation of the Small Ghetto

Mrs. Mosiewitcz is very good at acquiring new orders for her workshop and her Jewish workers. We work six days a week, often for over eleven hours a day, but are free to receive customers ourselves, carry out orders and deliveries without involving Mrs. Mosiewitcz or any Vorarbeiter as they are in other workplaces. Mrs. Mosiewicz knows that results are best if she does not interfere with the daily work of these highly qualified professionals.

Every morning we have to be at the exit of the ghetto at six o'clock. Our group, smaller than most, is fetched at 6.30 at the latest and are to be back in the ghetto by 7.30 in the evening at the latest. According to the circumstances, Mrs. Mosiewicz makes sure we have a decent amount of food and do not go hungry. She pretends not to notice that we take some back to the ghetto to spin out our evening meal and breakfast the next day, also for Rózia.

In the afternoon of June 23rd, 1943, Mrs. Mosiewicz says that the next day we ought bring necessities for several days to be able to stay at the workshop - she does not explain why. There is plenty of room when the workshop closes and no great problem finding twenty temporary sleeping places on the floor. We sleep there for two nights - but that turns out to be no help.

On June 26th, soon after nine in the morning, Mrs. Mosiewicz says the German police have told her - she mentions a name we don't recognize — that an escort is coming to fetch us in twenty minutes' time. We can see from her expression that she is worried when she says that within an hour at the most, we have to be back in the ghetto, all the Jews left in Czestochowa, without exception, and we have to attend the Appell that has already started. After a while she comes back and tries to explain. She has known in advance about the Appell and has arranged that we need not be present, but this promise has been taken back and she says she does not know what is to happen to us. From her way of questioning the workers on details of planned orders, I realise she is uncertain whether we shall be allowed to return to her workshop at all.

At the exit of the workshop, there are already four blue-clad Polish and two green German police, only one of whom I recognize — the thin, always restless Kinnel, and he is also the man in charge. They have been told to take the Jewish workers hitherto assigned to Mrs. Mosiewicz' workshop back to ghetto. Kinnel is polite and obliging as he speaks to Mrs. Mosiewicz, but not when he turns to us. He is in a hurry. The Polish police form up round us, refuse to answer our questions, and say not a word all the long way back to the Small Ghetto.

The Maple Tree Behind the Barbed Wire

It is the first occasion for a very long time I see the streets of Czestochowa at that time of day. It is a lovely summer's day with occasional thin white clouds high up in the otherwise clear light-blue sky. People look curiously at us as they pass, some in a hurry, others strolling slowly along. I see a number of women, a few with children in prams, or holding their hands — clearly out for a walk or on their way to shop. We and our escort, our shabby clothes and our appearance must seem very abnormal in this idyll.

We pass First and Second Aleja, then turn off to the left into ulica Warszawaska. There we are faced with a frightening contrast to the idyll as we approach the evacuated and closed-off streets round the ghetto. We see that on the short stretch of ulica Spadek are two eight-wheeled armored vehicles with their hatches closed, machine-guns and narrow cannon barrels menacingly protruding, the entire ghetto surrounded by German troops in full battle gear. In ulica Warszawska, near the corner to Ryneczek but out of sight from those standing in Ryneczek, are several manned positions with mortars and two motorcycle soldiers in helmets, their automatic rifles at the ready across their chests. Inside the narrow Wyjazdowa alley we can see a manned field telephone station - Kinnel greets them by raising his hand and one of the soldiers responds. I have never before seen such an array of battle-ready German troops in Czestochowa, and all this round our little ghetto. No such numbers of heavily armed German troops ever took part when the major Aktion, now almost a year ago, was carried out and we were ten times as many then. What has frightened the Germans into collecting round our little ghetto of 5,200 registered starving and cowed Jews such a large force in full battle gear? This is terrifying, but at the same time somehow flattering. We are frightened by what is soon to happen — some of us think it is the end.

In Ryneczek itself it looks like an ordinary Appell, no more ominous than usual. Several thousand Jews are already lined up in long rows. The Green police from Leipzig with their usual weapons — heavy pistols in their holsters — move easily round the square, the blue-clad Polish police standing more passively to one side, ready to carry out any orders given, and a little way to the left of the middle of the square are several German civilians, all in neat dark suits, white shirts and ties. They look like senior officials or men from a lawyer's office or a bank.

Our group appears to be the last to arrive at the Appell. Once Kinnel has reported to Degenhardt and we have joined one of the lines relatively close to the German civilians, nearby Jews tell us they have been standing there for what will soon be six hours. The Germans have unexpectedly appeared at dawn and started searching the streets and individual buildings for ZOB activities. The search is still going on. They have found a secret tunnel ZOB has dug from the cellar in

The Maple Tree Behind the Barbed Wire

Nadrzieczna 66 to an evacuated building outside the ghetto — the tunnel had been recently finished and was being used for communication with "the other side". In association with the tunnel, the Germans have found a hideout full of homemade weapons, petrol bombs and several grenades filled with explosives. They have also found a bunker used to shelter children, mostly boys in their early teens.

Captain Degenhardt and two of the German police officers, apparently relaxed, are chatting with the German civilians. A man in the same row as ours tells us that one of the civilians is Director Lüth - head of Hasag Industries in Czestochowa - and that he is a high-up in Germany. We can also see that in Captain Degenhardt's easy yet courteous, almost respectful behavior towards him. I have never seen Degenhardt behave like that before.

An occasional shot can be heard from the ghetto, as well as short salvos from automatic weapons. Small groups of Jews are still coming out from there.

About two hours after our group had arrived, at about midday we see a large group of young men and women coming out of the ghetto, one or two a little older, over thirty. They are surrounded by police and heavily armed soldiers with their automatic weapons at the ready — the Germans have captured the core of ZOB in Czestochowa when they went into the ghetto at dawn and surrounded the ZOB headquarters block in ulica Nadrzeczna.

I see that many, presumably all the Jews in this group have been beaten, perhaps tortured. Some are badly bruised, others have visible injuries, some are limping, and some need support from others in the group to be able to walk. Most have torn clothing, some no shirts, others lack shoes, and one of the young men has nothing on but short underpants. Despite their wretched condition, they try to behave with dignity, to walk with straight backs and heads high. They are taken to a special group which I see standing to one side of the rest of us and are being guarded by armed uniformed Germans.

Two large trucks with open backs come into Ryneczek, presumably having been standing ready in a nearby street, now driven right into the middle of the square, the rear flaps already down. Some of the many Jews in a separate group are now driven up on to the backs of the trucks, some refuse and with blows from rifle butts are forced on board.

When the trucks are full they start turning in the narrow square and driving slowly away with their human cargo. The young resistance men from ZOB start shouting loudly in the square, at first in a disorderly way, then more and more clearly and orderly, chanting first in Yiddish - then in Polish: "Vergess uns nys, nie zapomnijcie nas" — don't forget us, "myn tur nys vergessen" you must not forget, one must

The Maple Tree Behind the Barbed Wire

not forget, and when the trucks leave, still driving slowly through the narrow alleys round the ghetto, we hear them singing loudly the ghetto's battle song composed by the Chajutin brothers, and then Hatikvah - Song of Hope - which is to become the national anthem of Israel.

They sing more and more loudly, in strong voices. Many of us still standing the square are weeping uncontrollably, and some cry out a promise in loud voices: "we will not forget, ynz etmy nys vergessen, my bedziemy pamietac, my nigdy nie zapomnimy, we will never forget"
- no one bothers about the armed Germans all round us and more and more Jews call out aloud.

I think I call out, but am not sure, perhaps I just whisper. But I know that no one, not one of us will forget, no one can or may forget. If one single one of us is somehow to survive, that person must relate what we have all seen on this sunny day in Ryneczek in front of the ghetto in Czestochowa - these young men and women being taken away, what they make us promise to do, what responsibility they put on us as the last wish in their young lives.

Everyone has seen those trucks before, and we know they are used for taking Jews to the Jewish cemetery where they are stripped of their clothes, shot and thrown into mass graves, graves they have been made to dig themselves.

When the trucks come back for the next load, we see the backs are bloodstained — with fresh blood. The Germans clearly had to shoot some of those on the trucks when they refused to climb down by themselves. These now blood-stained trucks are driven into the middle of the square and loaded up with more Jews the Germans have brought out of the ghetto — a number of older people this time and two women with small children. How have they all managed to stay hidden for so long in the ghetto? How did they get food? At the same time, the Germans start taking out some from among those of us still standing in the square.

Captain Degenhardt himself carries out the Selektion, but he does not take out individual Jews, only a whole row, or part of a row. This is, he says, the punishment for the shots ZOB had fired and the handmade grenades they have thrown when their building had been surrounded that morning — he has never before justified his treatment of us. Even many of the Jews taken out at random are singing Hatikva as they are taken away on the bloodstained trucks. Even they cry out to us not to forget, that we must not forget, a challenge from those who without the slightest doubt know they are soon to be killed and their last wish is — not to be forgotten. I think there is a great difference in the way they were able to take us away at the major Aktion last September and the way we behave on this day, less than a year later.

The Maple Tree Behind the Barbed Wire

The Germans in the square seem worried. They are nervous and don't know what to do when Jews sent away on trucks can bring themselves to sing in chorus and with strong voices chant a message to us, a message the Germans perhaps do not understand. But what else can they do apart from killing us, and that is what they go on doing, in their methodical way — truckload after truckload.

Why are they so wrought up? They have heavily armed troops nearby, armored cars, mortars, are hugely superior in numbers to finish us off — and among us, these ragamuffins in ZOB, whom we have promised never to forget and who will forever remain our powerless but courageous heroes.

The Aktion of June 26th, 1943, is as good as completed. Those from the resistance movement the Germans have been able to identify are taken away, and with them many more Jews. The Germans in the square seem to have pulled themselves together and no longer feel threatened. Only a few Germans in green uniforms and a few Polish police bring out to the next truck the boys found hidden in the bunker in the ghetto. The boys from the bunker, over twenty, all between ten and twelve years old, at the most thirteen, all pale after such a long spell in the underground bunker. We can see from their spindly legs how thin they are and they must be undernourished. No resistance is expected from these emaciated children.

But the boys, for they are only boys in this group, suddenly turn as if at a given signal slip through the gaps between the surprised policemen and approach the German civilians in an assembled troop, chorusing "wir können arbeiten" - then turn to Lüth: "Herr Direktor, wir können arbeiten" - Herr Direktor, we can work. Captain Degenhardt, clearly annoyed at his men's carelessness, steps into the way of the boys and orders his police to bring the little group to order.

But Direktor Lüth leaves the group of German civilians and comes over to Degenhardt to speak to him. Degenhardt looks surprised and I see him gesticulating dismissively. But Lüth is peremptory, stubborn and firm. Later we find out from those closer to him that Lüth had maintained he wanted those boys in his factory for fine engineering work. Lüth looks neither at the boys nor at us other Jews in the square, just keeps looking steadily straight at Degenhardt, with authority and decisiveness. The boys realise something important to them is happening, so are quiet; from where I am standing I can see them standing quite still, waiting. All those in the square seem to be holding their breath and waiting.

Degenhardt hesitates — this is clearly not what he had intended. But we can see it is Lüth who decides and that Degenhardt gives way.

The square is absolutely quiet, not a sound except a collective sigh as everyone appears to breathe out with relief, or with surprised disappointment, when these lone boys who have managed to evade police Aktions for over a year, are taken off the last truck and hustled into the rows of Jews who have now stood in line for over six hours for the Appell.

A thin woman with chestnut-colored hair standing beside me is weeping copiously. "Oh God, oh God," she says. "Is this true? So there is a God in heaven." She has her arms folded across her chest, and with her hands on her thin shoulder she is rocking as if in ritual prayer or in a trance — "Oh God, oh God, oh dear dear God, thank you for existing", and I weep with her, not everyone is evil.. .

The Aktion and killing are over, for that day, June 26th, 1943. It has all been on the orders of the Governor-General himself, the ex-lawyer Hans Franck, that all Jewish ghettos are to be liquidated. The extermination of Jews in his Generalguvernement is to be reported to Berlin as successfully completed. If any Jews are left in Czestochowa, they are to be found in special German prison camps — and they don't count. So on June 26th, 1943, what was officially called Arbeitslager Tschenstochau, but which everyone, Germans and Jews, always called the Small Ghetto - das kleine Ghetto, was closed.

None of us may go back to the ghetto, not even to collect our belongings. Instead we are divided up into groups, the largest to go to Hasag-Pelcery - also called Apparatenbau. Bernard Kurland goes with that group with his assistants and what is left of the Jewish police with Parasol in the lead, and the twenty boys Lüth has saved. Three somewhat smaller groups are to go to the other Hasag plants in Czestochowa-Raków and their huge hot blast furnaces, Czestochowianka and Warta. All the other forced labour workplaces for Jewish workers are being closed, those previously allocated to those who survived the latest Aktion to be shared out among the various Hasag plants — these become prison camps for the remaining Czestochowa Jews. A small group consisting of twelve Jewish craftsmen however, are taken out and ordered back to Mrs. Mosiewicz' workshop; they are to complete earlier orders before that workplace can be liquidated. Pinkus and Sarah are included in that group and allowed to take Roman with them — but I, Ignas Katz, Pola Grün and a few more who have hitherto been working at Mrs. Mosiewicz' workshop are transferred to the prison camp. It all goes so rapidly I do not even have time to say goodbye to my parents or my brother.

Once the Aktion is over, Ryneczek is emptied and the armed German troops are withdrawn from the area round the ghetto — but not all. Left behind are the heavy mortars placed all round the ghetto. The next day, on the morning of June 27th, the ghetto undergoes several hours of shelling from grenade fire. This is to frighten anyone who just might be still there, hidden in bunkers, cellars and attics.

The Maple Tree Behind the Barbed Wire

On June 28th, German cars drive round the ghetto, and over loudspeakers offer jam, hot soup and amnesty to anyone still remaining hidden. They are given until June 30th — two days — to report at the exit of the ghetto.

Very few report. But when the Germans go into the ghetto after the mortar fire, they find over twenty Jews, mostly women, children and old people. All of them, even the children who can speak, are subjected to lengthy interrogation to make them reveal any remaining bunkers or hideouts for people, or for valuables. They are then driven to the Jewish cemetery, ordered to undress on the edge of a grave, then are shot and buried in the latest but unfortunately not the last mass grave. What is left of the ghetto is then closed to the outside world.

On July 20th, a unit of sappers temporarily withdrawn from the front, military experts who handle explosives come into the ghetto. They set dynamite charges in all the buildings and that same day all the low old houses in what was once our Small Ghetto are destroyed. Nothing but ruins remain of the buildings - all that is left after the war to bear witness to what happened to the large and active Jewish population of Czestochowa. But the gnarled old maple is still there when my daughter Lena and I visit Czestochowa many years later, as are the ruins of the Small Ghetto.

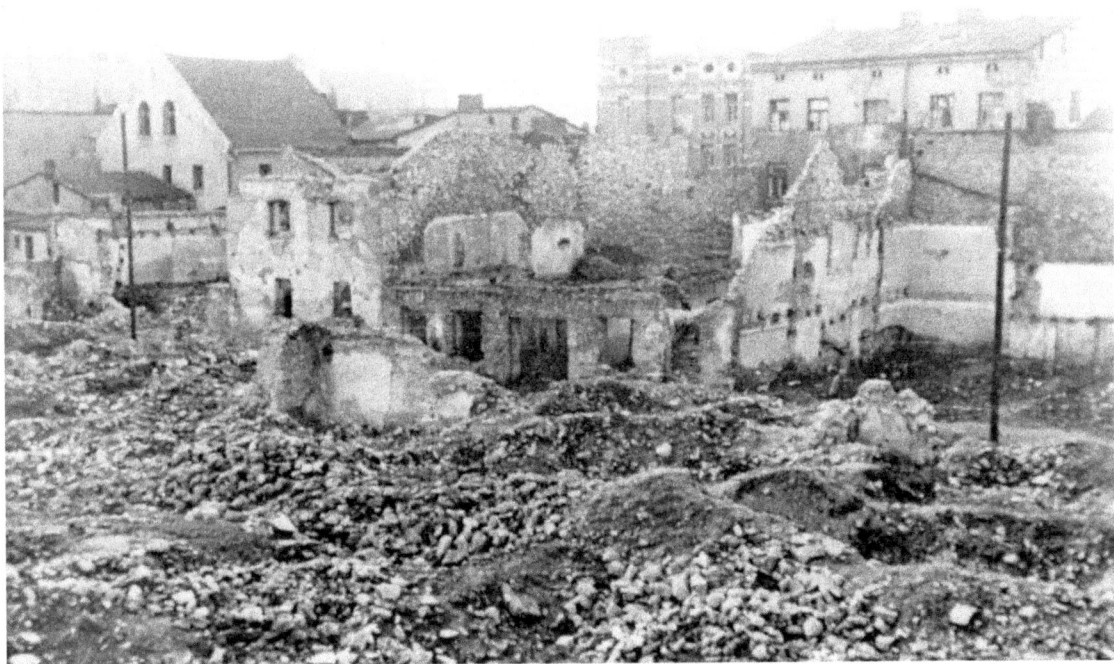

On July 20th, 1943, a section of military experts blow up the old low houses in what was once our Small Ghetto. After the war, nothing but ruins bears witness to what happened to the large Jewish population of Czestochowa

The Maple Tree Behind the Barbed Wire

The need to kill every single Jew is so great, the German armed forces put in troops and explosives, of which they no longer have a surplus, to make sure that Czestochowa is Judenrein and all the Jews exterminated. Those in the prison camp do not count.

But despite these efforts, they do not entirely succeed. Several ZOB groups remain hidden in the extensive and in places thick forests round the towns of Zlota Góra and Koniecpol, both quite near Czestochowa. One of the groups needs help to acquire ammunition and want to exploit the contacts which the nationalist AK - Armia Krajova - have with the Polish government in exile in London. But they are unlucky and contact the section of the ultra-nationalist NSZ. They are invited to a joint meeting and all are shot, on the spot, by Polish partisans. One single Jew survives, wounded. He manages to get a warning to the remaining ZOB groups in the forests, who instead seek and eventually contact a section of the smaller Gwardia Ludowa - the socialist People's Army, which has fewer resources and no contacts with the government in exile in London, but they do not murder Jews. They establish links with GL's Hanysch group, collaborate with it on several sabotage actions, mostly against German transports and transport routes. Several of these Jews were killed in the fighting, or in ambushes, but others are to survive the war and join those who enter the liberated Czestochowa together with the Hanysch group. The Country's Army - AK - and NSZ stay in the forest even after Czestochowa is liberated by Soviet troops.

CHAPTER V

PRISON CAMP AND LIBERATION
Hasag-Pelcery

I am prisoner number 3170 code: white/brown at Hasag-Pelcery, and live in a micro-world consisting of Hut 6, which houses 138 prisoners and me, and Maschinenbau, which is my workplace. It takes almost three days before we are finally let into our hut on the evening of June 27th, and I am allotted my workplace on 28th June.

My memories of the first three days and nights are blurred, but I do remember our clothes and our underclothes being taken away — for de-lousing, they said — then standing naked in a large empty cold hall with a concrete floor and otherwise totally empty. We had to shower twice, and again stand naked, enfeebled and dazed with exhaustion and hunger in an even longer queue for examination in a machine. Without knowing what the machine is for, we are pushed by a prisoner into a long narrow opening and pulled out again by another prisoner. They call out "breathe in", but never that we are to breathe out. Not until some months later do we find out from other prisoners that this is an X-ray examination of our lungs. The Germans do not want prisoners with tuberculosis at Hasag. I also remember the painful queues for the toilets for male prisoners, in a row in the yard, the booths separated from each other by low partitions which don't go all the way to the ground. We are always hungry, but not thirsty. Several barrels of fresh cold water are always in the main hall and we are allowed to drink as much as we like, but we are given food only twice during those first three days - 200 grams of black bread and a large helping of nourishing soup made from turnips and bits of under-cooked carrot which we can chew on and taste wonderful.

Supervised by a German in a grey-green uniform, I am finally enrolled by a prisoner sitting at one of the tables set up that morning in the big hall and am given my number as a prisoner - 3170 code white/brown.

The number is stamped into a six-by-six-centimeter sized metal disc, the top left corner painted grayish-white, and the lower right hand corner light brown. This is fastened to an equally wide, rounded at the top, four and half centimeter piece of soft hide with a machine-made vertical buttonhole to fasten the disc to a button on my clothes. I have to wear this disc always — in future it provides everything anyone needs to know about me — my registration number, in which workplace I belong at Hasag-Pelcery - and that I am a Jew, indicated with the sign of Zion, the Star of David, with its two triangles turned towards each other. I still have that disc with its black bit of hide.

Back at home in my study, I have a shelf of Swedish and foreign distinctions I have received over the years. In the middle of the shelf, surrounded by all the other awards, is my number disc as a German prisoner from June 1943 until January 1945, eighteen and a half months. It is my only relic from my days in the prison camp. At first the disc sat alone on the shelf, the other awards gradually accumulating over many years and placed round my old prisoner's disc. It is only chance that it ended up in the middle, but I actually consider that its proper place — for some reason I do not understand, I am more proud when I show it to people and explain what it means, than any of the other later acquired awards. Under any circumstances, I consider it to be the most important of the mementoes I have kept over a long life.

Some of the Germans guarding us over those three first days of becoming a prisoner are in civilian clothes, but most wear their grey-green summer uniforms with badges of rank on their dark green collars. They did not seem as artful or as threatening as the green Germans of the Leipzig police — later on I find out that the Germans in these grey-green uniforms are camp guards and are to be addressed as Herr Werkschutz.

After those first three days we find it a relief to be allocated our places in the huts, to be allotted our workplaces and daily routine can begin in a minor German prison camp linked to one of the Hasag factories in the Generalguvernement.

The prison huts at Hasag-Pelcery are not all the same. Ours is one of the smaller ones, has only two rows of three-story sleeping bunks and a long table down the middle.

Ignas Katz and I - we have nothing else in common except that our parents are still at Mrs. Mosiewitcz' workshop — try to stick together. We are allotted bunks next to each other, almost in the middle of the centre level on the left of the entrance to the hut. That our places are in the middle of the long shelf turns out to be a disadvantage during the summer when it is hot, but a blessing in winter when the cold whistles in through the thin wooden walls of the hut. Each prisoner has a straw mattress and a thin blanket — these mark out the prisoner's territory on the shelf as there are no partitions between sleeping places. There is an upper, a lower and a middle shelf along each side of the hut and there are 23 prisoners on each shelf, altogether 138 prisoners in each hut. There are no cupboards. Clothes and anything else a prisoner may possess is kept at the foot of the sleeping place or hanging on a nail — whenever a prisoner manages to scrounge one. Nearly all prisoners sooner or later acquire a nail and some have two or three hammered into the outer side of the long wooden plank at the foot of the sleeping shelf. I manage to get hold of two and that suffices. I have never heard of any thefts of clothing in our or in any other hut.

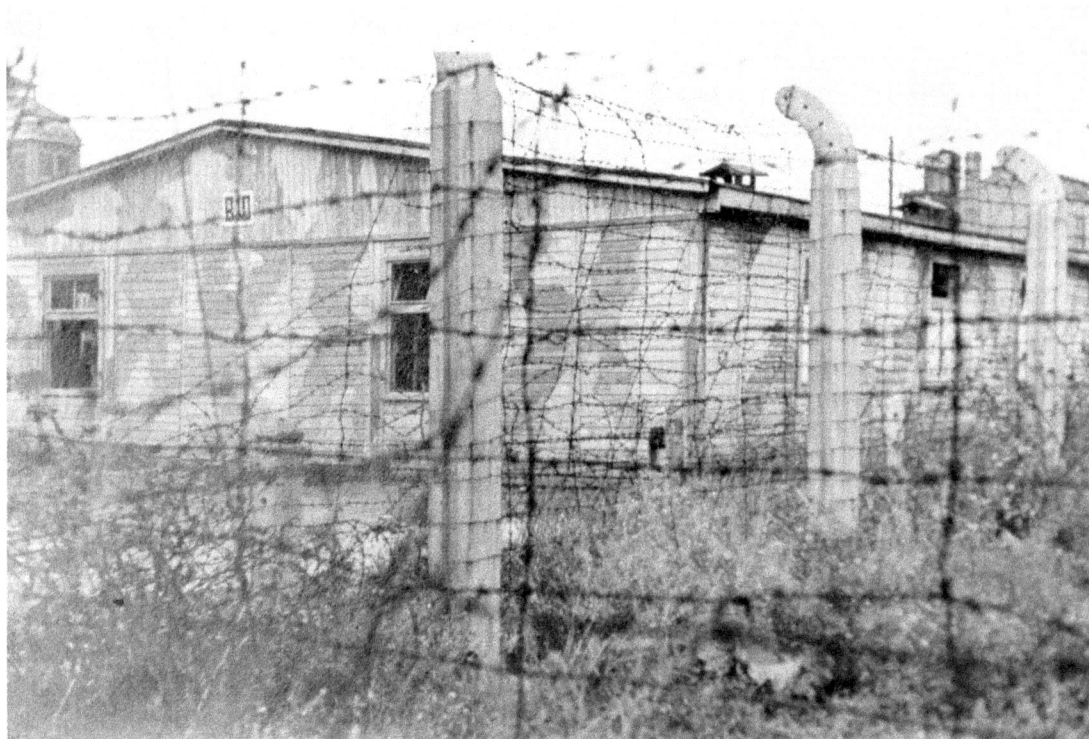

I am prisoner number 3170 code: white/brown at Hasag-Pelcery. My and 137 other prisoners' hut number 6 is next to the barbed wire fence. Each prisoner has a straw mattress and a thin blanket — these mark the prisoner's sleeping place on the shelf.

In the middle of the hut is a wide table of light roughly planed wood on four wooden trestles, and along each side is an almost equally long bench — that is the only freestanding furniture in the hut. During the short time in the day when the lights — three naked electric light bulbs — are switched on, many of the prisoners in our hut sit at the table mending their clothes or their socks, cutting up bits of cardboard to put into their wretched shoes, some writing with a pencil, others playing cards or just talking. The long wooden table with its two benches is the hut meeting-place for prisoners seeking company after work, the others occupying themselves on their bunks or going to bed early — nothing is allowed to be on the table when the lights are put out. I am the only one in our hut, presumably the only one among the over 5,000 prisoners in our camp, to spend his time on school books, the books I have brought with me to the camp. This is actually really

The Maple Tree Behind the Barbed Wire

quite strange, because at school I was not at all an industrious pupil.

At first, several prisoners ask me why I have brought these books with me, others ask whether I have nothing better to do? But after a while, with some indulgence, it is accepted that I spend every spare moment I have on my schoolbooks. Despite the number and the code — between us prisoners we are still individuals, each one with his distinctive characteristics. Spending most of the little time I have on old school books is what distinguishes me from the others.

All our clothes that have been de-loused in strong chemicals at a high temperature have changed color, everything previously white now smoky yellow, and after several de-lousing, they are smoky grey and even more fragile. When clothing prisoners have brought with them to the camp cannot be mended any longer, they are given clothes from a camp store, thus losing even more of his or their personal identity.

We work in two shifts, from seven to seven — two weeks in the daytime, two at night. Most prisoners have to work seven days a week, only a few free on some Sundays - that depends on the workplace. Before the shift can begin, there is an Appell - each workplace and shift has its own. The Appell is carried out by our guards together with a kapo and Kurland, Zylbersszac or Marzej Krause from the camp Jewish Arbeitsamt. It is to take half an hour at the most, but sometimes takes longer if something is not right on the first count or if our Werkschutz decides for some reason. If the Appell takes longer than half an hour, the Meister complains to the factory management.

Day and night shift have the same routine. Work after the Appell begins on an empty stomach. At nine o'clock, morning or evening, we have a fifteen-minute break for breakfast — a large mug of more or less hot surrogate coffee made of chicory and a hundred grams of black bread. At exactly twelve o'clock — day or night — we have a thirty-minute dinner break. Then we are given a large bowl of hot soup made of turnips and Swedes. What one is given in an aluminum bowl depends on how far down the ladle goes — the deeper the more there is to eat, the shallower the more watery the soup. In practice, breakfast and lunch may last a little longer. Our German Meisters have longer meal breaks than we have and most of them turn a blind eye if the prisoners also do. At the end of the work stint, for the second time every twenty-four hours — evening or morning — we are given a mug of chicory coffee and 100 grams of black bread. Some days we are given the whole of the day's ration of bread, 200 grams, in the morning, and then it is difficult to save half of it until the evening. Many prisoners cannot do that. Usually we are given something extra, a little margarine, a dab of jam, on Sundays perhaps an extra portion of bread and sometimes there are potatoes in the turnip soup. Then it is particularly important to have a helping from the bottom of the pan.

In the prison camp and at the factory, administration is partly German, partly Jewish. Lüth heads the hierarchy, making decisions in all matters. He is addressed as Herr Direktor and is the managing director of the entire plant. Apart from being one of the most senior members of the National Socialist Party, he is also a member of the Reichstag - the German parliament that has not met since 1934, not for nine years.

Apart from Lüth, there is also a technical director, Herr Bretschneider, and several civil engineers, the most prominent Francke and Arndt, who are also called Herr Direktor. These four make decisions for the factory, but we — the prisoners — see them only from afar. They never speak to a prisoner, only to our German Meister - the Germans in charge of the work. They are addressed as Herr Meister, or Herr Obermeister and there are a great many of them: Mathias, Niziolek, Hojzner, Körner, Schultz, Hochberg, Oppel - who often hit workers and when really annoyed may kill a prisoner with the heavy hammer always carried in their belts — and then Meister Herr, who kills himself with the help of his service weapon — many rumours go round about why. There are also two female Meister particularly feared by the prisoners. I don't know their names, but the red-haired one we call Marchew - the Carrot - and the other, who is noticeably fair and almost sickly pale, we call Pietrucha - the Parsnip. They are the cruelest of our Meisters. They beat prisoners and often send them, mostly women prisoners, "to the Guard". The kindest of all the Meisters is Otto Schiper, and he is called Fawys - a Jewish nickname. There are many more Meister and Obermeister, but I have not met them all — prisoners may not move around within the factory without a special reason.

To be sent "to the Guard" to atone for a misdemeanor is a much feared punishment. Many returning from that alive have been severely maltreated and some marked for life. Sarah's younger sister, Karola, is sent by Pietrucha "to the Guard" because as a kapo at an Appell, she was not able to account for why one of the prisoners in her group was missing. After mistreatment, Karola is admitted for almost two weeks to the camp sick bay — called by the Germans the Sanitesabteilung - and treated for what Dr Szperling calls internal bleeding. Karola never really recovers from this maltreatment and she does not want to say what really happened, but Dr Szperling says she will not be able to have children, which, unfortunately turns out to be true.

Karola's husband - Antek - is allowed to visit her in the sick bay and does so often, he tells me, profoundly worried that Karola is so apathetic or weeps. He thinks it would be good if Karola talked about it, but she refuses to, even when she is alone with him.

Karola does survive the war and suffers from her childlessness more than anything else that has afflicted her — her husband does not survive.

The camp is run by the Werkschutz - they also man the Guard. The Head Guard is Oberwerkschutzleiter Klemm, his nearest subordinate

The Maple Tree Behind the Barbed Wire

Werkschutzleiter Stiglitz, and the most notorious among the guards is the cruel Mors, who usually carries out the punishment of those sent "to the Guard".

Stiglitz is the only one of the camp guards who does not wear the grey-green Werkschutz uniform. He stumps proudly round in his brown SA uniform with the black swastika on a white field on his bright red armband. Few Germans wear the uniform of the SA troops. At the beginning of the Hitler days, they were the Nazi party's core troops. The SA - Sturmabteilung - were those to take Hitler into power, who carried out the Kristallnacht, the predecessors of today's élite — the black-clad SS - Schutz Staffel. Stiglitz proudly tells all who wish to, or have to, listen that he has membership number 126 in the party's Sturmabteilung. Other SA men who joined early and have such low numbers have either been killed in Hitler's great cleansing of his Sturmabteilung - he carried that out shortly after taking over power to improve his image with the German people — or can again be found among the highest ranks of government of the country. But that does not apply to Stiglitz.

Werkschutzleiter Stiglitz is a poor representative of the Nazi model of the German people and the Aryan race. Stiglitz is boastful, but there is nothing much wrong with his intellect. He is unusually open, almost frank in his dealings with the prisoners and he is not stupid. But in the National Socialist myth of the German people — the Herrenvolk of the Aryan race — the Aryans are to be tall, preferably blond and if possible blue-eyed. Stiglitz has grey eyes, darkish fair hair, but most of all is exceptionally short — almost dwarf size. The party has chosen to hide from the public the noticeably short, almost malformed Stiglitz deputy head of the guards of one of the smallest German prison camps.

But Stiglitz does not seem to be bitter, on the contrary, he is nearly always in a good mood, perhaps because he has been allowed to live although he is a cripple. In addition, he is proud of his high position in the Werkschutz - the party rewards the truly loyal and to be allowed to live is perhaps Stiglitz' reward.

I do not know what Stiglitz has achieved before in his SA career, but I have never seen him maltreat or kill any prisoner — he does not appear to be an evil man.

Responsible for the Jewish administration is Bernard Kurland, whom everyone respects. Kurland is the person to represent the prisoners at all communication with Direktör Lüth and Oberwerkschutzleiter Klemm and he also represents us with the Meisters. Unfortunately his representations rarely produce the desired effect, for Kurland has no power, only his impressive height, his proud bearing and personal authority, and perhaps also Lüth's confidence. The older of Kurland's two assistants is the lame Zylberszac, and the younger is Marzej Krauze. I think all the prisoners have undivided confidence in Kurland, nor have I ever heard anyone maintain the opposite — he is a good and unafraid man.

We also have Jewish Vorarbeiter at the factory — who have been appointed by their Meisters - and in the camp Jewish kapo, taken out at random by Klemm when we are divided up into the various huts.

In contrast to what turned out to be the case in some of the other prison camps, almost none of these kapo or Vorarbeiter are corrupted by their power. The majority of prisoners in our camp turn to their kapo or Vorarbeiter for help or advice — unfortunately they have few opportunities to help, but they could have done great harm, and they do not. The attitude of the Jewish administration contributes to the solidarity and a certain internal discipline among the prisoners.

It is rumored among the prisoners that ZOB is also active in the camp, but this rumor is not confirmed and no names are mentioned in that context. A week after our arrival at Hasag-Pelcery, however, when armed guards arrive and fetch two of the remaining Jewish policemen, Józek Winter and Poldek Wojdyslawski, the rumor is that they were involved in ZOB and arms have been found on them. Józek and Poldek are questioned and killed the same day, two of the finest Jewish policemen in Czestochowa.

We scarcely see the boys Lüth has rescued from the last Aktion at Ryneczek on June 26th. They are given food like everyone else, but are not involved in any fine engineering work at all. There is no such work at Hasag-Pelcery - had Lüth dared to lie to save them? No one harms these boys, but they have nothing to do and so have a somewhat impoverished and anonymous existence. Some are used as errand boys, primarily by the Jewish Vorarbeiter, by Kurland and his assistants, sometimes by a kapo.

Lüth has not visited the boys in their hut or spoken to any of them either on June 26th or since, not does he speak to any prisoner except Kurland and later on to Zylberszac. But all the same, he must be courageous and strong. What made him save these Jewish boys? For the moment they were found in a bunker at the liquidation of the ghetto they had forfeited their right to live.

The organisation of Hasag-Pelcery is difficult to describe. The largest units are called Abteilung - departments. I learn the names of most of the departments: my own workplace Maschinenbau, Rekalibrierung, Montage, Elektrotechnische Abteilung, Werkzeug-Abteilung, Baubetrieb, Transport and others. Some departments are large and have several sub-departments with their own names, others are quite small.

The largest workplace and the most dangerous for the health of the workers is the Rekalibrierung - where used cartridge cases are cleaned. This is done in a bath of strong acids to remove dirt and dissolve the rust, and fumes constantly rise from these acid baths, in which the water is to be at quite a high temperature and there is always an acrid smell there. For anyone to be able to stay in there, two of the walls of the main hall are open, and the roof is supported by thick pillars. When it is windy, the wind whistles through the hall — providing a change of air, but it is cold in winter. If there is no wind, the air mixed with strong acids seems quite still in the main hall of Rekalibrierung. When the frames of cartridge cases that have been lowered into the acid baths are raised, the water mixed with acid runs out on to the floor. The floor is covered with wide wooden slats so the water can run off between them, and the workers wear clogs with thick soles.

The cartridge cases then have to be inspected, which is done by specially selected prisoners, all women. They have to pick up every newly cleaned, often badly rinsed cartridge case by hand, see that it has the two prescribed openings, otherwise it is discarded. If a prisoner wants to protect her hands, she has to acquire some gloves herself. Few have them and the factory does not provide them.

That warm acrid smell is already noticeable outside the Rekalibrierung and it gets even stronger when you go into the big main hall. Those who work there are unusually pale even compared with other prisoners.

I am allocated to Maschinenbau, where generators fueled by wood are being manufactured during the first two weeks after my arrival. But the Italian company, which has ordered them is dissatisfied with the deliveries, and production is to cease. So they are planning the manufacture of another product - Panzerfaust - armored fist — a somewhat bombastic name for a long flame-colored pipe that is carried on the arm of a soldier and used to release anti-tank shots. Our Meister is very thorough at checking every example of Panzerfaust.

We prisoners are constantly hungry — even immediately after meals, yet the majority of us manage fairly well on the soup, bread and chicory coffee. But some do not, and those who suffer most in the camp are called Muzelmans - prisoners who owing to malnourishment or perhaps for other reasons cannot cope, who give up, stop washing in the mornings, don't mend their clothes, then we know that a Muzelman has not long to live. The name comes from a related word in Yiddish - a miser man - and has nothing to do with Muslim.

In my second week on the night shift, at the first break I catch sight of one of my ex-classmates, Mietek Jarzombek. He is standing there in his ragged clothes, a mug of coffee in one hand and a slice of bread in the other. I recognize him despite the fact that he has changed - a Muzelman. I try to talk to Mietek and ask him if he needs help of any kind, but he seems absent, his eyes flickering, though I can see he recognizes me and is trying to concentrate, but fails. He gives up and shuffles off away from the workplace after our nine o'clock at night breakfast — perhaps for the last time. The previously red-cheeked,

The Maple Tree Behind the Barbed Wire

constantly smiling Mietek Jarzombek cannot have much longer to live when I see him that night.

There are also occasional Polish workers at Hasag-Pelcery. They are not prisoners and in contrast to us, are decently paid, although some do the same work as we prisoners do. With the help of the Polish workers, sometimes some food can be got into our camp. There is still a little money left among the prisoners in the camp — not much, but some prisoners have saved for when times get worse, and others manage to make various small things, which may be of value to barter for food.

Trading is brisk at Hasag-Pelvery. You can order things from some of the Polish workers — they demand payment in advance, at the latest on the day of delivery. The prisoners buy primarily bread, a half kilo costing 80 zloty — a good profit for whoever negotiates the purchase. On the open market in town, half a kilo of black bread costs 12 zloty. Bernard Kurland finds out about this trading in the factory and goes to see Oberwerksschutzleiter Klemm and then Direktör Lüth; Kurland succeeds in persuading them to open a canteen in the camp. In the canteen half a kilo of black bread costs 24 zloty and is also fresher than the bread bought from the Polish workers. No one asks where the prisoners got their money from, but the canteen unfortunately is to open for only a few weeks.

On July 20th, 1943, at about nine in the morning, one of the prisoners in the kitchen of the Wirtschaftsabteilung - Cesia Borkowska - comes with our breakfast. Cesia tells us that a police car with Degenhardt and two other police cars have demanded to pass the Guard but have been stopped by Werkschutz who referred them to "Kolonia" - what we prisoners call the area outside the camp where the Germans employed at the factory live, and where the administration has its offices. I know Cesia - she is a few years older than I am, and we sit drinking our coffee and talking for a moment. Cesia has heard a rumor that Degenhardt was annoyed at having to wait with his assistants at the factory office to meet Lüth.

A visit from the German police from Leipzig arouses anxiety in any Jew from the Czestochowa ghetto — we have quite long and bitter experiences of their activities. I cannot remember that they had ever brought anything good with them to us Jews. The fact that they are here in Hasag is ominous. But when nothing happens for the rest of the morning, I forget what Cesia had told me.

Not until midday, just after twelve, when we are to have our usual soup for lunch, all the prisoners at Hasag-Pelcery are instead lined up for an Appell. The day shift is fetched from work, the night shift woken and escorted by the Werkschutz to the Appell.

It has rained that morning, so the ground it wet and dark low clouds still cover the sky. Although the daylight is reasonable, the powerful searchlights are turned on over the great yard at the entrance of Rekaliberierung, where most of the prisoners are lined up according to their workplaces. But it is not the German police — it is our Meister and Obermeister doing the Selektion this time.

According to a rumor circulating among the prisoners, there has been a misunderstanding. Oberwerkschutzleiter Klemm, but not Direktör Lüth, has been informed in advance that Degenhardt and his men are to come to fetch 500 prisoners, the remaining Jewish policemen and their families. Degenhardt seems to have started out from that it was enough to inform Klemm. When the German police arrive, Lüth does not allow them to enter his factory area and nor does he accept that we are 500 too many prisoners. When he comes to our group, our Meister says they have had orders to take out 300 prisoners for the next transport.

Captain Degenhardt and his policemen, on the other hand, are let into the hut area where the Jewish policemen live with their families. In the evening it is said in our hut that Degenhardt had made a speech to the Jewish police about their disloyalty and had taken with him all the 28 remaining policemen and their wives and children, 60 people in all, on top of the 300 our German Meisters had picked out — most of them Muzelmans. The Jewish police and their families are executed and buried in the Jewish cemetery, which becomes the last mass grave for the Czestochowa Jews murdered on the spot, escaping the long transport to the extermination camp - Treblinka.

In the evening, when I am back from the day shift, the prisoners in our hut tell us that Lüth had refused to hand over Bernard Kurland. Lüth is said to have maintained that he needed Kurland to keep up production. The camp telegraph is surprisingly well informed.

Two days later, on July 22nd, 1943, Degenhardt is back again in the factory management administration building in "Kolonia", this time with only his driver, Willi Onkelbach. They have with them a decree from senior German authorities. According to this decree, not a single Jew from the ghetto's previous police force or Judenrat is to be left at Hasag-Pelcery. Kurland is the last living member of the Judenrat - the Jewish Council - appointed by the Germans in October 1939. Bernard Kurland is summoned to factory management office and Degenhardt takes him to the Guard.

Rumours of all kinds go round the camp about what happens when Degenhardt meets Bernard Kurland for the last time and before Kurland is shot by Willi Onkelbach. The rumours largely come from the Werkschutz who were in the guard premises when Degenhardt and Onkelbach arrived there with Kurland - these scattered bits of information are however fairly unanimous.

In the presence of several guards, Degenhardt makes a speech to Bernard Kurland, containing the same accusations of disloyalty as in

The Maple Tree Behind the Barbed Wire

his speech on July 12th to the remaining Jewish policemen. Degenhardt stresses that Kurland knew of the presence of ZOB in the ghetto but has not informed the police. He then gives Kurland one last chance to save his life by revealing what he knows about ZOB's present activities.

But the German camp guards' stories pay more attention to Kurland's prophetic speech that is so much discussed among the prisoners. Kurland turns to Degenhardt and the others in the guardhouse hear him when he says: "The time on the clock of your destiny is now only five to twelve. You can kill me and other Jews, but you cannot stop the clock or escape the inevitable. Fate will catch up with you. You and others with you will be made to answer for what you have hitherto done to us and what you are to do in your remaining days." The German guards admit to a certain admiration for Kurland's dignified behavior at the end.

Bernard Kurland, previously a renowned athlete in our town, is tall, strong and unafraid. Degenhardt asks for help to have his hands tied and that is done, not with a rope, but with wire. Kurland is then driven to the Jewish cemetery in Czestochowa and shot by Willi Onkelbach - Degenhardt himself has never shot a single Jew.

We in the Hasag-Pelecery prison camp grieve for Bernard Kurland for a long time — many still grieve for this leading hero of the Czestochowa ghetto. He was a mature, courageous and unselfish man, who despite our misery and oppression managed to preserve his pride and an unbroken loyalty to his fellow-prisoners. He never yielded and for many of us became the symbol of maintained Jewish dignity during this war.

Kurland was the last of the Jewish administration in Czestochowa ghetto appointed the week after the Germans occupied our town. With him, the last of the Czestochowa Judenrat died and nor is there a single Jewish policemen now left. Accusations of violation and criticism against individual Jewish police actions in connection with certain definite events are later to be produced, among them against the second-in-command of the Jewish police, Parasol, and against the head of the billeting committee, Kohlenbrenner, because he had not been particularly accommodating. More serious criticism is to be directed at Dr Szperling, head of the cottage hospital in the ghetto and at Hasag-Pelecery. But the accumulated judgement must nevertheless be that they succeeded in resisting and were not corrupted either by the power they had over us, or by the activities of the Germans. This is to be admired, considering the circumstances, the persistent external pressures, the false promises of the Germans alternating with threats to their families, who in practice were hostages held by the Germans. The tradition Leon Kopinski, chairman of our Judenrat, together with Anisfelt, previously rector of the Jewish gymnasium and responsible

The Maple Tree Behind the Barbed Wire

for recruiting staff for the Jewish administration, set from the start, was to withstand the strains of the war. They did their best;, no one can ask for more.

The behavior of the Jewish administration helps those of us who are to survive to preserve our human value, to maintain our faith in human beings, and also helps us to survive less damaged and better than we otherwise would have been equipped to function properly under normal circumstances and in a normal peaceful society.

The remains of the ravaged ZOB survive, often with the silent support of brave people within the Jewish administration, both in the Large Ghetto and later in the Small Ghetto and — as it turns out — even in the prison camp. ZOB has little support from outside, for few wish to co-operate with them until they meet the Hanysch group in the forests round Koniecpol and then Zloty Potok. At least three groups of ZOB soldiers managed to escape from the Small Ghetto and Hasag. They cause limited but some damage to the occupation forces, primarily through sabotaging their means of communication. To judge by the forces involved in the liquidation of the small ghetto, they nonetheless give the Germans a considerable fright. They also help us keep our self-respect and give a few of us who are to survive something to remember and be proud of, although ZOB's presence among us means severe reprisals from the Germans. Presumably, we would have suffered reprisals anyhow but they were worse as a result of this presence. Not until long afterwards did we find out that ZOB's perhaps most important contribution in Czestochowa was what was carried out by the Jewish prisoners at Huta Raków-Pelcery. Their assignment was first to clean, then melt down missiles from the eastern front in the blast furnaces. In this connection they acquired the insignificant quantities of gunpowder still remaining inside these projectiles. For a long time it was largely through this gunpowder that the resistance movement all over the country - AK as well as Gwardia Ludowa - could be supplied with explosives.

Bernard Kurland's closest associate, Zylberszac, was appointed by Lüth as his successor. Marzej Krauze is now the only remaining associate in the prison camp Jewish administration. Both are good men and do their best in their exposed positions, but they lack Bernard Kurland's stature, courage and authority. Zylberszac, his wife and Marzej Krauze do survive the war — they are to die natural deaths quite recently, respected in their communities where they finally settled, Zylberszac in Toronto, Marzej Krauze in Chicago. Marzej's sister Renia also survives the war at Hasag-Pelcery and after much traveling and short stays in several countries finally settles in Buenos Aries, happily married to another ex-Hasag prisoner, Mietek Szydlowski.

My wife Nina and I have spent the last seven summers, 1991-1997, with Marzej's sister Renia Szydlowska and her husband in Flims - a

The Maple Tree Behind the Barbed Wire

small village in a lovely valley in the northern Alps in eastern Switzerland. Although it arouses anguish in us, we can't help talking about what happened during those years in the ghetto, the forced labour and the prison camp, the Jewish gymnasium where Renia was also a pupil, our teachers, of whom only two survived the war, about Lüth, Degenhardt, the German police from Leipzig, Klemm, Stigliz and our Meisters at Hasag, Leon Kopinski, Rector Anisfelt, Bernard Kurland, the Jewish police, about Zylberszac and Marzej Krauze, Renia's brother who died in 1994, and so many many more.

We, the tiny few to survive, are drawn to each other, united in our need to talk about what happened, to remember our Jewish heroes and the German rogues — for that is what they were in our eyes, almost all Germans we met during the war — but also about the few Germans who deviated from the mass. About Itcie - the only one of the German policemen from Leipzig to resist the pressures and never killed or struck a Jew - and Direktör Lüth, who never addressed us but who made our life bearable, probably saved many of us and anyhow saved over twenty orphan boys, who after the war were taken to Great Britain to continue their education.

Itcie showed that even an ordinary policeman can resist without being punished. Lüth showed that even among prominent Germans, there were strong and brave men with human emotions, that you cannot, may not treat a whole people in the same way, condemn a whole people — as the Germans did with us. You cannot even condemn all the members of a hateful political party. We have to look on every person as an individual, believe and hope that any older German we happen to meet today is not one of those who took part in the Exterminations of the Jews of Europe.

During the war, we have already heard about the Sudeten German who is saving Jews in Plaszow. But Schindler was to us an improbable legend and Direktör Lüth a tangible reality.

There are two versions of the fate of Captain Degenhardt.: According to one of them, his fate was sealed even more quickly than Bernard Kurland could have foreseen in his prophetic speech to him on June 22nd, 1943. After Degenhardt's last extermination Aktion against the Jews of Czestochowa, those still left in Hasag's three remaining camps, his assignment in Czestochowa is considered to have been satisfactorily concluded — he had demonstrated his efficiency. This contributed to him being transferred to Salonika in Greece for similar though in practice more difficult tasks than mass murdering defenseless Jews imprisoned in a ghetto. Through their contacts, ZOB has succeeded in informing the Greek guerilla in the mountains round Salonika of his activities in Czestochowa. Even for Captain Degenhardt, it turns out to be a much more difficult task to terrorize a population that can move about freely, or to exterminate a guerilla

The Maple Tree Behind the Barbed Wire

force which has the support of the population as well as help from the Allies and the Soviet Union by sea and air. Police Captain Degenhardt from Leipzig is murdered by the Greek guerillas shortly after his arrival in Salonika. A rumor of this reaches our camp.

I am quite definitely against capital punishment in all its forms. A human being has no right to take the life of another human being. I am aware that against this background, this is illogical, and I hope I may be forgiven that I think that what happened to Captain Degenhardt in Salonika was — well, let us say just. Which shows that it is easy to speak for abstract principles, but difficult to stick to them logically when you yourself are personally concerned.

According to the second version, it is Oberleutnant Überscheer who is killed in revenge by the Greek guerillas. After the war, Degenhardt, according to a version by a professor in psychiatry, was confused, and from the same professor he is given a certificate to say he is mentally deranged, so cannot be held responsible for his deeds. He is sentenced to preventative detention and dies many years later. His friend the professor of psychiatry is later revealed to be a forceful Nazi who himself had been guilty of war crimes against prisoners. He was dismissed and charged, but the trial of Degenhardt was never taken up again.

The Last Year of the War

Four days after the murder of Bernard Kurland and a month after my arrival at Hasag-Pelecery, on July 26th, 1943, I have my eighteenth birthday. I am alone, plagued with anxieties and longing for Pinkus and Sarah. We have no means of communicating with each other and I think and hope they are still at Mrs. Mosiewitz' workshop.

I find it hard to get up when we are woken just after five in the morning. I like to stay under my warm blanket for a little longer, fall asleep again, so I don't have time before Appell to get into the queue to wash in cold water at the long zinc trough outside our hut. It is humiliating after a few days when the prisoner nearest to me points out rather harshly that possibly for the odd day it is all right to skip washing, but I should not do so every day. Ignas Katz agrees — "we can smell that you have not washed". This painful criticism does, however, have an effect. I get up every morning at least an hour before Appell and am among the first to go and wash, although this could hardly be called enjoyable in the semi-darkness and the cold, the water icy and the piece of brown soap issued to each prisoner hardly lathering, then drying on a thin rag still damp from use the day before. I feel better, even slightly proud when I see I can manage, and in future I wash properly every morning.

The Maple Tree Behind the Barbed Wire

Now it is the second week in my third two-week period on the night shift. At first I find it difficult to get used to working at night and sleeping in the daytime, but one advantage is that I am free from work for a couple of hours of daylight. At about five in the afternoon I am sitting on a wooden box in the slanting sunlight at the entrance of the hut area, presumably a rather pitiful sight.

Since my arrival at Hasag, I have had several opportunities of noticing Helenka Majtlis - before the war she lived in the same building in Katedralna Street as Bela and Ignas Enzel. Helenka is a trained nurse and works at the camp Sanitetsabteilung. She is motherly, dark-haired, cultivated, and despite the semi-starvation in the camp, she is still quite a plump woman in her thirties, her light complexion an attractive contrast to her longish raven-black hair. Helenka always wears her black, rather shabby nurse's uniform, but this afternoon I see she is not wearing her nurse's white cap. She stands a little way away, looking at me, then comes slowly over, asks me if I remember her and whether she may sit down.

I am pleased and surprised, shift over and she sits down on the box beside me, ruffles my hair, and then puts her left arm in a friendly way round my shoulders. We just sit there together on that wooden box. After a while, Helenka says: "Are you lonely, Jurek? — using my diminutive nickname, otherwise only used by parents, family and friends, but no one in camp. "Are you missing your parents?" Then she adds in her deep calming voice: "That is natural. Do you think I can help in any way?"

I am tremendously grateful and touched by someone as good as Helenka Majtlis taking an interest in me. At the same time, she reminds me of what there has been between Rózia and me and I am slightly ashamed that she arouses my youthful fantasies, which are wholly unrealistic considering Helenka's intentions, and in addition in a prison camp where there is no space for any kind of private life. Helenka Majtlis comes to see me several times over the following weeks and on each occasion is just as friendly, warm, understanding and close, but at the same time with no other intentions — those are only in my fantasies.

All this — managing to get up and wash every morning, studying regularly with the help of my school books, feeling more at home in the hut and at work, being an object of interest to lovely Helenka Majtlis, perhaps even the youthful fantasies she arouses in me when as she comes smiling towards me in her black nurse's uniform — all this contributes to my pulling myself together, beginning to accept the situation and adapting to life in the camp. When the autumn of 1943 comes, Helenka Majtlis stops coming to see me. But I think about her sometimes, her soft femininity, her friendly interest, how lovely she is and that does me good - I know I can go and see her should I need to.

The Maple Tree Behind the Barbed Wire

When the winter of 1943 comes to the camp, it turns out that even the attempt to make Panzerfaust at the Maschinenbau at Hasag-Pelcery has failed. We find out that a group of experts from the Wehrmacht, the German army, has visited the Hasag works in Germany where the construction has been taken to and they had carried out a series of test firings, but rejected all the selected examples our Meister considered the most successful. The Wehrmacht experts judge the firing range too short and the accuracy too poor. This hardly comes as a surprise to us prisoners making this simple construction on a conveyer belt.

As the Maschinenbau neither has nor expects to have any more orders from outside, the workforce is reduced to cover only the factory's own needs for making machines and carrying out repairs. Our Jewish Vorarbeiter - Heniek Hofman - asks me if I would like to go over to Wirtschaftsabteilung and to be transferred to Bautrieb - the factory-building department. "It would be outdoor work," he says. "That can be troublesome in winter, but they have no night shift, Sundays are often though not always free, and they have a Polish foreman who functions as Vormeister." I gratefully accept as I am keen to make a change and go to the Baubetrieb.

One morning at the beginning of November, an hour after our stint has begun, a Polish worker I have never seen before comes to the place where our group is working that week on the outskirts of the factory area. He is a stocky, dark-haired man of ordinary appearance. He moves clumsily but at the same time gives an impression of purposeful efficiency.

The Polish workers at Hasag-Pelcery also maintain a solidarity between them — he goes up to our Polish foreman - Adam Wawrzyniak. Adam seems to be pointing at me, then I see him nodding in confirmation and he stays there watching while the stranger comes over and asks me to step aside with him.

We go behind a shed our group has recently built as a temporary store for our tools and he hands me a brown paper bag. "It's from your father," he says. Then he adds: "Be careful." When he sees how surprised I am, he puts the paper bag into the pocket of the thin coat I have taken out of the camp clothing store against the November cold, then turns briskly round and leaves without giving me a chance to say anything. I start going after him, but realise that is pointless, so stop. But I am overwhelmed with relief. A sign of life from my father.

Not until an hour later, in the breakfast break, do I have an opportunity to go into the tool shed and open the bag — in it is a little white loaf.

I can't remember when I last saw white bread it seems so long ago. To me this is not just any white bread, it is double the size of an

The Maple Tree Behind the Barbed Wire

ordinary roll, slightly oblong, quite coarse, with some seeds in it — perhaps sunflower seeds. It seems well baked and not like the black bread we get in camp, not properly baked as it is and moist with water to increase the weight . I break a little bit off this little loaf that in some miraculous way Pinkus has managed to get to me, crumble it up and spread the crumbs on to the dark camp bread we have been given for breakfast. All this must have taken quite a time, for my black chicory coffee has cooled, but all the same, I think it is the best breakfast I have had for a long time.

The rest of the white bread lasts for three days. Small crumbs on black bread for breakfast and in the evening, a little piece with my soup at twelve o'clock — it doesn't matter much when by the third day it is not quite so fresh.

I have had confirmation of what I have been trying to convince myself all this time; my father Pinkus is alive and can reach me even in Hasag-Pelcery where we are so efficiently cut off from the outside world.

Hasag-Pelcery is not a mass-extermination camp like those in the eastern parts of the Generalguvernement - Belzec, Majdanek, Chelmno, Sobibór and Treblinka - where practically all newly arrived prisoners are killed with cyanide gas in large sealed gas chambers the day they arrive, then are cremated. Nor is Hasag-Pelcery like one of those large combined prison camps with their own gas chambers and crematoria of the type at Auschwitz-Birkenau - in which two million people, mostly Jews, Soviet soldiers and gypsies are reckoned to have been killed — or like one of the enormous prison camps in Germany itself, where the majority of prisoners die within a few months, camps such as Gross-Rosen, Buchenwald, Sachsenhausen, Bergen Belsen, Dachau, Dora, Mauthausen, Ravensbrück, Stutthof, Neigamme. German doctors are allowed to carry out scientific, fairly meaningless but cruel experiments in those camps, mostly on women prisoners.

Instead, Hasag-Pelcery is one of the smaller German camps in the Generalguvernement intended for Jewish prisoners and located in association with some form of German manufacturing industry. Hasag-Pelcery is part of the German industrial company Hasag AG, which had four, but now three plants left near the industrial town of Czestochowa.

Deep down in my memory are details of camp life - I remember the huts where I slept, the daily routine when I worked the day or the night shift. The Appells, the long rows of outdoor privies with their scarcely metre-high partitions, and also individual events that have become etched on my mind. But however good you are as narrator, reporter, actor or film director, I think it is impossible to transmit to anyone who has not gone through what the everyday life of a prisoner was like in a minor German prison camp towards the end of the

The Maple Tree Behind the Barbed Wire

second world war.

It was a difficult existence. I was hungry and felt threatened, a constant awareness in my subconscious of that unconditional sentence to death. But despite this, it is not all-just misery. Reasonably healthy people, perhaps particularly the young, are able to go through things that have to be regarded as positive. Although it is hard to imagine, there were actually moments of joy, even happiness. You make friends, fall in love, feel attraction, are disappointed or encouraged by a look, a few words, and a touch. I am pleased when I see a ladle of the thicker soup from the bottom of the pan, when the soup in cold mid-winter is unusually hot, when the extra portion one Sunday is particularly generous. Temporary sports teams are formed, linked to the different workplaces, matches are played, and I go and cheer on my team, which perhaps wins. We are happy and start singing when one evening the clever Chajutin brothers play to us in our hut, to cheer us up. You can become truly elated when you are one of the lucky ones, someone who after several long weeks of knowing nothing, has had a message from his father, and then for three days is able to ration the crumbs of fresh white bread.

The things that happen to us Jews during the Second World War are shocking, profoundly frightening experiences that change a human being — some of us for the worse, but others, at least in some respects, for the better. Which it becomes depends on many factors?

One factor is the character of the camp, for instance if the hunger is so great that it breaks almost everyone. Another is the individual prisoner's personal predilection to accepting the situation and adapting. But there are also other circumstances, an important one the attitudes of prisoners to each other. One decisive difference is if prisoners given some responsibility and with that some power over us others, then identify with the Germans, or if instead there is some kind of unbroken solidarity and a feeling of mutual confidence between prisoners. It makes a huge difference if you are feeling lonely, alien and constantly suspicious of the other prisoners, always having to be on your guard against everyone, or whether there is a feeling of mutual confidence between prisoners — that we have a common enemy — the Germans - and a common aim — to survive.

I think one condition for survival as a prisoner is to be able to maintain hope for the future, for us at Hasag, the hope of being rescued and surviving, however unrealistic it may have seemed for a Jew in a German prison camp in the winter of 1943-44. It is also a great help if you manage to acquire what may well be a false but well-meaning myth that there is someone protecting you — in my case, it was Pinkus. For some it is God, but for others God will not do in that role in a prison camp. Many who had been religious before the war and become so again after it, deny that a God that allows what we are forced to go through exists — and not many want to believe in a God

The Maple Tree Behind the Barbed Wire

who is not good or is powerless in face of the Germans.

I know that my values and attitudes, my personality and my daily dealings in future have been marked by the experiences of almost six years when I was growing up. I know I am damaged — but also strengthened. I like to think that from those experiences I have become less frivolous, more considerate and in some respects perhaps a better person.

We are effectively cut off from all contact with the world outside. I can no longer even imagine what life is like outside the gates of the camp and the factory. I have no idea whatsoever how the war is going — except that I realise it is not over and as long as it is not over, there is hope. Anyhow, how the war is going is not what is most important — for the day. A prisoner has much more pressing problems overshadowing everything else — to survive the day and the week.

We have got ourselves into a harsh and demanding routine, in a continuously whirling treadmill, and to manage this daily routine uses up all our energy and all our strength. Getting up early in the morning darkness to have time to wash before morning roll call, work from seven until seven, with the longed-for short breaks for breakfast and lunch, then evening roll call at the workplace, chicory coffee with no sugar to the other slice of dark bread in the evening, and finally the paltry two hours at our disposal before the two unshaded lights are switched off in our hut.

It has turned very cold, the solitary stove in our hut incapable of providing the warmth needed during the cold nights of the winter of 1944. At the beginning of February, when the stubbornly persistent winter plagues us most, old Katz and my father — both still at Mrs. Mosiewicz' workshop — succeed in getting something to help Ignas and me. One evening, when we come back from work, lying on our bunks in the hut is a note summoning us to the camp office. There is Zylberszac and we are given a warm quilt each. Zylberszac says the quilts have come with the ordinary daily consignment of necessities for the camp, but on them was a note to say that they are intended for us and came from Mrs. Mosiewicz' workshop. That is all Zylberszac knows.

I am in the same camp as my aunt, Karola, but nevertheless have few opportunities of meeting her as it is forbidden to enter the women prisoners' huts. On one occasion I manage to find what I like to think is a legitimate reason for going into the Rekalibrierung hall where she works.

The otherwise happy, extroverted, neat and tidy Karola seems apathetic, her hair straggly and her complexion grayish. It is the lunch break and she says in a dull voice that she is pleased to see me. I feel helpless when I see how sluggish and uninterested she is, what a bad way she is in, yet there is nothing I can do for my only surviving aunt and the only one of Sarah's sisters still alive.

One evening a prisoner asks us if we had seen small insects in the timbers of our hut; several confirm that they have. After a week we realise the bugs have gained a foothold, are very fecund and spreading rapidly. They are everywhere in our bunks and at night when it is dark even in our bedding. I realise we will never get rid of them once they have got into the deep cracks in the poor quality timber. The fact that things are much the same in the other huts does not make it any better.

I think it is horrible. I feel exposed and defenseless against the lice when I go to bed at night and the lights go out, with no chance of switching on the lights in the middle of the night to see what is happening in my bed. In the end I fall asleep from exhaustion and scratch in the morning at real or imagined bites.

I don't know whether the lice contribute to the typhus epidemic that breaks out in the camp that late winter of 1944.

Those who fall ill with a high temperature are quickly isolated by the efficient staff in the camp sick bay, the sick just disappearing from the huts. Four men fall ill in our hut, Motek Birenbaum the last — he sleeps on the middle shelf, only three bunks from me. Stiglitz, who is still the most communicative of our camp guards, tells us — with little noticeable emotion — that our camp, with us too, is going to be liquidated if the epidemic is not quickly limited. This perspective frightens us more than the actual disease.

But the epidemic is brought to an end by the intensive efforts of the camp Sanitetsabteilung, headed by the tough but efficient Dr Szperling and his staff. The sick are swiftly isolated, efficiently, and well cared for considering the circumstances. But the rapid intervention by the Germans is of significance. By delousing every garment, blanket, pillow and mattress, forgetting nothing, for once we and the Germans have exactly the same aim. Every hut is closed off and the vermin I thought we would never get rid of are smoked out in thirty-six hours, all doors and windows effectively sealed.

Several victims of typhus recover, surviving thanks to the good care they are given. They come back from sick bay emaciated, some with no hair on their heads, but nonetheless alive - Motek Birenbaum is not one of them. He never comes back.

The Maple Tree Behind the Barbed Wire

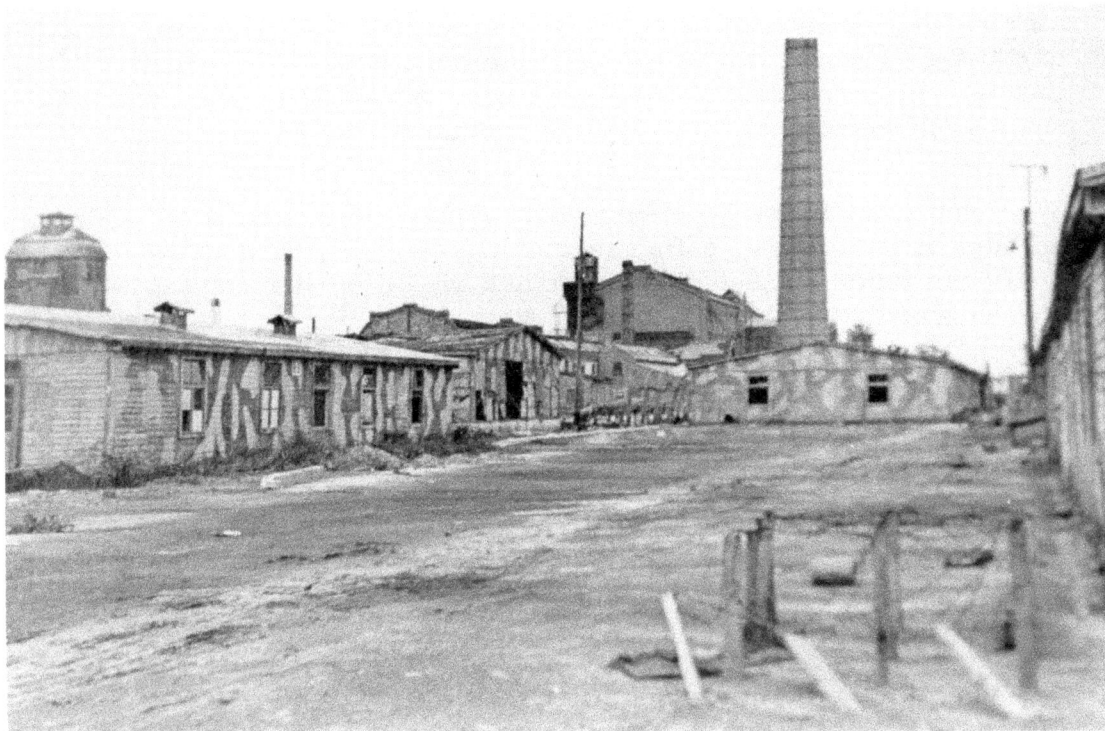

A forest of small simple fireplaces appears on the big space between the huts for female and male prisoners. The camp guards take no notice, perhaps because we are in the middle of a typhus epidemic.

An enterprising woman prisoner sets up a simple fireplace made of nine bricks in the wide space between the women's and the men's huts. The guards ignore them, perhaps because of the typhus epidemic. Several prisoners follow her example and a number of small fireplaces appear in the great yard. They boil water on them for washing clothes, for personal hygiene, some prisoners heating their daily ration of soup on them, perhaps spicing it or spinning it out — if they have anything to spice it with or something to add to the pan. There are plenty of bricks and combustible waste at the factory, so within a week or two a new trade flourishes in simple food that can be boiled and eaten, the Polish workers the main suppliers, at greatly increased prices.

At the beginning of March 1944, the same Polish worker again comes, bringing white bread with him to my workplace. Again he exchanges a few words with my foreman, Adam Wawrzyniak. As Adam has no objection, the Polish worker quickly heads straight for me, takes me aside and once again hands me a brown paper bag — the third gift from my parents. He does not have to tell me to be careful. I am perfectly aware of that, and also that it is pointless asking questions - I would not be given an answer, anyhow. I open the bag during the next break, I open the bag and in it is a white loaf, the same size as before, but also a single medium-sized onion.

If you have never experienced the monotonous diet of our camp, perhaps it is impossible to imagine what a delicacy a thin slice of onion can be on a piece of coarse black bread, or how good it is with strips of fresh onion in hot cabbage soup. The onion lasts a long time, varying my simple meals and making eating more enjoyable, and as long as I have this slowly diminishing little bit of onion left, I have a feeling of that I myself am deciding on how to vary my meals.

I remember that wonderful taste of a slice of onion on bread so vividly, I can still eat fresh onion in almost unlimited quantities, on bread, but also to various hot and cold dishes — to Nina's dismay, though she tolerates this bad habit of mine, because she knows I like onion and she likes me.

Already by February, after six months in camp, I begin to find it less meaningful to go on improving myself with the aid of my schoolbooks. At the beginning of March I realise I have already learnt all I can get from them, that I have already solved the calculus examples several times over. There is no prohibition of schoolbooks in camp and no one bothers about it, but it is not possible from inside to acquire any more books and I am still obsessed by my hunger for education. To satisfy this need I manage to acquire a new and what perhaps could be called an intellectual occupation which I like to think will be useful in the long term — to increase my Polish vocabulary in various ways and practice speaking the language well. If needs be, this can be done without books.

It all begins when I am talking to an older and particularly well-versed man in the camp and notice that he uses a few words which I recognize and understand, but do not use myself. In order not to forget them, I jot down these words in a thin little pocketbook with stiff light brown covers Sarah has given me for important addresses. From then on I write down new words I happen to hear. I also seek out prisoners I notice have a wide vocabulary, ask them, or in some other way try to extract new words to write down. On the last pages in the notebook are sentences I have made up, which I think are original and apposite, like this, for instance:

If suffering ennobles, then all we Czestochowa Jews must be very noble.

I still have that little notebook among my war souvenirs. When I leaf through it, I realise that the sentences are trivial, not particularly clever or profound, but I also realise that then, in the winter and

The Maple Tree Behind the Barbed Wire

spring of 1944, this occupation was of value to me. Perhaps it was my way of defying the hopelessness and preparing for the future — a future after the war. For in a prison camp, an extensive vocabulary is not much use; for the language used there is very simple and straightforward and it would be considered peculiar if in everyday life I used sophisticated words or tried to speak in sensible sentences.

Spring comes early in 1944, some warm days even in April, and for the first time hitherto, I have a most relaxed and pleasant day in the Hasag-Pelcery prison camp.

On the first Sunday in April, a match is played between two newly formed football teams, one from the Transportabteilung, the other from the Maschinenbau. The initiative for the match has been taken by the prisoners themselves, but they have asked the Werkschutz and have been given permission. The early April sun is shining from an almost cloudless sky and I am standing in the unexpectedly large crowd, my face turned up to the sun.

Many of us in the crowd, and presumably the players too, forget for a moment the reality we live in and are carried away by the excitement. I yell myself hoarse as I cheer on the Maschinenbau - my previous workmates. The temporary football pitch is too small, the lines unclear and the goalposts not according to the rules, but nonetheless I think it is an excellent football match. Several of the players on the pitch have played in third and fourth division football teams before the war, one or two in the second division. Transportabteilung's team is getting the worst of it and start playing rough, which makes for increased sympathies for the team from the Maschinenbau. The referee is also good and has pre-war experience of games in higher divisions, so knows his job, keeps the players under control and punishes transgressions. The Maschinenbau team wins.

I feel a temporary but unadulterated joy, as if I myself had contributed to winning the match. I notice my face is smarting from the sun and realise I am getting sunburnt. I have no access to a mirror, try to imagine how good I must look with fresh sunburn and become even more excited. I want to have some time to myself, but finding a private place where you can be yourself in practice is impossible for a prisoner in a camp. All spaces are communal — the huts we sleep in, where we wash, the communal shower room with several showers and hot water we are now allowed to use every other week, even the toilets. Just as I am about to give up I catch sight of a big grey trailer a truck has for some reason left behind. It is alongside a large windowless storeroom, a little to the left of the provisional football pitch. I go over to it. There is no one around and I climb up on to the trailer — surely that is not forbidden?

The Maple Tree Behind the Barbed Wire

The round clock above the entrance to the Kolonia says it has gone four in the afternoon, the sun — still slightly above the horizon — shines on me as I lie on the floor of the trailer. I take off my shirt so that the sun shall also warm my torso as I make myself as comfortable as possible on the wooden floor. I fold up my crumpled shirt and with both arms behind my head, turn my face to the sinking sun and fall into a relaxed semi-torpor as I think how good things are at that moment. I start fantasizing about the future.

For the first time for a long time, I again think about the soldiers who are going to come to rescue those of us left in the camp and the people at Mrs. Mosiewicz'. I have long since stopped being absorbed in what will happen after our liberation, and nowadays think only about the events round our actual rescue — how happy we will be, what the soldiers who come to chase away the Germans will look like, what I will say to those soldiers — and then I fall asleep.

As I climb down again almost two hours later I feel rested, relaxed and for some reason full of confidence — that has always worked hitherto, I do not know how, but somehow things are going to sort themselves out in the future. I think about how sunburnt I must be, bringing back memories of happy times before the war, what awaits me when the war is at last over — all wars must come to an end sooner or later. Now it is a matter of staying alive, being there still and being allowed to experience it.

Like most other units in the Baubetrieb, my group is largely occupied with fairly meaningless tasks. As a result of a decision that turns out to be a hasty one, we are digging the foundations for a hut that is never built, then we fill up the hole in the ground and level out the soil — that type of occupation is not uncommon. Road maintenance inside the plant is more meaningful, sometimes making new bits of road, or building a new hut or a store, but we are far too many in the Baubetrieb for this limited requirement to occupy us sufficiently.

I realise that for the management of the Baubetrieb it is important that we are kept busy, that all the achievements of the unit are recorded. But it is obvious that no one follows up or evaluates the usefulness of our contributions, or else no one can be bothered. This presumably contributes to why our Polish foreman sees no reason why he should press us into working more quickly or stop us talking to each other. He is also indulgent towards the fact that — sometimes leaning on my spade - I am occasionally sunk in my thoughts. Once when I took out my brown notebook to note something down, Adam Wawrzyniak, perhaps slightly suspiciously, asks me what exactly I am doing. He shrugs with surprise when I tell him about new words and sentences, but he does nothing to stop me.

The Maple Tree Behind the Barbed Wire

My impression is that the achievements of the whole company - Hasag-Pelcery - cannot be particularly impressive. Both the hitherto tested projects within the Maschinenbau have turned out to be failures and the department, previously considered the most promising in the factory, is now mainly working for the internal needs of the factory. The same applies to Werkzeugbau, Technische Abteilung and several other units within Hasag-Pelcery. Rekablibrierung, as far as I can judge, is able to report the best results, but even they receive a great many complaints — large boxes, sometimes whole consignments of cartridges are returned by the recipients for a second cleaning. Despite this inefficiency, activities are kept going and more transports of prisoners are also beginning to arrive at the camp.

The first is a trainload of women from Piotrków at the beginning of May 1944. Shortly after that, 500 men and women from Lodz, the German Litzmanstadt, arrive. Things speed up and we have more meaningful work to do at Baubetrieb as we have to erect two huts for the women — the men from Lodz ghetto are spread around the existing huts, largely to places left by prisoners who have died. The new arrivals from Lodz are said to be professionals in the Hasag area of interest, but they are in a rather bad way and also terrified — they have not known where their transport was to end up, and they look like the most emaciated of our prisoners at Hasag.

I go to see some of the men newly arrived from Lodz, but none of them knows anything about my grandparents, either Szyja or Szprynca. When I tell them how old they are and describe their way of life, the men I talk to find it difficult to believe they might be still alive - Chassids of that kind no longer exist, a tall thin, very tired man with a shock of tangled hair tells me.

Two weeks later, the prisoner who brings lunch for us to our workplace tells us that those working in the last Jewish plant outside Hasag - Mrs. Mosiewicz' workshop — have arrived at our camp and have been recruited into the workshops of Wirtschaftsabteilung. When I tell our Polish foreman, Adam, he thinks that this is an unusual event and sends me off on a minor errand for him to the Wirtschaftsabteilung office. After ten months I again see Sarah, Pinkus, Roman and the other workers assigned to Mrs. Mosiewcz.

Sarah weeps and says: "Look how thin Jurek is", and I get a lump in my throat. Romek has grown, Pinkus seems tired but otherwise unchanged — he keeps repeating in Yiddish. "Mein Josele, mein Josele." They think I have changed, but I don't ask in what way. Sarah says that I have "zmeznialen" — matured.

For the past ten months, the people from Mrs. Mosiewitcz' workshop have been in contact with a great many customers and so have not lived in isolation from the outside world as we have. On the other hand, they have been separated from the rest of Czestochowa's Jews.

The Maple Tree Behind the Barbed Wire

In many ways things have been better for them than for us, which can be seen by their better clothes, they are healthier than the majority of us at Hasag-Pelcery, but they are pleased to be back with more of us — and we four are happy to be together again.

As usual with the Germans, everything has been planned in advance for how the new arrivals are to be spread round existing workshops for skilled Jewish workers within Wirtschaftabteilung. Some are give new workshops of their own — the old master-tailor, Pinkus Einhorn, is one of those.

The workshops are in the Wirtschaftabteilung's own building, close to the guarded gate between the factory and the Kolonia. As the workers make clothes, underclothes, shoes and other things personal to them living in the Kolonia, the Germans do not want them to be in the camp huts. So in the Wirtschaftabteilungs building are some living quarters behind the workshops - Pinkus, Sarah and Roman are allocated a room of that kind. The room is small, but they have access to a common kitchen, a washroom and two water closets for all the workers — all indoors.

I have never been in the Wirtschaftabteilung building before and am given only a brief spell of time to meet my parents before I have to return to my workplace. But the Baubetrieb also belongs to the Wirtschafteilung and is over-manned, so it is not difficult for me to move to the workshops, all of which happens three weeks later.

To be with Pinkus, Sarah and Roman again is like coming home. To be allowed to move into my parents' room behind the workshops is to me like coming into a palace equipped with sophisticated luxury. To have access to all these comforts which in peacetime we took for granted will never be again be self-evident - I can appreciate them to the full, for I have missed all this for a very long time.

Every newly arrived prisoner is plied with questions. A prison camp isolated from the outside world is seething with eagerness to find out anything that has happened to their vanished relatives and close friends. I have not yet heard mention of any case in which such enquiries led to anyone finding out anything about anyone.

The very next day after her arrival at Hasag, Sarah goes to see the women who have come on the transport from the Lodz ghetto. Sarah knows a lot of people in Lodz, but none of those she speaks to have met or heard anything about her parents.

On the next transport to Hasag-Pelcery are several Jews from Plaszów - they confirm the unlikely rumor about a Sudeten German who saves Jews, tell us his name is Schindler, that he wears civilian clothes and is a member of the National-Socialist party. In the middle of the summer, in July, yet another transport of Jewish prisoners arrives from a camp somewhere near the town of Demblin.

The Maple Tree Behind the Barbed Wire

At the end of October 1944, as another severe winter in camp is approaching, the hitherto largest ever transport of Jewish prisoners arrives from another of the Hasag company's plants which I did not know existed — the plant is Skarzysko-Kamienna, halfway between Warsaw and Czestochowa. They tell us that their camp has been wound up quite calmly. They say the reason for this was that the Soviet front was coming closer. The new prisoners are very numerous and as no new huts are being put up, our camp becomes even more overcrowded. On the same transport are the guards from the prison camp in Skarzysko headed by Oberwerksschutzleiter Bartenschläger. Among their Werkschutz is one Dzierzan and his trained Alsatian dog. Bartenschläger is a major, senior in rank and with more years of service than Klemm. He takes over the command of the Camp Guard.

Oberwerkschutzleiter Bartenschläger is an imposing, rather powerfully built man, taller than average, with thin rimless glasses, dark-blond hair, almost crew-cut and with light brown slightly watery eyes. He is neatly dressed in his tailored uniform and, when it is cold, an elegant uniform greatcoat. Bartenschläger moves lithely, apparently restless, as if constantly striving for excitement, so the authority he undeniably radiates seems unpleasant and frightening. In camp, he often walks around with a loaded pistol in his hand. Rumor has it that on the day of his arrival, after inspecting the camp, he made it known that: "Things need tightening up here, a new order," which he promises to bring about — he considers what exists is slack and he does not like it.

The day after his arrival, Captain Bartenschläger issues his first order — the prisoners' fireplaces are to be destroyed immediately. He personally kicks several over with his black jackboots. The next day a group of prisoners is ordered to remove all the bricks from the area.

After a few days, Barteschläger picks out a woman prisoner - Debora, a pretty young Jewess employed in the kitchen — and with his pistol in his hand he takes her out of the camp. The hut kapo at evening roll call is told by a Werkschutz that Debora has been reported by the chief guard as shot. The prisoners from Skarzysko camp are not surprised. They tell us that Bartenschläger had on previous occasions selected out young women prisoners in the Skarzysko camp and shot them in a nearby forest glade. Various rumours had gone round about what he had done with the prisoners before killing them, but these rumours were unconfirmed — none of the selected women had returned alive to tell them.

Dzierzan is another of the camp guards from Skarzysko. He is a humpbacked, strongly built, rather fat man with a noticeably short neck and unusually long arms, his hands almost coming down to his knees — he seldom says anything and no one has ever seen him smile. Dzierzan has a dog he has trained to answer to the name Mensch - man. When Dzierzan has chosen a victim, he gives the dog the command "Mensch, nimm den Hund" - Man, get that dog. The powerful well-trained dog silently leaps to the attack, rearing on his strong hind legs, snarling and biting until his victim falls, then the dog clamps his great jaws on to the victim's throat and waits for Dzierzan's order. When Dzierzan gives it, which he does sooner or later, the dog bites - Dzierzan's command is the equivalent of a death sentence. Most prisoners are too weak to offer any resistance, and for the Alsatian Mensch, they are easy prey and easy to injure. If he does not succeed in killing the prisoner, Dzierzan finishes him off with a shot, firing one single shot, straight into the prisoner's face, then leaving the body lying on the ground — not even checking whether the person he has shot is dead.

Dzierzan the guard is kind to his dog and praises him after the killing and the young Alsatian leaps round his master, wagging his tail with delight. Dzierzan's dog is really trained to track down escaped prisoners, but no one has succeeded or even attempted to escape from Hasag-Pelcery - there is nowhere to escape to and Dzierzan has found a way of his own to keep the dog alert.

The huge area of prisoners' huts is surrounded by barbed wire fastened to strong concrete posts, an opening in the wire to the factory area, which in its turn is surrounded by a high wall with sharp bits of glass cemented in along the top. Between the factory area and the Kolonia is a gate constantly manned by several guards and which is the only exit. But the prisoners are allowed to walk freely from the huts to the factory area, which is effectively cut off from the outside world. Part of Bartenschläger's "new order" is to limit the prisoners' freedom of movement even more. He issues orders for a barrier to be erected between the huts and the factory — a gate constantly guarded by a Werkschutz. This order is never carried out, for Lüth throws Bartenschläger out of Hasag-Pelcery, though for quite a different reason.

No one could say our old Werkschutz have been accommodating. With iron discipline, they have made sure everything functions, ruthlessly punishing the smallest transgression or the slightest suspicion of a transgression without taking the trouble to investigate what has really happened. However, there has been a certain distorted camp justice which has been fairly predictable.

The camp guards from Skarzysko are more brutal and less predictable. Quite openly and for no reason whatsoever, they maltreat a prisoner and no one knows why. Dzierzan selects his victims to amuse himself and his dog. Bartenschäger makes examples of people, as with his constantly drawn pistol he shoots a passing prisoner to whom for some inexplicable reason he has taken a dislike.

Several of the factory Meister have admitted to their Jewish Vorarbeiter that they dislike the new order. The Skarzysko guards take liberties which upset the work, leaving individual Meisters with no control any longer over which prisoners are to be punished. This affects the running of the factory as prisoners are suddenly absent without warning from their workplaces. But no one intervenes to stop Barthenschläger's new order — until the furniture transport from Skarzysko arrives.

Scarcely a week after the prisoners and their camp guards from Skarzysko have arrived at Hasag, the guards' furniture and other belongings they have not been able to take with them on the passenger train, arrive at Stradom station — the siding to Hasag-Pelcery. Bartenschläger and twenty of his guards file into the hut area, wake up the night shift, who have only two hours earlier gone to bed. Shouts can be heard all over - Raus, raus, schnell, schnell - Dzierzan's dog barks but does not bite, shots are fired, though no one is injured. Although it is already cold outside, the prisoners are not given enough time to dress properly and they are herded off to the station with blows from sticks and set to unload the guards' heavy luggage. Then the guards stand in two lines along the roadside, striking with their sticks the prisoners who have to pass with their heavy packs along the long stretch up to the Kolonia.

It is said that it is our old assistant chief guard - Stiglitz - who together with a German Meister goes to fetch Director Lüth. Lüth arrives in an elegant dark-blue leather jacket with a grey fur collar. He stands for a while on the other side of the camp gateway watching what is happening, chain-smoking all the time as he does when he is indignant. I watch this entire course of events through the workshop window. Lüth takes a puff or two on his cigarette then throws it down, stamps on it and grinds it into the ground and lights another. After a while he sends a Polish fireman to fetch Bartenschläger.

The new chief guard is standing with his feet astride in his smart uniform greatcoat, a stick in his left hand and a drawn pistol in the other. He waves away the Polish fireman, who stands his ground and points at Director Lüth. Lüth waits no longer, but comes through the gate — the guards salute — and goes over to Bartenschläger and says quite calmly but sufficiently loudly for the other Werkschutz and the prisoners to hear what he is saying: "Dies ist keine Kinderstube, Herr Bartenschläger, es ist eine Fabrik. Die Gefangene müssen heute Nacht arbeiten..." — this is no children's nursery, it is a factory — these prisoners have to work tonight. Who has given you permission to wake the night shift? And Lüth goes on without waiting for Bartenschläger to reply. "I must ask you to cease these childish games and instead speak to the Obermeister at our Transportabteilung. He will then arrange the unloading in a smoother and better way than in this unprofessional manner." Bartenschläger is pale but says nothing, and Lüth goes on: "Within my plant, it is not the business of the Werkschutz to see to the transports." He turns on his heel and goes back to the Kolonia. He does not wait, knowing Bartenschläger will comply with his request.

The loads the night shift prisoners are already hauling are carried out to the Kolonia, but without any more beatings from the Skarzysko guards. Then the night shift is allowed to return to their huts. Unloading is completed by prisoners summoned from the Transportabteilung with carts, supervised by their Jewish Vorarbeiter. A fairly passive German Meister looks on, some of the Werkschutz from Skarzysko equally passively staying to supervise that their furniture goes to the right places in the Kolonia.

The next morning, Bartenschläger and other Skarzysko guards are stopped from coming into the factory area. Standing just in front of the big gate, the previous chief guard, Oberwerkschultzleiter Klemm maliciously tells Bartenschläger that this is on the orders of Director Lüth, and that further orders can be found at the factory management office — several prisoners are able to see what happens.

According to the Polish fireman, also standing by the gate, Klemm has said that the management of the Hasag Company has decided that Bartenschläger and other guards from Skarzysko are to be transferred to a place where they are needed more than they are here at Hasag-Pelcery. However, the Polish fireman does not understand much German, so what Klemm actually said to Bartenschläger is not certain. But however it happened — we never need see Bartenschläger or any of the Skarzysko guards again at Hasag-Pelcery. Bartenschläger, with him Dzierzan, his dog Mensch and the other guards from Skarzysko are transferred — though unfortunately to Warta, another of Hasag's smaller plants.

Lüth has great personal authority, which is a help in various situations, but he is also very influential — clearly a few telephone calls to the company head office had been enough.

Although the winter of 1944-1945 is not a severe one, some of the prisoners do not manage that last winter of the war.

The previous already meagre food rations were reduced even further, the bread ration unchanged but the soup even thinner, the weekly handout of margarine or jam ceased altogether. Some of the Germans maintain that they are also short of food, but this is not noticeable.

There is no longer any fuel for the stoves in the huts, which are now heated only by the bodies of the prisoners. The cold and the wind penetrate through the thin wooden walls, to everyone's misery, but most of all those with bunks nearest the walls. A prisoner at Hasag has to count on his workplace as long as he is alive and is not taken to the camp sick bay, but more and more prisoners — long since undernourished and inadequately clothed — find it difficult to cope with outdoor work or in premises now cold through and through. Some give up from undernourishment, others in their exhausted state find it hard to resist what are otherwise banal illnesses, some give up altogether and become Muzelmans - specters who die, perhaps from

The Maple Tree Behind the Barbed Wire

cold and hunger, or maybe from apathy and hopelessness.

We who work in the Wirtschaftsabteilung workshops receive the same food and freeze like all other prisoners, but we can wash indoors, have two communal indoor toilets, and we have some kind of private life.

In the second week of January 1945, unease begins to show among the Germans at Hasag-Pelcery. From misdirected benevolence, Stiglitz has a way of in a calm and uninvolved tone of voice bringing us the most frightening news — perhaps he knows no better. This time he comes to the Wirtschaftteilung to tell us that the whole camp is shortly to be evacuated and we are to be sent to another prison camp, presumably in Germany. He talks about "die schrecklichen Russen" — those terrible Russians causing all these problems. But we do not need to worry, he assures us, there is plenty of time and that they — the Germans - are to take us with them and not hand us over to "die schrecklichen Russen". He says the Germans in the Kolonia have already begun packing.

The Germans pack everything they want to take with them — and that is a great deal — and the prisoners have to help. Large crates are made in the camp carpentry shop, and although we prisoners are ordered to work for fifteen hours a day, we fail to complete all the orders. The Germans coming to our workshops ask when their shoes, shirts, suits, coats and everything else they have ordered will be ready. They take prisoners back to their homes to help with their packing and more prisoners than ever before are let into the Kolonia. A German is allowed to take one prisoner out of Hasag-Pelcery with him for help with his transport. Previously, taking prisoners out of the plant has rarely occurred. The usual strict German order still prevails, but the departure has meant breaking several of the regulations. At the same time, several factory departments is are wound down and some cease altogether.

Early in the morning of January 15th 1945, a long goods train comes into the siding to the factory — those who have seen it say they recognize the much-feared cattle wagons for transporting humans — in the middle of the day the Germans squash 3,000 prisoners into it. It all happens fairly calmly. No Selektion of individual prisoners as in the autumn of 1942, but instead whole groups taken out — apparently at random — everyone in a certain hut or everyone at a workplace. There does not seem to be any significance in how the groups are chosen. We are all to be sent out anyhow, but there are not as many wagons as on the previous transports — in 1942.

The selection however is not a matter of indifference to the prisoners. Many of those taken to the train try to get away, probably in vain for the guards are relentless when a prisoner has already ended up in a group taken out for the transport.

With this first transport go the majority of the prisoners placed in the Maschinenbau. Both the German Meister in the Maschinenbau want the Jewish Vorarbeiter Heniek Hofman, who is much appreciated by everyone, to stay with the six prisoners selected for cleaning up the main hall and packing the tools. Heniek Hofman is relieved, as he wants to stay, but several of his workers from the Maschinenbau appeal to him and say they want to stick together, that they feel safe if he is there. Honiek Hofman declines to stay, goes with his group to the long train and travels in the same goods wagon as his workmates — with the first transport from Hasag.

The train with its human load chuffs off just after three o'clock in the afternoon. Shortly after midnight, another, equally long train with similar wagons arrives, stays all night at Stradom station and waits for its load.

As the train is leaving, I am sitting in the workshop with a pair of light brown trousers over my right knee, sewing on buttons and thinking. Departure from what has become habit is being prepared for us and for the Germans, but the contrast is striking. We are sent away in cattle wagons, not allowed to take with us even the barest necessities, while the Germans take great crates, furniture, even pianos — some perhaps from Jewish homes. The thought of what awaits us fills me with anxiety. We are to be sent away — but to what? I do not even dare think the thought through - I am afraid — very frightened.

Early the next morning embarkation of Jewish prisoners goes on, and on January 16th the second goods train leaves shortly after twelve o'clock with its load of 3,000 prisoners. We in the Wirtschaftsabteilung building do not see the transport. Not until an hour or two after its departure do we hear that Karola's husband has been sent away, but not Karola.

At about four in the afternoon, Rutka comes to our workshop, weeping, to tell us that her father Maurycy, Pinkus' brother, was also on the day's transport. Rutka is now alone; in her profound despair, she accuses Pinkus of not doing enough to save Maurycy. Pinkus does not defend himself. He is miserable, for this is his only brother. Sarah tries to console Rutka, but Rutka is upset, shakes off the hand Sarah has put on her shoulder and runs out of the workshop.

When the war is over, we find out that the train of prisoners that left on January 15th was destined for the Buchenwald concentration camp and those on the train on January 16th were to be divided between the camps in Gross-Rosen and Ravensbrück - all camps in "das Reich".

Many of the Czestochowa Jews die in their new prison camps in Germany, others are sent out on death marches — that happens several months later, when the Allied troops are approaching the western front, but before the British and American troops rescue those still remaining when the German western front collapses in April-May, 1945.

Only a few hundred of the over 6,000 prisoners on these two transports survived, among them Heniek Hofman and Samuel Janowski, who had been sent away from Hasag-Warta on the train on January 15th, 1945. Samuel marries another surviving prisoner from Hasag in Czestochowa - the pretty Marysia Bialek. They both become our closest friends in Sweden - even after all these years, the surviving Hasag prisoners still have a sense of belonging, we have so much in common.

Neither Karola's husband nor Pinkus' brother survive. We who by chance are still at Hagas-Pelcery on the afternoon of February 16th, 1945, after the two prisoner transports had left, fortunate, have enormous luck, which no one could predict.

For once the Germans failed with their thoroughly made plans, but it is also an unusual and therefore unexpected wartime event that is the reason.

The Maple Tree Behind the Barbed Wire

Chosen to Live

In the late afternoon of January 16th, 1945, we hear the rumble of distant detonations. Shortly after, Lolek Taubenblatt, a thin dark-haired prisoner who has been out in town with his Meister, comes back to the camp, tells us that there are Soviet tanks in the suburbs of Czestochowa and that it is at them the Germans are shooting. His Meister has pointed at a burnt-out tank and said it was a Soviet one. Not everyone wants to believe Lolek, but the rumor he is spreading and the shots we hear give us a spark of hope — is it possible? I dare not think any further.

At about eleven that night, Werkschutzleiter Stiglitz comes to the Wirtschaftsabteilung. I have not seen him, but others tell me that he has come to say goodbye.

Many of us in the Wirtschaftsabteilung building stay up all night, speculating and waiting. In our room, we lie down and try to sleep. It is late and it becomes an uneasy night — however, I do manage to go to sleep.

Early the next morning, January 17th, I am woken by shouts and excited voices. I dress quietly and go outside. Some of those who have spent the night there are already outside.

The Wirtschaftsabteilung building is near the entrance to the Kolonia. The gates are wide open, guarded by some Polish firemen simply standing there, apparently not caring who goes out or comes in. I see no German Werkschutz, so ask those nearby and passing prisoners; and they all say the Germans have left during the night, fleeing in panic and leaving behind a lot of food and other things in the Kolonia. Sarah and Pinkus come out to ask what has happened.

I look at the lively traffic in and out of what for us has been a closed gate. Can it be possible that the Germans have left so quickly and not had time to take us — the remaining prisoners at Hasag-Pelcery - with them? I remember what I had heard just before we went to sleep, that Stiglitz had come to say goodbye, and what Lolek had previously said about Soviet tanks in Czestochowa - so it could be true. I ask around whether it is definite that all the Germans have gone. Some reply with happy smiles "yes, all of them", others are in such a hurry they don't even answer.

A cautious expectant joy rises in me. Although all this time I have been hoping something would happen to rescue us, I find it difficult to believe it is happening right now, that this is the moment I have been waiting for, that all the Germans have disappeared and we are still here — free. I had not thought it would happen like this — where are the soldiers who have rescued us?

The Maple Tree Behind the Barbed Wire

We go back to our room to decide undisturbed what we should do. Sarah is practical and starts taking out everything we might need should we leave the camp, but I want to know more and go out again.

The Polish firemen in their blue uniforms with red stripes, one with his brass helmet in his hand, are still at the gate, as they have been ordered — but they seem uncertain. Do they still have to obey German orders? They look bewildered and just stand watching as more and more prisoners pour in and out through the open gates.

The hastily abandoned German houses in the Kolonia are the prisoners' first targets — they are looking for the bare necessities they have gone without for so long. Some come back to camp in peculiar clothes — one in an elegant double-breasted jacket over his prison garb, another in a smart dark-brown leather jacket and his ragged camp trousers. Several are carrying shoes, bedclothes, rugs or foodstuffs. One man on his way back to fetch his starving friends confirms that there is a lot left in the Kolonia. He talks excitedly about lots of margarine, butter, meat, oil — all to be found there — food we have not tasted or even seen for a very long time.

After being malnourished for so long, plagued by hunger and overwhelmed by all this surplus, many prisoners try to eat their fill, stuffing themselves with everything they can get hold of, not least the fat-rich food we have lacked for so long. Several at once get severe diarrhea and fall ill; one dies a day after liberation.

I am less interested in all this back and forth now and realize I just want to get away as soon as possible. At the same time, I feel a surprising sense of loss when I realize this will also mean that I am to be parted from the other prisoners.

Our room behind the workshop, usually so neat and tidy, is in disarray, Sarah, Pinkus and Roman already dressed. They have put on the best they can find from their rather worse-for-the-wear clothes — we want to get back to Czestochowa as soon as possible, to see what is left of what was for so long our home in Aleja Wolnosci 3/5. Everything we possess has been laid out on the beds - I am surprised how much a small room can hold, with its two double bunks along each wall and hardly any free floor-space in between.

Sarah still has her corset with the precious stones sewn into the seams - I don't know if she has taken any out and sold them. Pinkus has his green cloth bag with the life insurances from Winterthur in Switzerland. He reckons they can be turned into money — they are his security in face of this new future. I take my tattered schoolbooks and Roman also takes a few books. We have only small bundles with us as we set off in the direction of the still open gates. A group of prisoners hoping to get back to Czestochowa has gathered there; together with the four of us and a few more who have joined us, we are over thirty people about to start the trek to town.

The Maple Tree Behind the Barbed Wire

One in the group is Mosze Szydlo from the Transportabteilung. He is slightly older than I am, sturdy and dark-haired, and the impression he gives is not only one of toughness but also of reliability. Some of us are appalled when we find Mosze has a gun and says there is a ZOB cell at Hasag-Pelcery, as well as similar cells in the other two Hasag plants in Czestochowa - he refuses to say anything more — we are still uncertain about what might happen. When my unease over any Jew being armed has subsided, I realise that Mosze's gun gives me security — but how has he succeeded in keeping a gun hidden in camp?

Just before nine in the morning of January 17th, 1945, full of dread, we set off on our uncertain trek. Everyone in our group is in fairly decent shape, not too exhausted, a few having managed to acquire some warm clothes from the Kolonia. I had not thought of that, or perhaps had no desire to wear German clothes. To keep warm, I have on several layers of shabby clothes I have had in the camp, two pairs of much-mended socks, and thin-soled brown shoes lined with bits of cardboard to keep out the cold.

As we start off, the January sun has already risen above the horizon, but it is bleak and cold. No one stops us as we leave the camp and the factory.

I think of it as a wonderful warm morning -- which it cannot have been - southeast Poland has a markedly inland climate and mid-January is bitterly cold. But I feel neither the cold, fatigue nor hunger, although I have had nothing that morning except a glass of cold water and a piece of dry bread Sarah has saved and shared out between us.

A still cautious but more and more noticeable sense of relief washes over me as we walk. I begin to realise the significance of what is happening — maybe we have been rescued! Not as I had imagined, so what is happening is not perfect, but all the same — the dream we never dared believe in is about to come true.

We do not know what or whom we are to come across in Czestochowa, or what the town looks like, but the Germans have gone. For reasons we don't comprehend, as if by a miracle, they have suddenly vanished and left us unharmed. I am to be allowed to live, perhaps for many a year to come, to go to an ordinary school, perhaps have children of my own, even be allowed to grow old — life is to go on.

That I am able to go where I like, across fields and along streets, to move freely, that alone is the innermost core of personal freedom. I lengthen my stride and join the small group with Mosze Szydlo and his revolver in the lead.

As we walk through a residential area we are alone in the sunlit but ghostly streets. Not a single human being in sight — only us — the shops along the street are all closed although it is a weekday. All those living there stay indoors, presumably afraid to go out. But we are not afraid — what is there to be afraid of?

The Maple Tree Behind the Barbed Wire

Individual prisoners say goodbye and leave our group; I am feeling melancholy. Do we really have to part? I don't say so aloud, for I realise that would be meaningless, would probably sound foolish, but I think those who just quickly say goodbye and leave the group just like that are emotionally cold. We have been through difficult times together, so can't we go on building up new lives together? I have spent almost six years of my youth being shut in, but also with a growing fellowship with those shut in with me, and I am plagued by an unexpected anguish faced with leaving this deceptive security the fellowship of the persecuted produces. But I say nothing, reluctant even to let anyone know what I am thinking.

We are nearing the town centre and are still about twenty prisoners. There are now a few people around in the streets, and they gaze at us in amazement as we stride purposefully along. They must be thinking how thin and pale we are and how shabby our clothes are — that is when I take off my metal number plate and put in my pocket.

We pass men in civilian clothes wearing red and white armbands - Poland's national colors - on their upper arms. They are in pairs and are the beginnings of the new militia - the four militiamen in the two patrols I have seen hitherto are all wearing leather jackets. They are presumably armed, perhaps with handguns under their clothing; despite this, it seems unsafe that no soldiers, not even uniformed police, are to be seen on the streets.

Aleja Wolnosci 3/5 looks just as I remember it when we were moved to the large ghetto — that seems decades ago. We ring the caretaker's doorbell on the ground floor and the caretaker's wife opens. She has aged, but we recognize her — she looks terrified, repeatedly and rapidly crossing herself - Jesus Maria, Jesus, Maria - Boze kochany, ja nic nie wiem - My God, I know nothing, she says before we have time to ask. For some reason she is afraid of talking to us, that is clear - as if we were ghosts, and we were, really. When Sarah asks, she finally tells us that no one lives in our old apartment on the first floor up in the front building facing the street, then she closes the door and I hear agitated voices behind it.

We go upstairs through the kitchen entrance, try the door to our apartment — it is closed and no one opens when we first knock quietly, then thump harder. We ring the bell of our Polish neighbors — the same old nameplate that had been on their door before we moved is still there. Mrs. Górska opens and looks at us standing there at her door in our shabby clothes. She is clearly surprised and does not ask us to come in, but is not as speechless as the caretaker's wife.

The Maple Tree Behind the Barbed Wire

That's right, says Mrs. Górski, no one lives in your apartment. There is a restaurant for officers and civilian German employees inside. It is usually rather messy until late at night, she adds.

We go down into the courtyard, then up through the main entrance, but that door is also locked and no one answers when we ring the bell. But we must get in - where else can we go? This is our old apartment and no one is living in it. My skill at opening locked doors comes in handy, though it is not as easy as it had been when I was clearing up in the large ghetto — the door is strong or I have not the same energy, but in the end it works.

We feel at home in our old apartment, although the walls in all the rooms have been papered in pastel colors. The only furniture in it are close rows of tables painted black, the majority with white cloths on them, and chairs of the same kind of wood with pale brown comfortable upholstery — the chairs and tables look as if they are all ready for guests, and they fill all the rooms except our old workshop.

The door to what had been the workshop is closed, but it is easy to break down. It is now full of wooden shelves, on them in good order innumerable bottles of alcoholic drinks, a great many bottles of vodka, but also rum, cognac and various sorts of wine, mostly red wine — our workshop has been turned into a well-supplied store of spirits.

It must be worth a fortune. But Pinkus says we cannot stay and we must leave at once for a lot of people are sure to know what is in the apartment, and there will be fights when they try to get at the drink, so it would be dangerous to stay. We get ready to leave the apartment, although we don't know where to go. I think taking the risk and staying would solve many of our problems. We could keep ourselves going for quite a time, get hold of food, clothes and the furniture we need in exchange for whatever valuables the Germans have left behind when they fled, and no one owns. But even I realise that would involve risks perhaps not worth taking.

Pinkus looks doubtful when Sarah takes three bottles of cognac with her; she has put them into a paper bag she found in the store. But Sarah forestalls him, saying: "We have no money — we must have something to exchange for food and houseroom." We leave the apartment with its broken door, then are again back in Aleja Wolnosci and rather aimlessly continuing along Second Aleja.

Sarah asks a militiaman with his red and white armband if he knows of anywhere we can stay the night. He looks apologetically at us, asks us where we have come from, then consults a colleague and says in friendly tones that at Garibaldi Street 19 there is an office block the militia have requisitioned for refugees and Jews from Hasag.

It is afternoon and there are more people in the streets now. We walk on through the town to Garibaldi Street. It is true, there is a building there for homeless refugees and we are allotted two rooms with a sofa bed — it is almost like being back in the camp again. We meet other

The Maple Tree Behind the Barbed Wire

prisoners who have been directed to the same building. They tell us what has happened and why the Germans had fled during the night.

A number of Soviet armored vehicles, heavy tanks with no infantry support, have been far behind the retreating German front and have made an unexpected and unusually forceful breakthrough. The Soviet armored unit is said to be still by one of the bridges across the River Warta. The Germans were afraid their retreat might be cut off and have fled headlong from Czestochowa and our camp — they had had to leave most things behind, just as they had previously made us do. But there are only thirteen tanks responsible for the breakthrough and so far no troops have arrived behind them. They are still by the bridge over the Warta, in a semi-circle, their guns turned outwards and they are not allowing anyone to come anywhere near.

They also tell us that the militiamen are mostly from the left-wing guerilla GL - the People's Army. When the Germans had fled, the guerillas had left the forests round Koniecpol and come into Czestochowa, among them some Jews from the remnants of the ZOB groups which for almost a year have been part of the Hanysch unit within Gwardia Ludowa. Among the militiamen are also some from socialist and communist underground movements in Czestochowa; they have contacts with the advancing Soviet army and are organizing a new police and security service. The blue-clad Polish policemen have had their authority taken away for collaborating with the Germans and their activities during the war are to be investigated. The militia want people to report to them if they see any Germans who have stayed in Czestochowa, or any collaborators. The militia has arranged for food, clothing and bedclothes in the building in Garibaldi Street. What we need can be taken from the common store on the ground floor, but there is nothing but the barest necessities there. The Armja Krajowa loyal to the government in exile are still in the forests.

We are aware that a few militiamen with hand guns cannot stop the Germans should they return to Czestochowa, and several people in the building in Garibaldi Street are uneasy about this. But I am beginning to get used to the idea that the impossible has happened and I begin to think about the future. By then it is evening and we arrange for the night with blankets from the store on the ground floor.

I wake early the next morning, but stay lying there for a while in order to think and plan for my first day of freedom. I dress and, despite Sarah's protests, set out to take a look at the Soviet tank unit that has frightened away the Germans and saved us. On the way, I pass a tank — burnt out — otherwise there is no sign of any military activity.

The Maple Tree Behind the Barbed Wire

A crowd has gathered by the eastern abutment of the bridge across that narrow river, and there, in front of us in a semi-circle, their guns turned outwards, is a group of blotchy dark-green Soviet tanks. I had no idea a tank could be so large; they are huge, but there are not many.

The hatches are open and we see several Soviet soldiers standing around smoking, others walking round their tanks. They look warlike in their black hide helmets with bulging black rubber ear-protectors, but they do not behave in a warlike manner, on the contrary. One of them has climbed down from his tank and he waves at the crowd gathered in the street.

Gratitude to these soldiers and their monster tanks overwhelms me — it is good they have guns, ammunition and look warlike, for that was what had frightened the Germans away. If their breakthrough had come a day later, or had not penetrated so far behind the German front, we would have been taken away on that train already standing waiting at the station and we would still have been in German hands, at their discretion — left to the mercy of Dzierzan and his dog, to Bartenschläger, or other German guards wherever we would have been taken to. Those places and guards now seem tremendously distant.

They have rescued us, these Soviet soldiers in their black leather helmets, men, perhaps also women, whom I have never met before and will perhaps never see again. They and their huge armored vehicles are standing there right in front of me and have saved us with their surprise breakthrough. They have done it, and no others.

I dearly want to go over and explain what they have done for us, what a near thing it has been, how grateful we are, shake hands — as I had done in my imagination. But they do not want anyone to come anywhere near them — heavy armor is excellent for a breakthrough and a swift advance, but vulnerable with no infantry backing. They must see we are friendly-minded, but they can take no risks. They have their terrifying tanks, as large as a smallish house, and their menacing guns, but the soldiers are few and can only wait until the Soviet infantry arrives to occupy Czestochowa.

An elderly woman with a black kerchief over her head — she has been standing in the square for a long time — tells me that the commander of the armored unit, a young officer had come over to the civilians in the square, shaken hands and in broken German asked some questions. He had two of his soldiers with him, though they had stood at a distance behind him. He wanted to know if there were any German troops left in Czestochowa. A man standing listening nearby maintains that the Soviet officer had said that the troops' commander had been killed in one of the tanks the Germans had succeeded in setting on fire. The woman in the black kerchief and others who had long been there deny that the officer had said that — in the discussion that followed, these varying opinions on what the Soviet officer had said were blamed on that he spoke such bad German.

It was good that I was allowed to see them, our saviours and their huge tanks, if only at a distance. They are not anonymous to me; they have faces, although I have seen them only at a distance. For regardless of what the aim of the breakthrough had been, whether it had been that kind of senseless advance that sometimes occurs war, or a planned, unusually daring breakthrough to protect the bridge across the Warta, these young men had saved me and the other five thousand the Germans had not had time to take with them when these soldiers in their enormous tanks had broken through the German front, driven up to Czestochowa and into the proximity of our camp.

Not Americans, as I had imagined, nor British troops, nor the government-in-exile in London with General Sikorski - it became these young Soviet soldiers who had done it. Several of them in tanks that were burnt out, perhaps even their commander, had sacrificed their lives for this risky advance, but they had saved all of us left in Hasag. They had not come riding on white chargers, nor did they shake hands, nor hand out chocolate, talk or ask questions. But these soldiers, who do not even want to talk to us, who do not want our thanks, it is they who work the miracle we have all hoped for have been unable to imagine how it would happen — and they have done so at the very last moment.

When the infantry and supply troops arrive two days later and re-fuel the armored vehicles, they leave to go on harrying the retreating German army, perhaps rescuing more prisoners in other camps.

When I get back to Garibaldi Street, it is nearly midday. Sarah has managed to get together a lunch and food on the table. Sarah says that Roman is somewhere with neighbors, and she is worried about Pinkus.

My otherwise vigorous father is slumped on a chair with his head on one side, staring at the cloth Sarah has put on the table, presumably without him seeing anything. Sarah says he has been there all morning while I have been out. Why have I been away so long? I am also worried and try to speak to him - Pinkus slowly raises his eyes and looks at me, smiles rather harassedly, and says: "Yes, yes, Josele", but then stays sitting in the same position.

He has been living under constant pressure for several years, putting everything he has into helping his wife and two boys survive, into helping his employees, his remaining relatives. He has been as strong as a granite rock, outwardly calm, never giving way, always giving us a feeling of safety — and we have learnt to take it for granted. Now when rescue has come, reducing demands on him and the tension lessening, he is as if in an apathetic torpor. It is true there is a lot to do, but we are no longer threatened, and now he has no strength left, nothing more to give to solve the new and difficult problems of everyday life. Now Sarah - I too, perhaps, will have to take the decisions.

Nothing much happens for the rest of that first day after our liberation. We have no energy to join in on the hectic szabrowanie as a little compensation for everything we have lost.

To us — until recently prisoners — and all others who have been plundered by the war and are now returning empty-handed to Czestochowa, this is a period when we are fully occupied acquiring somewhere to live, furniture to make it habitable, clothes, food, cooking vessels, cutlery, suitcases, everything needed to live a more or less normal life. We who have been in camp have no money to trade with, so we have in some other way to acquire what is most necessary. A new expression is created to describe this hectic activity — szabrowac.

Szabrowac in our situation is nothing reprehensible, not plundering, or stealing something belonging to someone else. The Germans have taken everything we possessed, have stripped us bare and we who have survived have nothing left — except our mangled lives. In this situation, taking something you need which the Germans have left behind is legitimate and reasonable. But I - undoubtedly the most appropriate one of our family to acquire some of all the things we need — cannot bring myself to do it. Nor does anyone make such demands on me, but I am aware of our needs and the possibilities, so feel pitiful and inadequate for not contributing.

Instead Sarah goes to Mrs. Plowecka, and is told that it is all right to come and collect all the things we have asked them to store for us — there are some honest people, Sarah says with relief.

But all I can think about is getting myself a proper education. Occupied as I am by this, or perhaps using it as an excuse, I contribute nothing to equipping our home. Instead I go round various schools to find out if they have opened again, whether I can register with them, but all the schools I go to are closed. Towards evening I go down into the clothing store in Garibaldi Street, find an almost unused, loosely fitting soft suède jacket in a light dull brown color, which is to be my main garment for a long time ahead, and a pair of shoes with thicker soles than the worn-out ones I had brought with me from Hasag.

On January 19th, two days after our liberation, we make another attempt to return to our old apartment — we ought not to wait too long or someone else might move in. Sarah makes sure we take blankets and bedclothes from Garibaldi Street, the little we had brought from Hasag, and Sarah's three bottles of cognac. We have no problems carrying everything we possess as we again set off for Aleja Wolnosci 3/5. We go in through the street entrance and up the wide stairs. The door to our apartment is just as we had left it, but the rooms are not so clean and neat as they had been two days ago. Some wild partying must have been going on there, for all the drink has gone.

Sarah at once starts cleaning up, Roman and I helping — we are worried about Pinkus. Sarah's anxiety is so great she speaks sharply to Pinkus and that helps. Pinkus begins to haul himself out of his apathy, hunting out his cloth bag with the life insurances and asking Sarah how things had gone on her visit to Mrs. Plowecka. He says we ought to give her some of things they have kept for us as a reward, perhaps one or two pictures, some cloth.

That same afternoon, Sarah and I collect our old pictures, two of Sarah's best tablecloths, the small porcelain figures that had adorned our home before the war and the two small green rugs that as long as I can remember have always been beside my parents' beds. We have to go several times to bring back all Pinkus' cloth — not everyone has tried to profit from our difficult situation during the war. Mrs. Plowecka does not want to keep any of our valuables, for she thinks our need is greater. She says they understand how important it is for us to have in our home the objects that had adorned it before the war, and that Pinkus may need all his cloth.

My parents were to take several of these things with them when they emigrate to Canada three years later. Some of them are still in Roman's home in Burlington and in our home in Danderyd.

Not until the next day, January 20th, do I see the first Soviet soldiers at close quarters.

In the middle of the third day of my hopeless, far too premature search for a school that is functioning, I see a camouflaged military vehicle — no larger than a German Volkswagen - it stops at the beginning of Second Aleja. An officer gets out of the rear door, wearing a thick grey-green military great coat with four small stars on the red shoulder-flaps. A soldier stays in the car, neither of them in battle gear. The officer looks round before striding across the wide street towards the entrance of the nearest building — he is quite tall, seems young and has on long uniform trousers and low black shoes.

I hesitate for a moment, but he seems relaxed and inoffensive and I don't want to miss this opportunity either — so I take the few steps necessary to get in his way. With my hands open slightly away from my body, the palms facing him to show I am unarmed, I slowly say one of the few words I know in Russian - dobryj den, good-day — then go on, just as slowly and over-explicitly in Polish: "Mysmy dlugo na was czekali" — we have waited for you for a long time. He seems neither dismissive nor surprised, but is clearly in a hurry. I think he smiles as he walks past me and says something in Russian I don't understand, then pats me on my right shoulder — he is wearing thick green woolen gloves — and disappears through the entrance. The car and driver stay where they are in the street.

Not until that moment, as with my own eyes I have seen a Soviet soldier not in battle gear, do I feel safe - Soviet troops are here in Czestochowa. We must be quite a bit behind the front, so the Germans cannot come back. At that moment — to me — the war is at last over.

I know there is still a front with soldiers fighting, but to me the most important event of the war has already occurred. May I be forgiven, but I am only vaguely interested in Marshall Ivan Konev's 1st Ukrainian front advancing on Leipzig - home of Captain Degenhardt and our green German police — or Marshall Gregorij Sjukov's 1st White Russian front starting its 170 kilometers wide wave of attack from its bridgehead by the River Oder. I think that is good, but to me the most important thing is not that over 1.5 million Soviet soldiers, 4,000 tanks, 7,000 planes, 16,000 artillery pieces, innumerable caterpillar-track gun carriages, armored cars and mortars are beginning the offensive that is to end in Berlin. I don't even think it particularly exciting when over 300,000 German soldiers surrender to American, British and French troops in the Ruhr area. May I be forgiven, but to me the minor detail above all else in this world war that is being fought on four continents is that the town of Czestochowa with our camp has been captured by Soviet troops, and those of us still at Hasag have been saved. May I be forgiven, but I am only vaguely interested in what is happening on the fronts in Europe and Asia, but instead am overwhelmed by the intoxicating feeling of being allowed to move freely, to go wherever I want to, at last able to do what in the summer of 1942, from the bay window in Aleja 14 I saw other people doing, and which I have so fervently longed to do — to be allowed to stroll down a street.

It is rather strange that you have to go through a long period of being shut in, the defiant hope and daydreams of those condemned to death, to be able to appreciate what is perfectly obvious to most people — to be able to move freely, not to be shut in. To me, this is not something obvious. To me it is always to be an inestimable privilege.

I realise I am being selfish in my still unclouded happiness — for we are so few that have been saved. Of all the approximately 5,000 saved at Hasag in Czestochowa, about 2,300 are Jews from other towns and camps in Poland, who were evacuated to the large ghetto in Czestochowa established in 1942, or transferred to the Hasag prison camp as the Soviet army advanced. Only 2,718 survived out of Czestochowa's 39,000 Jews - and yet people say we were lucky.

The Maple Tree Behind the Barbed Wire

The remaining prisoners in our camp saved that January 17th, 1945, by an unusually early stage of a local collapse of the German army, are in relatively good shape. The Germans have not had time to take us with them on their notorious death marches with no food in the cold. We escape having to go through the last weeks of other camps when prisoners die of starvation or are indiscriminately murdered.

After the war, by those who experienced other camps, Hasag-Pelcery came to be known as Hasag-Zdruj - Hasag-Brunn(Well) - and the macabre comparisons made in these contexts are perhaps reasonable. The miraculous rescue in January 1945 of an only partly evacuated concentration camp in which the prisoners were not too bad a way — in all this insanity, with hindsight makes it reasonable to call our camp Hasag-Brunn.

I myself am also a privileged person among the privileged, chosen to live and also granted after liberation not having to suffer the loneliness that tormented the vast majority of Jews who survived the War of Extermination. There must be more, but I know of only two other remaining Jewish core families who survived in German-occupied Poland. One of those is Toska Roller and her family, whom I am shortly to meet.

I am one of the few by chance chosen to live, but I am also changed and damaged, like all other Jews in the hands of the Germans during the one thousand one hundred and fifty-three long days and nights of the Second World War. For five years and four months, I was condemned to death and went through how that sentence was carried out on other Jews all round me, methodically and icily coldly, with not a trace of regret. All of us Jews who found ourselves in the 300 German prison camps, just as are all those who tried to hide themselves with false identities on the "Aryan" side, are severely spiritually damaged "in their souls". After the liberation, we were simply let out and had to manage as best we could. No one told us to be careful when you start eating after lengthy starvation; there is no time for any therapy or other forms of sophisticated help — there is a war on.

A few decades later, psychologists and psychiatrists are to begin to become interested in how badly damaged we were, to study and describe — as if they had made an astonishing discovery. But even for us it takes a long time before old memories and new ideas declare themselves.

Actually it is wrong when I write that to me the war ended in January 1945 when the Germans fled, or when three days later somewhere behind the front I exchanged a few words with a Soviet officer in long trousers and low shoes. For us, the war did not even end on May 7th, 1945, when General Alfred Jodl signed the

The Maple Tree Behind the Barbed Wire

unconditional surrender, or on September 2nd, 1945, when the Japanese capitulated.

For we, "the Chosen," have to live with our memories. Perhaps what is most unexpected is that these memories crowd in with increased strength after fifty years have passed. One reason is that we know that our days are soon at an end, that for each week that passes there are fewer people left who can testify. So in our old age we feel a need to produce our testimony, which we hope will be difficult to deny. Some do it by writing a book, others by talking on the radio or television, some by giving lectures in schools — children may remember it longest.

I hope that when all of us who survived the Holocaust have gone, there will still be people who will stand up and say - I have seen one of them, I have heard one of them and I believe what they have said.

CHAPTER VI

AFTER THE WAR

Schooling

A week has gone by since our liberation. A few days ago I had decided to aim for Traugutt's second state gymnasium. Before the war it had been considered the leading school for boys in Czestochowa. Once upon a time, it had been Sarah's dream that her sons should go to that school, and when I was in the concentration camp, that had been in my mind as I worked on my schoolbooks. Traugutt's gymnasium is still there, but the only person I see on my daily visits is the school caretaker — a middle-aged man, imposing and authoritative, but kindly under the surface — just as a good caretaker in a good school in Poland should be.

My polite but persistent daily visits in the end arouse the school caretaker's sympathies. As before, he stresses that the school has not yet opened, that I cannot be registered, but he will nevertheless let me in to see the teacher preparing for the re-opening and at last I am able to see the almost empty school from the inside.

The fact that the premises of this much coveted temple of learning of mine are shabby — like most buildings in the previous Generalguvernement, except those used by the Germans themselves — does go to that school, and when I was in the concentration camp, that had been in my mind as I worked on my school books. Traugutt's gymnasium is still there, but the only person I see on my daily visits is the school caretaker — a middle-aged man, imposing and authoritative, but kindly under the surface — just as a good caretaker in a good school in Poland should be.

My polite but persistent daily visits in the end arouse the school caretaker's sympathies. As before, he stresses that the school has not yet once elegant but now shabby suit, a white not very well ironed shirt and a grey tie. He looks serious, but friendly.

The first schoolteacher I meet after the war looks wearily though perhaps a little curiously at me. He does not introduce himself, but says he is a teacher of mathematics and this is the office of the future rector, though no one has yet been appointed. He is pleased to see my eagerness to learn. "That's not particularly common these days," he adds. But I should cool down, for they will tell me when the school is reopened and the registration of pupils begins.

The Maple Tree Behind the Barbed Wire

When I ask him, he looks at my marks and is clearly surprised to see the leaving certificate from my class in the Jewish gymnasium. But I am more interested in his opinion of the more informal handwritten certificates from three years of teaching on the secret courses. This elderly teacher says there are sure to be many with certificates from various informal courses — and in his opinion, marks that are so complete and signed by such competent teachers as mine will be approved. I may come back, but should not do so for at least a week — it takes time to assemble a staff, sufficient numbers of pupils and to organise the teaching.

On my way out, I meet the school caretaker. He is waiting for me at the school gate and wants to know what the result of our conversation has been.

Traugutt's second state gymnasium opens about a week later with plenty of pupils and excellent teachers.

Anyone in Poland hoping for further education after six years in elementary school, may go on to a four-year gymnasium, and from there on to a two-year lyceum, then take the student exam. When the school opened my marks from three years of secret courses were approved - I am allowed to start in the first year lyceum class. However, pupils who have not taken part in the school's own courses are informed that the extent of hat we know will be monitored in connection with the ordinary teaching, and that moves may be necessary.

On my first school day after the war, January 31st, 1945, I find myself in class wearing the light-brown suède jacket I had found in the store in Garibaldi Street, and thick grey trousers — very badly dressed in comparison with my classmates. The school day starts with a morning prayer. Like all the others, I stand up, but say nothing, for I do not know the Catholic prayer and anyhow it is not my prayer. After that, our class supervisor starts the first roll call.

At roll call, details lacking in the register of pupils are to be supplied, among them what is still obligatory in Poland, information on your faith. The majority of pupils are Catholics, one Protestant, and when my turn comes, the teacher says aloud as he fills that in - Roman Catholic. No, I protest in a loud clear voice, "wyznanie mojzeszowe" - I am of the Mosaic faith. For a brief moment the teacher is speechless, then pulls himself together and enters my faith into the register, which means one of his pupils is a Jew. Many of the others look at me with both curiosity and doubt in their eyes, but I don't care that they are staring, or what my future school friends think about having a Jew in their class.

To me, a period of a hermit-like existence now begins as I live in a kind of self-imposed isolation. I cannot avoid meeting people, but am not particularly polite when I do and quickly try to put an end to every

The Maple Tree Behind the Barbed Wire

conversation, at home as well. My parents are indulgent, perhaps even sympathetic as without any noticeable awareness of my surroundings, I bury myself in schoolwork, my only interest school and my teachers.

I do not sleep much, eat quickly when it suits me, may get up to work at my books in the middle of the night, then go back to bed for a while in the morning before going off to school. Sarah is there all the time, quietly and considerately offering any practical assistance without my having to ask her. Her patience is endless, although she is trying to build up an enterprise of her own at the same time.

My teachers notice my knowledge is uneven, but in some subjects I am obviously considerably better than the rest of the class. I am one of those our class supervisor calls into his little office for a solo talk — that is when I first tell him about my lonely plodding through old school books in the ghetto and the prison camp. At his request the next day I take the schoolbooks I had had in the Small Ghetto and the concentration camp with me to school. He quickly looks through the tattered pages, full of underlining's' notes and my own comments — all in pencil — then after a few questions says he will come back to me.

As the teachers at Traugutt's gymnasium had predicted, quite a number of pupils are transferred to other classes once there has been time to assess the extent of what they know, the majority transferred having to move down to a lower class. I am again called into the office and am told that the teachers are agreed that I have better knowledge than the average in my class and I am asked whether I would like to move up to the second year of the lyceum. The teacher adds that it may be hard for me, as my work is so uneven — and did I want time to think it over? I need no time for that, and the very next day, a week after the beginning of term, I move into the school leaving class.

In this new class there is less fuss at morning roll call when I happen to mention I am of the Mosaic faith. Rumor has already gone around that one of the pupils in the lycée is a Jew.

Before the war, Traugutt's gymnasium had been a school for boys. The new education authority has decided to accept pupils regardless of gender, so we have a mixed class — mostly boys, but among the pupils are a few girls. During break after the third lesson, I happen to be alone by the blackboard and a girl comes over to me. She is pretty, noticeably well groomed, her blond hair carefully done, and she limps slightly. She seems rather shy, but also purposeful — her name is Marysia. I see that Marysia does not really know how to start the conversation and I help her. In the end Marysia asks me tentatively and in a singing southern Polish Lwow dialect, whether after moving up to her class I have the necessary textbooks. Then she looks straight at me and asks quite clearly, straight out, if I would like to do my homework with her.

The Maple Tree Behind the Barbed Wire

I have no desire or plans to become involved in mixing with my classmates - I have not come to school for that, but I am flattered by this open and unexpected invitation from a pretty girl. Why just me? But my long slumbering, though by no means enfeebled male vanity is the only natural explanation for why she was interested in me as a man — it could not be anything else.

In future, Marysia and I meet, not particularly often but fairly regularly, several times a week. We may go to the cinema, or to one of the newly opened still rather shabby tea-shops with their meagre choice of pastries and hot and cold drinks, or perhaps we just talk during breaks, on walks, or on one of the green benches again put out when spring comes on Second Avenue's wide centre promenade.

I find that Marysia Lewicka is a thoughtful, wise young lady, her presence always pleasing and she finds it easy to keep an interesting conversation going, so I am never bored in her company, not even when we are both silent. After a while Marysia gives me a feeling of a quiet, equable and infectiously pleasant well being, but I also sense a sorrowfulness beneath her light-hearted surface. Very quickly after her first resolute approach, my attitude changes and I realise Marysia is a serious-minded but also open person, who for some reason feels genuine sympathy for me, which I also reciprocate.

Despite this serious note, our conversations are fairly superficial. I have told her some things about myself but Marysia never says anything about herself. Over the almost three months we have known each other, she has not been to our still not particularly well-ordered home and she has never invited me back to hers, or told her parents — though during our conversations it has appeared that they exist. But that does not worry me. I am not that inquisitive and have not asked.

Moving up into the leaving class is a challenge, and I am stimulated by my success into doing nothing but chasing after the highest marks. Whenever I am not sleeping or eating, I spend all my time at school or at my desk at home with textbooks in a state of disorder only I can keep track of; I have no other needs.

My father Pinkus is marked forever by his experiences, by the unbroken chain of demands he has made on himself and the constant tension he must have lived under during the long war, but he has recovered from his semi-torpor. Pinkus is one of the oldest, perhaps the oldest survivor of the Czestochowa ghetto and Hasag prison camp. Although he is over sixty, Pinkus is trying to build up a new professional life for himself, but it is difficult to find the right associates, acquire the necessary aids, cloth, accessories, and customers. I realise Sarah is feeling rather insecure and feels the consequences — she starts up a practice and a dental technical laboratory in our home.

The Maple Tree Behind the Barbed Wire

Sarah has the necessary training and the formal qualifications, and she has made sure that they still apply. Dental technicians in Poland must have authorization to practice their profession, but they also have the right to open their own laboratory and a practice for patients. Sarah has not worked in her profession for over twenty years and lacks experience of new methods of treatment and modern aids. So she installs a dental technician who had qualified just before the outbreak of war and together the two of them open a laboratory and a practice, Sarah managing it; it is also Sarah who visits and finds potential customers. She goes out early, her pleasant manner and attitude incurring respect, particularly towards the town dentists, so she easily recruits customers, and her business grows. Sarah also succeeds in conjuring up the necessary equipment, aids and materials a dental technician requires - which helps in the competition - not all dental technicians are successful at that.

Sarah soon learns the new methods. I can see that she enjoys her newly won professional independence, but that doesn't stop her from giving Pinkus, Roman and me the same affectionate and what is for us comfortable basic care. We three take it for granted, which is of course neither right nor even reasonable, but Sarah is like that and we are like that — three "male chauvinist pigs". Here is an example:

One Sunday I happen to be having lunch — or as it is called in Poland -- second breakfast — together with my parents. Roman is not at home. Pinkus loves eggs and can eat several for lunch. It is Sarah who takes four eggs, boiled for five minutes and still hot, out of the big glass bowl in the middle of the table, shells them and hands them to Pinkus. He munches up an egg in a flash. After the third, Pinkus says: "No more, thank you", but Sarah starts shelling another newly boiled egg. Pinkus says again: "Sarah, I said I didn't want any more." But Sarah goes on shelling, and after a while says quietly: "It's for me". With his embarrassed smile, Pinkus has the grace to show he is ashamed — all three of us are really spoilt male chauvinist pigs.

Pinkus also succeeds with his workshop, employing a few assistants, though not so many as he used to have in his flourishing business before the war. He does not advertise, yet customers come once the rumor gets around that Einhorn is alive and has reopened his workshop — his good reputation means that increasing numbers want to have a suit made by the old master-tailor. The cloth kept during the war at Mrs. Plowecka's is not plentiful but Pinkus manages to buy up more, though not as good quality as his prewar stock. The business grows although Pinkus does not want it to — he says he doesn't know if we are to stay in Poland.

To me, any implication of that kind is frightening and threatens my new existence. I have no intention of moving from Poland. I wish to stay where I am. I have already begun to build up my future. One forced departure is enough and I don't want another — even voluntary.

When the subject is brought up again, I say quite definitely I do not wish to leave and start again in another country. I have my whole future staked out in Poland - student exam, university — though I don't yet know which subject I want to read or what I want to be. I find it hard to choose and do not want to be distracted by any talk about leaving the country. To my annoyance and dismay, a great many other Jews are planning to leave the country — that worries me.

In the autumn of 1945, there are 2,167 Jews in Czestochowa - some have survived the war in Poland, others have come back from the Soviet Union, some are school friends from the Jewish or Axer's gymnasium, some from my own or an adjoining class. I start going to their meetings, if only rarely at first. I realise the majority are thinking of leaving Poland and others already have advanced plans to do so. Some want to go to Palestine, others to the United States, Canada, Australia or South America - depending on where they have relatives or acquaintances — several just want to leave but don't know where to go. Many think that we Jews have no future in Poland, others want to leave this country in which they had previously had parents, siblings and large families, and where they are now alone — for them it is like living in a large cemetery. Some think that Soviet communism will take over Poland and they don't want to live in a communist country, many bring up the way the Polish population has behaved towards us during the war during the period of the ghetto and the Holocaust when frighteningly many spontaneously expressed their sympathies for the German extermination Aktions, a few busily informed on Jews, and the great majority were passive, although some brave Poles dared to help us although that entailed punishment.

These recurring discussions give rise to an unpleasant feeling in me but do not affect my profound conviction that I shall not leave the country — under any circumstances. I say so over and over again to my parents. After a while the subject is dropped at home, at least when I am present. I also notice that it is far from all Jews who want to leave Poland. Among those intending to stay are Heiniek Ufner, who shared my desk at school, and Sevek Grindman, though they do sometimes waver in their conviction.

Among others from our old Class IIB at the Jewish gymnasium to survive the war are Bronka Mass and Hanka Bugajer - the two beauties in the class. But Hanka is living under a false name in Saska Kempa - a suburb of Warsaw. She has survived with false papers on the Aryan side, refusing to admit to being a Jewess, and has no contact with any of us — the instinctive terror of being recognized as Jewish is still deep in those with false papers who have managed to survive. Różyczka Glowinska from our class is also alive - I have not met her — and it is said that Pola Szlezynger has survived in Belgium.

The Maple Tree Behind the Barbed Wire

That is all I know — not many from a large lively class of a young age in which relatively more Jews survived than in any other age group. Other classmates of mine whom I knew so well, whom I liked and with whom I felt great fellowship, have gone. But I don't really give much thought to that, which is perhaps just as well.

One day towards the end of April, Marysia Lewicka says I have been invited by her parents to visit them on the following Thursday - she makes this out to be a major event, which I think is an exaggeration. On the day, a cloudy but warm spring day, when we go to her home, Marysia is unusually composed and serious — she seems tense.

The Lewicki family live in a small two-roomed and kitchen apartment on the ground floor of an old building on Aleja Kosciuszki, cramped but pleasant. I am offered very strong tea, a freshly made apple-cake with whipped cream, and I meet Marysia's parents.

Mr. and Mrs. Lewicki are sympathetic, pleasant people. It can be heard from their speech that they come from Lwów - easy to recognize from the pleasing singsong dialect which with some success I had tried to learn. The atmosphere in this cultivated home is good, they are widely read and find it easy to talk and they are clearly interested in talking to me about my parents. But I notice they seem slightly bothered — as if wanting to say more, but do not. My visit to their home is a brief one.

Marysia comes halfway back home with me. She asks me what I thought of her parents, then whether I had noticed anything special. I tell her I think her parents are very sympathetic people, otherwise I had not noticed anything in particular. Marysia stops, looks round at me and says: "But don't you understand?" "No, what am I supposed to understand?" "We are Jews!" Marysia has difficulty in getting it out, then once she has said it, she looks troubled. I am astonished. Why hasn't she ever told me so on one of the many occasions we have met.

I am profoundly distressed and feel sorry for this nice family. Several months after the war they are still living in their self-imposed lie, unable to dare admit their suppressed identity. What suffering it must be to lose your identity, not to be able to recognize who you are. I was right during the war to refuse to save myself over on the Aryan side, and I am pleased Roman didn't stay there long. The price Jews have to pay for surviving on the other, the "Aryan" side is terrifyingly high. But it turns out there are Jews in Poland who even today live with this lie. The Lewicki family members are not to do that. After a while they revert to their old Jewish identity and adopt their family name - Roller. Marysia's name is Toska and her father goes back to his pre-war profession. He had been a well-known pediatrician in Lwów. They do not stay in Poland.

The Maple Tree Behind the Barbed Wire

The school year at Traugutt's gymnasium in Czestochowa has begun — it is the end of January—1945. So that we shall catch up the school has no summer holiday. We work non-stop all the year round with one day a week free - Sunday - and we take our exams in mid-September. The school — and we who have taken the exams — have then caught up, finishing the school year before the next academic year and the autumn term at the university are to begin.

I am probably the most surprised in the class when we get our final marks, but Marysia Lewicka says she has always known I would come out top. My parents are inordinately proud when, at the ending ceremonies in church, I am chosen to give the traditional speech of thanks from pupils to their Alma Mater - our school — and the staff.

Despite my ignominious failure at Zofja Wygórska Folwasinka's school, in the end I was allowed to go to the Traugutt's second state gymnasium and also come top of the graduating class. Despite being a Jew, the way is now wide open to whichever university and whichever faculty I like to choose, but for that to happen, there had to be a war and all that that entails.

Naturally I do occasionally think about what my life might have been like if I had not had to live through the second world war in a German-occupied country and the German war of extermination against my people. No one can know that, of course, and speculations of that kind are really rather pointless, but sometimes it is hard not to think along those lines.

When the war started I was a fairly light-hearted, boastful and immature young man, not very interested in my education except possibly during my last ordinary school year before the outbreak of war. Presumably I would have matured even if I had not had to live through a war, just as my father Pinkus had said. But I am convinced that my over-ambitious, almost pathological hunger for education, the driving force during the war and several years afterwards, would never have happened to me without the experiences of the devastating war.

The Maple Tree Behind the Barbed Wire

Nina

No country wants war; all countries maintain they want peace, that war is something they have been forced into by circumstances over which they have no control. Later on in the history books, who is considered the aggressor depends not only on which side wins the war, but also on which country's history book is read — the difference can be hair-raising. I am to find this out as I search through Swedish history books for a description of the great battle of Czestochowa.

In Poland, that battle is extensively described in the history of the country, at least a whole chapter in school textbooks. Polish schoolchildren have to learn that a miracle occurred when the vastly superior forces of Swedish troops, with fourteen cannons supported by two regiments of Polish defectors led by Lieutenant-General Burchard von der Lühnen, in the autumn of 1655 were thoroughly defeated by Czestochowa's scarcely 300 defenders led by Augustin Kordecki, the unbending Prior of the monastery, and under the protection of the picture of the famous Black Madonna painted on cuprous wood. In Poland, the battle is described as a turning point in the Swedish invasion of the continent of Europe. In Sweden, it is described as an insignificant skirmish that had to be ended when King Karl X Gustaf ordered the army back to camp for the approaching winter. Who is right? Both sides — for each country writes its own history.

When, often several decades later, independent historians analyse the event without prejudice, they nearly always come to the conclusion that both sides are guilty of creating a situation which made war inevitable, but the established historical dogma of a country is nevertheless not re-evaluated. In school history books, unfortunately, only pitch-black rogues and dazzlingly white heroes are to be found. Napoleon Bonaparte is a hero in France and Poland, an imperialistic warmonger in England and Russia. But there are exceptions.

If the profoundly unjust Treaty of Versailles is ignored — all history books would agree that Germany under the leadership of Adolf Hitler and the National Socialist Party, bore the responsibility for the outbreak of the Second World War. All honor to the Germany of today for unreservedly admitting it.

Great Britain and France were guarantees of Poland's self-government, integrity and independence, so the invasion of Poland was the introduction of a world war. When after vast human losses largely among the Soviet peoples, the Allies finally found themselves on the winning side of the war; they abandoned Poland's independence, integrity and self-government. The dying Theodore Roosevelt, weakened by large doses of painkilling drugs, settles in February 1945 with the healthy Josef Stalin in the town of Yalta on the Crimean Peninsula.

The Maple Tree Behind the Barbed Wire

It was the Soviet Union, which broke the back of the apparently invincible German military might. No one questions that the Soviet people had to bear by far the greatest loss of human lives and property. But was it reasonable to repay that by sacrificing the independence of eight countries, among them the faithful allies of the western powers, Poland and Czechoslovakia and their total of seventy million inhabitants?

In this betrayal of Poland, Great Britain was given the role of the executioner. The Polish armed forces which fled to England - air force pilots, infantry and naval forces, largely during the early years of the war made a significant, according to some independent opinions, a decisive contribution, and the Polish government in exile in London was an important ally. At the end of the war, they are completely at the mercy of the British and their goodwill.

The newly elected Labour government after the war under Prime Minister Clement Attlee persuades the reluctant head of the Polish government in exile in London, Stanislaw Mikolajczyk, leader of the Agrarian Party and a couple of known politicians in exile to go to Poland to partake in the Warsaw government set up by the Soviet Union with Osóbka-Morawski as Prime Minister. Mikolajczyk was forced to accept the ceremonial post of Deputy Prime Minister and the unimportant assignment of Minister of Agriculture.

With that done, the western powers have good reason to approve the puppet-government in Warsaw, now reinforced by Poles in exile. The problem from their point of view is therefore solved and the task completed, although they must have been aware that in practice they had formalized the handing over of that ravaged country to the Soviet Union, which controlled the army, the militia and Sluzba Bezpieczenstwa - Bezpieka in the vernacular — the well organized, much hated and feared secret police. They save face and wash their hands, but can hardly wash away the historical shame.

No more than two years pass before, at the last minute before his arrest, Stanislaw Mikolajcyk manages to escape to England, then on to America. What is traditionally a large and popular Social Democratic Party, PPS, is forced to join the smaller Communist Party and together form PZPR, in practice the Communist Party of Poland. All is revealed when a Russian marshal who happens to have a Polish-sounding name - Rokossowski - but does not know a word of Polish - changes uniform and becomes the Polish Minister of Defense and the Commander of the resurrected Polish armed forces. The first measure taken by the new commander is an order to supply his forces with only a very limited amount of ammunition. The government and the new parliament of Poland take measures that tie the country to the economy of the Soviet Union. The pre-war once rich but now impoverished country is in future ruthlessly exploited by the Soviet Union and further impoverished. The appointment of Rokossowski is described in the media as advantageous; Mikolajczyk as a traitor and the order to reduce the supply of ammunition to the Polish units is not mentioned. Armja Krajowa, the underground movement loyal to the government in exile in London and with that to the western powers, is obliterated.

I follow these tragic events only distractedly - I have problems rather closer to me to think about, important decisions I have to take.

It is still possible to leave Poland if you have a valid visa to enter another country, but acquiring a visa to a free country is an insuperable obstacle for most people wanting to leave Poland. If you have no valid visa, nor can you acquire a passport. For the large majority of Jews nothing remains but to leave the country illegally and become a refugee, with all the risks and disadvantages that entails.

From the bitter experiences of the Nazi period and the war — at a time when no one wanted us and our lives were under threat — many Jews want to contribute to the formation of a Jewish country which could accept all persecuted Jews and where Jews have the right to provide for their own defense. But Israel does not yet exist and Palestine is more or less closed by the British Mandate to all legal Jewish immigration.

The academic year of 1945-46 begins in Poland at various points in time at different universities - either early or late autumn 1945 or early spring 1946, depending on when premises and a more or less complete teaching staff to start the courses become available. Poland has a significant lack of academics, for none qualified during the war, so the teaching begins although resources are insufficient. I apply to all the universities accepting applications from students, the problem being that I still have not decided what subject I am to read.

With much anguish, I at first exclude an agronomist course, as I have experienced several years of starvation and I ask myself whether there is anything more important than being part of the earth providing us with sufficient food. But I still find it difficult to choose between the two remaining subjects tempting me: biochemistry and medicine. Medicine means looking after life, but biochemistry is the basis of all natural sciences. As I find it difficult to choose, I apply to both faculties and hope that fate will decide — but fate refuses to.

In October 1945, I am told I have a place at the Schools of Medicine at Wroclaw, Gdansk and Lódz, and for studies in biochemistry at Wroclaw and Lódz.

At first I am pleased to have so many places to choose from, but that does not last long for then anguish sets in. It is bad enough if a young person is not offered anything, good to be offered several, but best of all to receive only one definite offer so that pondering and choosing is unnecessary. In the end I choose Lódz, perhaps because even before the war, Lódz was in Poland, Wroclaw in Germany and Gdansk a free state, or perhaps because Lódz was nearest to Czestochowa.

The entrance exam is surprisingly easy and I start in both the schools of medicine and biochemistry. No one stops me. But within a week I realise my inability to choose has put me in an untenable situation - I cannot keep running between compulsory lectures in two subjects that are not co-coordinated, so I give up biochemistry.

Processes when making a difficult choice are often complicated, the basis of our motives complex and the noble reasons we like to imagine to have been decisive often faulty. I like to think I have chosen medicine because I want to look after sick people — a noble reason, but it is possible that the final decision is that the cap medical students wear is the smartest. Whatever the reason, I acquire the university student's square white cap with its broad red ribbon of the School of Medicine - the decision has been made - I am to be a doctor.

We have an extended free spell at the next weekend — from Thursday to Tuesday morning. I have been in Lódz for almost three weeks, and have at last, anyhow for the moment, made an important decision, so justify taking a well-earned breather and going back home to Czestochowa.

As I walk though the door to our home in Aleja Wolnosci 3/5, it is like coming from a dry desert to a wonderful oasis of luscious greenery, swaying palms and mirror-bright water — in reality an oasis of good food, a comfortable bed and profound mutual appreciation and human warmth.

My parents share my delight in starting at university, but they worry over that I look pale, thin and tired — and I am. In Lódz I live in a shabby, temporary student hostel, eat irregularly, mostly bread with not always fresh things on it and have very few hot meals. I dutifully protest, but am grateful when Sarah comes with me back to Lódz on the Tuesday to arrange my life.

I am given a large comfortably furnished room at the home of some acquaintances of Sarah's, the newly married Zylbermans. Sarah agrees with Mrs. Zylberman that I shall have my main meal with them — an arrangement I make use of while Sarah is there, but not after she has left.

Sarah also makes another valuable contribution — together with some woman acquaintances we go to the town's best dance restaurant — the Tabarin. Spending an evening in this subdued atmosphere, listening to calm, rhythmical dance music, I discover that new tunes have been composed and I dance, mostly with Sarah but also with other ladies in our company. Knowing I do this well arouses memories, opens my senses to another world I had forgotten existed. There are several young people there and I discover that there are other pleasures in life apart from insane twenty-four hour studies. I realise I have got to a stage when I ought to grant myself time for other things.

The Maple Tree Behind the Barbed Wire

In 1946, when as a student in Lódz I go back home to Czestochowa, it is like coming to an oasis of mutual appreciation and human warmth

Not that I begin to live an ordinary student life, but I do leave the Sleeping Beauty slumbers of exaggerated ambitions overpowering a semi-awake student, and explore inquisitively the possibilities around me. I occasionally allow myself a visit to the cinema, or to the Tabarin - when I have company — and even privately mix with my contemporaries. This means I find that in Lódz there is a Jewish student club, which largely meets in various private homes, and it is through this club that the most decisive thing is to happen in my life - I meet Nina Rajmic, or rather, Nina meets me.

The Maple Tree Behind the Barbed Wire

We are second year medical students at the newly formed University of Lódz - the first begun in the spring of 1945. There is a great shortage of doctors in Poland - many were killed during the war and none qualified over the long six-year German occupation. The poorly equipped medical faculty accepts over 800 students in my year — after a month or so, we are about 600, the rest not appearing or perhaps realizing they would not be able to keep up, but 600 is already a large number.

It is hard to get hold of textbooks and not all the planned compendiums exist in print. There are no laboratories, no seminar rooms and the teaching is exclusively in lecture form. On the other hand, only the professors lecture — for good or bad. The poorly ventilated lecture hall is always crammed full with students thirsting for knowledge, there are insufficient seats and I learn to get to lectures in good time.

Lectures are compulsory — there is an efficient check on your presence at the door of the lecture hall — but otherwise nothing much is efficient. Sometimes I make my way through the crush to the source of knowledge — the professor at the lectern — and wait in the queue to ask a few questions, but otherwise there is no space for individual teaching.

On my last visit to Czestochowa, Sarah tells me she has decided to give up her dental laboratory and practice, that she has already begun the process and is doing so with no sense of loss. If she is to go on with it, she would have to invest more in it, which she could do, Sarah says slightly hesitantly, but there are other reasons as well. I realise they have not dropped the idea of leaving Poland.

One after another, our Jewish friends and acquaintances are leaving Poland, most of them illegally, among them Sevek Grundman - he has decided to make his way to France. Sevek, Heniek and I meet, not often but regularly. On the last day before Sevek's departure we spend a nostalgic afternoon and a long night together. During the afternoon, we go to a photographer and have a photograph taken, then we each keep a copy of these three friends, promising we shall keep in touch with each other. Regardless of where we end up, we are to write to each other at least once a year.

Nina and I have visited Sevek in Reims when motoring in the south of France and were warmly received. But Sevek does not appear to be happy there, where he is a part owner of his father-in-law's clothing factory.

The Maple Tree Behind the Barbed Wire

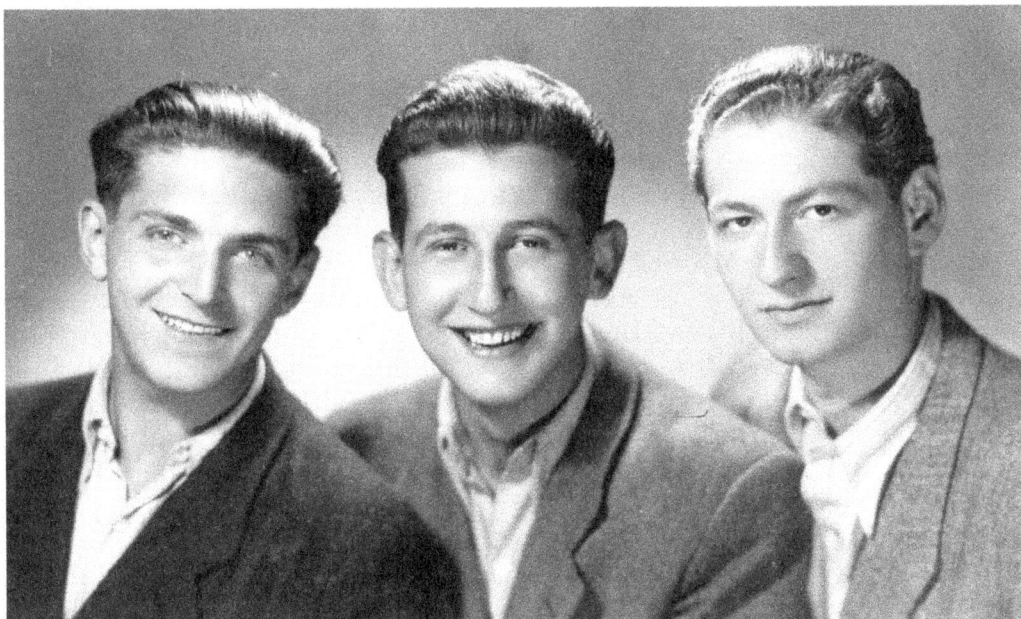

We are three friends and survivors from class IIB - Sevek, Heniek and me. We meet for the last time on January 20th 1946. The next morning Sevek is to leave for France. We have our photograph taken together, keep it and promise to write to each other at least once a year.

Nina and I have also met Heniek Ufner several times. He is just as cheerful and extroverted as he was at school and still finds laughter easy. Heniek is a successful businessman. He and his wife have created a warm, secure home for themselves and their three children, now all married. Heniek and I enjoy each others company just as much as we did at school.

Shortly after that, Bronka Mass comes to my home in Czestochowa to say goodbye — it is her last day in Poland. The next evening she is making her way illegally across the Czech border, a guide already arranged and on the Czech side a man, Michal Igra, is waiting. They are to marry and go to Australia together.

Michal Igra and Bronka are not suited to each other — he is a closed, dominating person, Bronka extroverted, always cheerful and does not allow herself to be dominated. Bronka later becomes a skilled dentist and marries a Polish Jew, also a dentist and a university teacher. They live in San Francisco and we meet occasionally.

Of the others in my class I have on a few occasions met Różyczka Glowinska, who lives in Israel. We have also recently met in Flims in eastern Switzerland, where she, Nina and I happened to be on holiday. I know that Pola Szlezyngier lives in Belgium, but we have had no opportunity of meeting. The beautiful Hanka Bugajer, who went on living for a while under a false name in Poland, also eventually moved to Israel. She married Professor Talmon, a well-known historian at the Hebrew University in Jerusalem. For some reason she has kept her first name from her false identity arrangement during the war and today is called Irena Talmon. We meet occasionally.

That is what has happened after the war to the few surviving pupils from our large class IIB at the Jewish gymnasium in Czestochowa. Nor should be forgotten one of our two surviving teachers - Poldek Pfefferberg. After the war, Poldek opened a handbag and suitcase store in San Francisco. He was the man who met the Australian journalist, Thomas Keneally, and told him about the destinies Keneally described in his book - Schindler's List. I have had no opportunity of meeting Polek since the war, so remember him as our young strong gymnastics teacher at the Jewish gymnasium in Czestochowa in the tailored sub-lieutenant's uniform of the Polish army reserve.

We find out that the Swiss insurance company Winterthur is to open an agency in Warsaw - new clients are tempted with advertisements about "security in a Swiss insurance company".

The insurances that Pinkus had taken out with Winterthur before the war would now be a great help to us. My parents take the insurance policies Pinkus has dragged with him all through the war and go to Warsaw. They want me to go with them, so I am present when Pinkus and Sarah meet the Pole living in Switzerland, but is at present visiting Warsaw to investigate the conditions for establishing an agency in Poland.

The director of the future office in Warsaw looks rather surprised when Sarah and Pinkus appear with their old insurance policies — when Sarah had telephoned, he had thought they wanted to take out new insurances. He seems troubled when he tells them that he has no responsibility for old insurance policies, nor has his head office in Switzerland. Sarah is upset and asks who is responsible. "No one, really," he says. The agency in Poland before the war was an independent subsidiary company, now wound up. Pinkus quietly asks whether the insurances taken out now, after the war, really do provide "security in a Swiss insurance company". The director, even more troubled now, assures us that they certainly do, but at the same time he points out the small print about force majeure — a war is a force majeure, the director explains. Sarah protests that Switzerland was not involved in the war but Pinkus realizes that any further talk is meaningless and the director clearly indicates that our visit is definitely over. To get rid of us, he says we should write to the central office in Switzerland, for he represents only this new subsidiary office.

The Maple Tree Behind the Barbed Wire

Pinkus takes it surprisingly calmly that the insurances he has reckoned on as security are useless - he is a stoic. On the other hand, Sarah shows how upset and frustrated she is, perhaps most of all that she feels she has been defrauded. I don't understand finances and even find it difficult to keep my own in order, but I still sometimes wonder how all that money Pinkus has earned through his own hard work over several years and quite legally paid into a Swiss insurance company can now have disappeared.

All through the war, Pinkus has carried with him that cloth bag of Swiss insurances and neither he nor Sarah has been able to throw it away. Not until Sarah dies in Toronto in 1989 do Roman and I throw them into the garbage. They are not souvenirs of the war either of us wants to keep.

When I go for the second time to the pleasant Jewish student club meeting, those there are mostly boys. It is not dull, but fairly calm when two girls come rushing in late - Helenka and Nina - they get the whole meeting going. I have not met them before, but several of the others have and they gather round these high-spirited girls - I stay where I am, leaning against the round old tiled stove, looking on at what is happening.

Helenka is noticeably good-looking, a light-skinned beauty with straight black hair, markedly black eyebrows, red lips and serious, dreamy, slightly sorrowful eyes.

Nina, or Ninka as I hear several people call her, has a pretty, round face, which many would call piquant, others would say interesting, quite short dark brown hair, a glittering laugh and a watchful look in her grey-green eyes — she is high-spirited and I think really rather noisy, but she seems sympathetic and arouses in me a not insignificant, nevertheless airily absent interest. I notice she is looking at me.

Several people in the room gather round Helenka, who is made to tell them something interesting. I am not quite sure whether it is Nina who comes up to me or whether I go over to Nina, but somehow we have the opportunity to make each other's acquaintance for a moment.

I switch on my stereotyped girl-bewitching charm, which surprisingly often has an effect. Nina mentions the British film "The Man in Grey". I ask teasingly if she would like to go with me to the cinema to see it. She replies, yes, why not? I enjoy Nina's company. There is an undertone of warmth in our rather superficial conversation — but nothing more.

The Maple Tree Behind the Barbed Wire

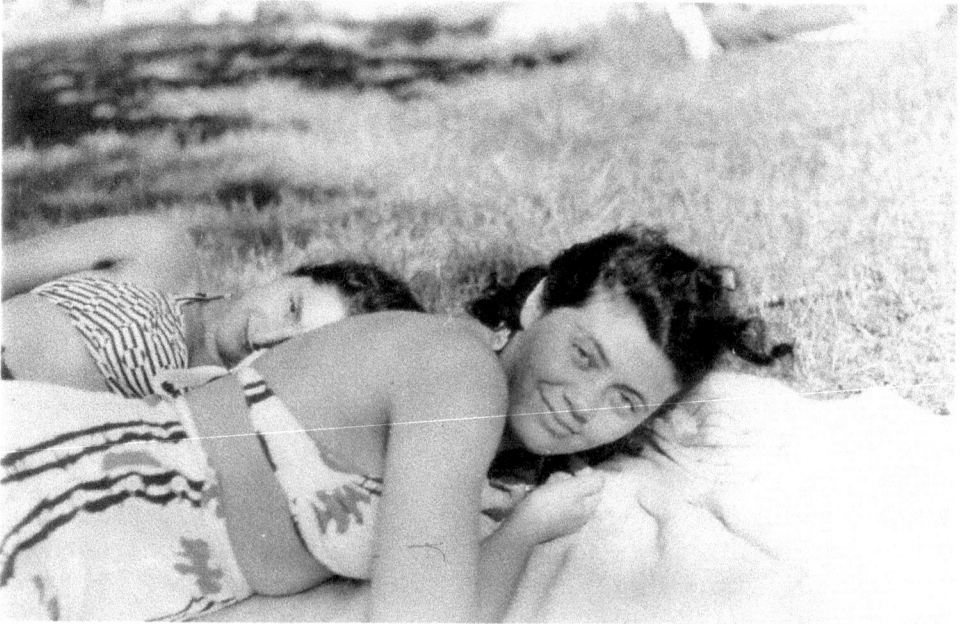

Nina has a round pretty face some people would call piquant, others interesting, quite short dark brown hair, a glittering laugh and an open look in her clever grey-green eyes. She is the best thing that ever happened to me in my life.

Self-absorbed as I am, I forget my invitation to go to see "The Man in Grey" with Nina - but Nina has taken it seriously, expecting me to fulfill my obligation and is disappointed when she hears nothing from me. But as luck would have it, I have another opportunity to meet Nina to ask about the previous year's textbooks — yes indeed, she still has them, and I may borrow them if I like. Nina has started at the university in January and is now in her second year of medical studies at Lódz. Perhaps it is good for the development of our future relationship — and lucky for me — that Nina is not there when I arrive at her home to borrow two of her old textbooks.

Both Nina's parents were killed in Warsaw during the war, her mother during the very last days. Nina herself went through the Warsaw ghetto, the Selektions at ulica Mila, but on one of the last days before the extermination of the ghetto managed to escape from the workplace she had been sent to in the Schultz and Töben workshops — the Warsaw equivalent of Czestochowa's Hasag. She had to hide at the home of a Polish officer's family in a villa outside Warsaw, went through the Armia Krajowa uprising and was saved on several occasions by her only brother, Rudolf, eleven years older and whom she calls Rudek. She lives with him in their old quite large pre-war apartment in ulica Zeronskiego 85 - Rudolf is a lawyer and not much later becomes an Associate Professor in the faculty of law at Lòdz.

The Maple Tree Behind the Barbed Wire

When I arrive at their apartment I am met by an older woman - Aniela - who has worked in the home since the two of them were small, and whom they rescued after the war. Just after the end of the war Aniela had been dying of pernicious anemia. She found out that Rudek and Nina had survived and sent a message to ask whether they could help. Nina had learnt how to make shoe-cream in the ghetto and after the war she made shoe-cream in two colors in a room in their apartment, sold it on the streets to get money for Aniela's blood transfusions — and when she improves, for the recently discovered life-saving vitamin B12. But there is no sign of this when I first meet her — this apparently robust and austerely friendly woman appears to be fighting fit.

Aniela does not send me away. Nina is not at home bit I am nevertheless allowed into Nina's not particularly orderly but rather pleasant room and Aniela asks me which books Nina has promised to lend me — both of them are lying there, clearly left out. Aniela thinks I should take them with me, as Nina had promised, and I leave with the books under my arm. Not until many years later does Nina tell me that Aniela had said to her: "I think you should marry that polite student who came here to pick up your two books." Nina has never told me what she replied.

I don't know whether this event is of any importance to my future destiny. Nina lost her parents early and has great respect for Aniela. At the same time, many years later Nina was to maintain she fell in love with me "from the very first moment" when she saw me leaning against the round tiled stove at that meeting of Jewish students at Wiktor's home.

Nina and I meet several times. It is usually she who discreetly takes the initiative, though sometimes I do — or at least I think I do. I am fairly light-hearted in my relations to girls I meet, but I instinctively realise that if I take up with Nina, then it will be serious and without consciously doing so, I take the consequences of that insight. Despite meeting repeatedly, I make no attempt, not even an intimation of physical approach, which is probably sensible, but not only that. To avoid any eventual misunderstanding, I clarify the situation, "put my cards on the table" in my stupid insensitive way, quite uncalled for, and for no sensible reason.

Nina tells me there is going to be a student ball in the Pontiatkowski Palace, the upper class wealthy Polish family property that has been nationalized and become public property, in reality a state property. I ask her if she would like to go with me to the ball and she says she would. Then she says there are only a limited number of tickets and adds candidly yet shyly that she has reserved two. Nina understands people, and me, and she looks ahead.

The Maple Tree Behind the Barbed Wire

I put on an elegant dark blue suit Pinkus has had made in his workshop for his elder son who has got into university, and we dance. I am a good dancer, especially to languishing tunes — that is thanks to Sarah. Nina does not draw back when I occasionally put my cheek to hers; and I don't think this is going too far. I offer Nina a soft drink and we go out into the spacious well-maintained grounds, which are rather overgrown with bushes and trees — she lets me hold her soft warm hand. The air is fragrant with the promise of spring, the stars twinkling in the clear sky, we find ourselves in fantastic surroundings and it is a wonderful evening, which I then spoil.

"You know," I say as we stroll along the narrow path, hearing loving couples in the bushes. "I won't marry until I'm forty," and I develop this theme with my father's example — it takes time to build up your future so you can be sure of supporting a family, and I want to do that before I marry. Nina is just twenty-one, I will be twenty-one in a few months' time. She says nothing whatsoever — as if I had not just said something abysmally stupid, insensitive and uncalled for. She does not even take away the hand I am still holding, and I think that all is well — although Nina has never even implied that she wanted a steady relationship with me, not to mention marry me.

We go back into the big salon of Poniatowski Palace, the six-man orchestra is playing, we go on dancing, then after some more soft drinks I escort Nina home and we thank each other for a pleasant evening. I have an impression that the atmosphere towards the end of the evening is somewhat cooler — think perhaps she is tired.

I was to manage to commit many more blunders in my time with Nina before she made me grow up — or perhaps I was programmed in my genes to mature all the same, as Pinkus had foreseen, without him or anyone else knowing then that there existed genes governing our lives to such an extent.

But Nina could not know that I would mature. Even today, at the end of the summer of 1999, I cannot understand what this clever, joyful and pretty girl, liked by everyone, with unusually fine legs, could see in me during those early years after we met. What was there to like in this handsome but immature, horribly self-absorbed and spoilt young man. Perhaps what was decisive was that she saw through me and realized that beneath the boastful surface I was uncertain and lacking in independence, that someone had to take care of me and the task attracted her. Or had she perhaps anticipated that in me was a certain potential and that with good management, I might achieve something sensible with my life.

The Maple Tree Behind the Barbed Wire

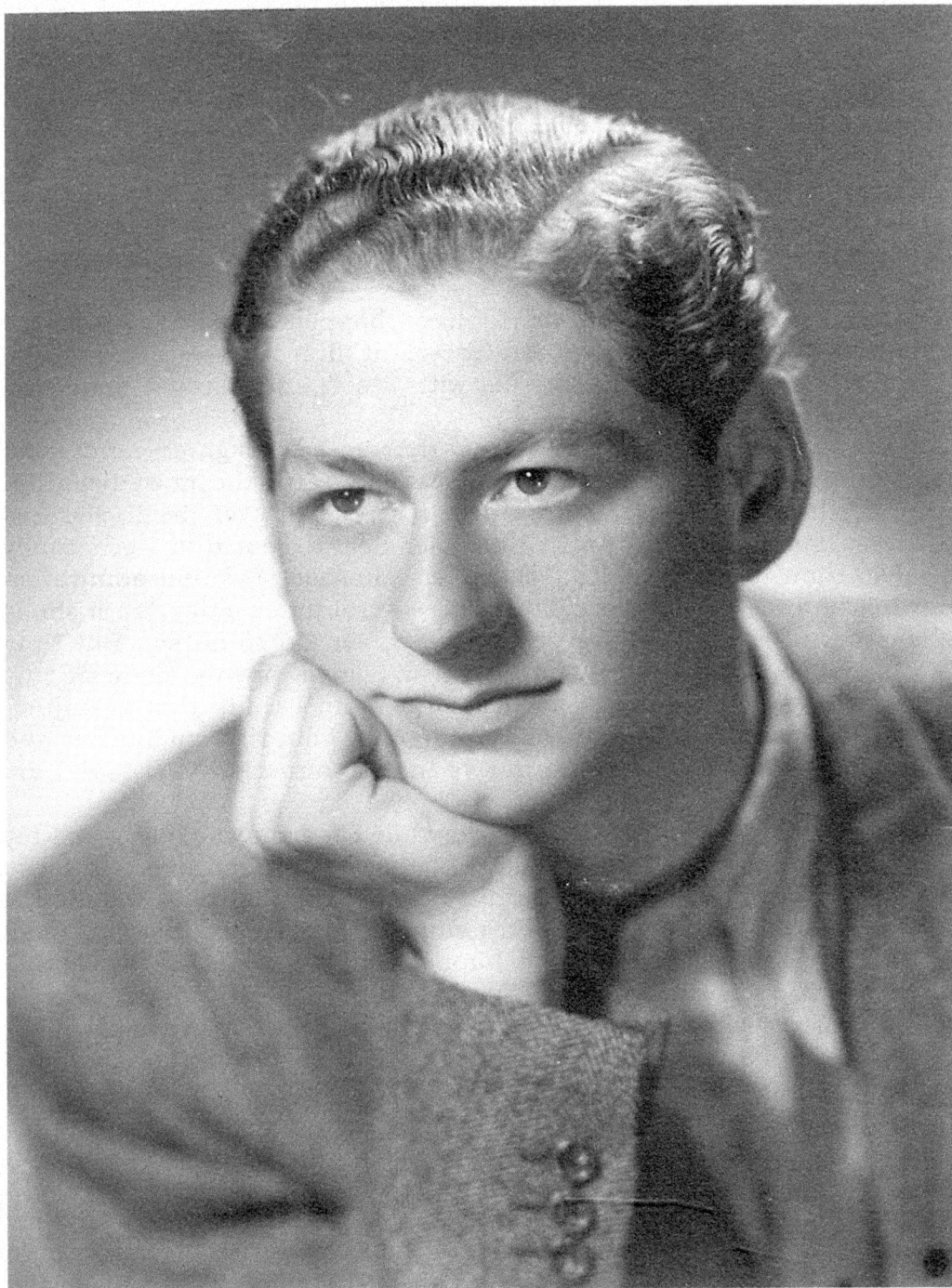

Many years later, Nina is to maintain that she fell in love with me "at the very first moment". Even today I am unable to understand what this clever girl, much liked by all, could in 1946 see in this handsome but immature and horribly self-absorbed young man

The Maple Tree Behind the Barbed Wire

Nina does not deny the description of my personality during my Lódz period. She says she had not at all thought along such complicated lines, but had simply fallen in love when she saw me standing alone, leaning against the tiled stove, and apparently not noticing her. In that case, it is the best thing that has ever happened to me in my life, that she fell in love before she got to know me — things like that can happen even to the best of us - and that she later stood by me despite my obvious defects and all the unpleasantness I must have caused her before gradually realizing the best thing to do was to tell her I loved her and propose.

Nina is the best thing ever to have happened to me. From the moment we met she has been there, at first in the background, discreetly steering me and my life with a soft and devoted hand and always for my own good.

I think my Nina is the cleverest, the most far-sighted, and most discerning and kindest creature on earth — also the most beautiful woman, friend and lover I have ever met or will ever meet. She has done so much for me, and I so little for her. Except that I eventually realise I am insanely in love, that I also harbor profound admiration for her and tell her so every day, often several times a day, until she is pleased and says, laughing: "Stop it now, you do go on so." But Nina becomes embarrassed whenever I can't help openly showing my feelings — "You embarrass me", she says and I think that is unjust. We have been married exactly fifty years and I am right to like her and talk about what I feel for my wife. Is that so strange? Nina says I am still rather childish.

Nina would good-naturedly look on while I raged away and gored my horns off. I am lucky that Nina quickly decides and is then faithful to whomever she chooses. Also, perhaps Nina would not have wanted me if I had not been as I was — and I shudder at the very thought. I like to imagine that everything that happens after we met at the Jewish student club's second meeting in the autumn of 1945 and before I proposed on October 1st, 1948, was nothing but a preparation for what was to occur between Nina and me. When I think back today, I see myself as an out-of-tune violin which Nina takes into her soft warm hands, tuning it, then playing on it throughout our entire life together, constantly extracting the best sound the violin can produce.

In connection with my next visit to Czestochowa, Pinkus wants me to go with him to Dr Nowak, a Polish Jew with a practice in Stockholm. Nowak has come to purchase art that is cheap in Poland at the time, and at the same time he orders two suits and a winter coat, which Pinkus is to deliver, I go with him, and with Pinkus look at lovely pictures by old Polish artists Nowak has already bought or is considering buying, but I am more interested when he talks about Sweden - a well-ordered country, the Swedes reliable people. I ask him

The Maple Tree Behind the Barbed Wire

whether it is true, as we had learnt at school, that in Sweden people don't lock their doors and leave their bicycles unlocked.

On the way home, Pinkus says to me that Sweden is a fine country, then adds that is where they award the Nobel Prizes. According to Pinkus, the Nobel Prize is the highest award a person can be given.

I would never even get anywhere near receiving a Nobel Prize. Yet it is a pity that Pinkus never saw his son being one of those who for over twenty-five years has been one of the judges deciding who is to receive one of the Nobel Prizes - that in physiology and medicine. I think that would have delighted my father. At Nina's and my home, every year we honor the memories of Pinkus, Sarah and Nina's parents — by lighting a candle that burns for at least twenty-four hours. On that occasion I try to tell Pinkus that I have not been awarded the Nobel Prize, but am one of the distributors.

My father, Pinkus, lived until he was seventy-four and died of cancer in 1959. Sarah was younger. She was to live on for thirty more years and see me as both a member of the Nobel Foundation of the Nobel Committee and as head of the Radiumhemmet Cancer Centre. But my impression is that she did not think much of this Nobel Prize or Radiumhemmet business — as long as we, our children and grandchildren were healthy. Sarah was so proud of managing to be a prababka — a great-grandmother. She was too old to travel to see her great-grandchildren and my grandchildren too small to go to her, but Sarah was happy when she was able to see her great-grandchildren on photographs my daughter-in-law Susanne had taken.

Denmark

The academic year 1945-46 at the University of Lódz is coming to an end, the demanding examination period beginning. In various ways, I have managed to acquire the necessary textbooks and my compendiums are full of notes, I have copious notes from lectures and am fairly well up on the work. Despite this, I refuse all distractions, even going home to Czestochowa, again spending days and some nights at my desk, neglecting meals and social contacts.

So I do well in the written exams and the orals afterwards, in which the professors in each subject themselves, examine each student and award our marks. This is a formidable achievement for we are many students, although some choose to postpone being examined. I am probably one of the few or perhaps the only one to ask the surprised teachers to be allowed to re-take the two subjects in which I have the next but highest marks, in order to get the highest mark in all subjects — a five, actually of no practical significance. At this stage Nina makes her first contribution to guiding my life.

I am disturbed when someone rings the doorbell; this time it is Nina in the hall talking to my landlady, Mrs. Zylberman. Mrs. Zylberman is a friendly but firm, uninhibitedly dominating lady with strong calves and long hairy legs I cannot help noticing as she walks around in exceptionally short skirts. Nina comes into my room and breathlessly tells me why she is in such a hurry.

An invitation has come from Denmark. Two hundred students at the University of Lódz can have places for laboratory work in chemistry during the summer vacations, priority is given to second year students, so Nina's year have had this message first, but surplus places are to be offered to first year students. Nina has put her name on the list and is going to Denmark - if I am interested, I have to decide quickly — that morning over a hundred and fifty have applied and there will be fierce competition for the remaining places.

I had had no vacations the previous year, but have no thought that that would stop me. Of course I want to go.

This is an adventure. I have never been abroad in my twenty-year life - I eagerly ask Nina where I should apply. Just like the tickets for the ball at Pontiatowski Palace, Nina says with some embarrassment that she has already applied for me — to be sure, but complementary information is required, and she wants to hand that in as soon as possible. I do not even give a thought to why this pretty girl is doing all this for me, just hand over the information required.

My parents are also indulgent when I tell them I have been given an opportunity to go abroad — to Denmark. They don't even mention the plans they have made for the summer — of course I must go if I think it would be interesting as well as useful.

The Maple Tree Behind the Barbed Wire

Sarah packs for me, while Pinkus has a pair of elegant pale brown summer trousers in light gabardine made for his son. They also give me a real silver cigarette case - I don't smoke but they say I can sell it in Denmark if I need money. Roman is away from home when two weeks later, Sarah and Pinkus see me off on the train to Lódz - the journey to Denmark is to leave from there.

I do not have to arrange any formalities myself. Our group has a single joint passport made out to the group leader, our sympathetic professor of endocrinology - Beer. Fastened to his passport is a long list of names of those travelling with him, all seventy-two medical students going from Lódz. One of the professors in the chemistry faculty has a list fastened to his passport of the accompanying chemistry students - one of these is Marysia Lewicka, now called Toska Roller.

On our arrival in Denmark, we are overwhelmed by the hospitality. Members of the Women's Voluntary Service in their smart pale grey uniforms serve food on the quay and there seems to be no limit to their goodwill. On the way to where we are to be billeted — a school vacated for the summer, in Klampenborg - our coaches make a detour round through the streets of Copenhagen to show us something about this great city. I am surprised by the lush June greenery in the parks, and the large individual plots. Everything is orderly and well maintained in this prosperous country, no damaged buildings, no burnt-out houses, torn-up streets or derelict parks. Denmark was also occupied, but we do not see the defects that must exist, for we come from a much more devastated country. This beautiful capital appears to be quite undamaged.

Our life in Denmark is trouble-free, luxurious and pleasant. The friendly, always smiling women volunteers are our hosts — no one could imagine better ones. Everything is well arranged to make our life easy and pleasant — food, laundry, daily transport to the university laboratories. We have Danish-, German- and English-speaking lecturers under the direction of Professor Rosenthal, and are given very generous pocket money to enable us to amuse ourselves on our own in Copenhagen. Our group is an appreciated element on the streets of Klampenborg and Copenhagen. People greet us and cheer when they recognize us in our characteristic square student caps.

One moderately warm Saturday at the end of June, two Polish students - Zbyszek and I - take the local train in to Copenhagen to try out on our own the cheapest amusements the capital has to offer. By the window in the same compartment is an ideal beauty out of some fashion magazine.

The Maple Tree Behind the Barbed Wire

Everything is perfect about this amazingly beautiful cool young woman gazing absently out of the window at the passing view, which she must have seen on many other occasions. Her thick, quite long wavy hair is fair and held together by a crocheted ribbon of white angora wool, her fair but not pale complexion faultless, her even white teeth, which she likes to show as she smiles slightly, her calm blue eyes, her gracious neck, her long legs crossed under just the right length pleated pale pink skirt - I ask myself whether I have ever seen such a perfect woman. Her soberly elegant clothes make me wonder why she is on a simple local train among us ordinary passengers, but that does not prevent me from moving along so that I am sitting immediately opposite her. I turn on my girl-hunting charm, nowadays enriched by the nerve of a young medical student who has just completed his first year's studies and thinks the whole world is his, and for the first time in his life, he is abroad.

As she slowly turns to look at me, I can see deep down in her great eyes - I have no need to make any effort to show my genuine admiration. At first I try out my diffident English and am surprised and flattered when she does not at once fob me off. She has no objection when we switch to German - a language the Danes are otherwise unwilling to speak — perhaps because I am not German myself. Her voice is melodious, occasionally slightly veiled, and she speaks both English and German distinctly, so is well educated and does not swallow half her words as so many Danes do, even when they are speaking a language apart from their own.

She lives in Klampenborg and knows we are billeted there. I don't lose the thread when she takes over the conversation, questioning me about how things are for us, why we have come to Denmark, whether we are being well looked after, what I think about Denmark, then probing further — what are things like in Poland? She takes a lively interest in recent events in our country, the prevailing circumstances in Poland, and what the student situation is like. The conversation is serious and she smiles indulgently when I tease her a little now and again. In the end I boldly ask her if she will come and visit us at our billet. She smiles her attractive smile, says solemnly that she would very much like to, and asks if she may bring a girlfriend with her. She gives me a cool hand, says her name is Bodil and tells me her surname before getting off the train a couple of stations before Copenhagen Central Station. Bodil catches me watching her walking along the platform in her high-heeled white sandals.

The very next day — a Sunday -- Bodil and Margaretha come to our billet; I am enormously proud when Zbyszek and I are able to show off these two elegant young women. Margaretha is critical of our Danish hosts allowing so many — over ten — to sleep in the same room and because we have to keep everything we possess in our cases under the beds. Otherwise there is not much to see or show. As we sit talking on

The Maple Tree Behind the Barbed Wire

a bench in front of the building, Margaretha asks whether we would like to go home with them home for coffee; they live within walking distance from our billet. I can see from Bodil's expression that she is astonished at this clearly unplanned invitation to their home, but she does not protest.

Bodil and Margaretha live together and that night neither Zbyszek nor I go back to our lodgings.

I do not spend many nights at our billet in the school in Klampenborg after that. Zbyszek is sometimes with me — usually at weekends. Bodil initiates me into secrets pertaining to perfect relations between a woman and a man — with her gentle manner she is a wonderful teacher.

Bodil stays at home from work more and more often. I come back in the evenings after my laboratory work and am just as welcome each evening. I eat with them - Margaretha usually gets the breakfast and Bodil the dinner in the evening. One morning, when only Margaretha and I are at breakfast in their big kitchen, she tells me with mild reproach that Bodil stays away from work too often and will probably soon lose her job — they have been good friends for a long time and work for the same firm. Bodil has told her not to worry; she will get another job.

This is not love. We both know it and we have only a limited time to be together, but there is undeniably genuine warmth in our relations and also in me genuine admiration and profound gratitude. It is shameless of me that I leave her earlier than planned without saying goodbye, perhaps even more shameless and selfish when later and unannounced, I again trample into Bodil's life for a brief interlude.

We are developed by the people we meet and can be damaged or enriched by our experiences. I was lucky to meet Bodil that Saturday morning on the local train from Klampenborg to Copenhagen. Bodil has meant much to my development as a man and also as a human being. She has given me a little more self-confidence, taught me to be less superficial, to listen to people and show consideration and concern, including in my relations to women. Bodil also gave me a brief spell of light-hearted happiness just before another difficult period of my life. I hope that I brought something positive into her life.

I am well aware that this Danish idyll cannot last, but have no idea that fate is to deny me the promised respite until the day of our departure from Denmark in mid-August, 1946. In a brutal way, I become aware that there are many people who still hate the few Jews that have survived, those who consider there is no place for us on this earth, most of all in post-war Poland - people who, right in the middle of the Nürnberg trials, are prepared to continue the extermination of the last few remnants to survive. Rudolf, Nina's brother, is the first with the bad news.

The Maple Tree Behind the Barbed Wire

Nina receives a telegram in which without mincing matters he says she must not go back to Poland, but he does not explain why. The post is slow and several days go by before Nina and I, on the same day, each get a letter, Nina from Rudolf, I from my parents. A few days later, Helenka Zymler also receives a letter with the same content, from an uncle, her only surviving relative still in Poland.

The first ill omen was that someone has broken into a Jewish student's room in Lódz and in a bath full of water cut his throat; it is not clear whether he bled to death or drowned. In a very visible place in the room was a note put together with letters cut out of a newspaper saying that there was no room for Jewish students at Lódz University and the same fate would befall those who ignored this message. Where there should have been a signature are cutout letters spelling "What Hitler did not manage to complete, we shall accomplish." The police had not succeeded in identifying they guilty parties.

A day or two later, on July 4th, 1946, there was a pogrom in Kielce - the governor's town in the county Czestochowa is in. Forty-three Jews were dragged out of their homes and workplaces, maltreated and tortured in the middle of the day, in closed rooms and on open streets, then finally murdered. Those murdered are nearly all of the Jewish inhabitants of Kielce - the majority had been rescued from German prison camps and some had survived the war in the Soviet Union. Only two of the Jews in Kielce escaped, one into a Polish home she was by chance visiting, the other a badly maltreated and mutilated man lying in the street beneath his new wife's bloodstained body, pretending to be dead. Such large crowds took part in the pogrom, the police lost control of the situation and were unable to stop the daylong winkling out and murder of Jews - no guilty persons had yet been identified or arrested, but the investigation is continuing.

My parents write in their long letter that Poland is no longer the same country as I had left in June. I must not go back, and they themselves were to leave the country soon. The hatred of Jews released by the pogrom in Kielce is now noticed in other places in Poland, not least in Czestochowa. Jews were murdered in Sokoly Boleslawiec, Biala Podlaska, Lublin, Polaniec, Turek, Piaski, and Skarzysko-Kamienna. Attempts at pogroms were crushed by the police in other places such as Kraków, Radom, Miechów and Rabka. Jews were leaving Poland en masse, my parents write — as if there were masses of Jews left in the country.

Almost two weeks have now gone by since the pogrom in Kielce. We cannot read the Danish newspapers, and no one has told us, perhaps just as well, for as a result we have been given respite in friendly Denmark where nearly all Jews, in one single night, were rescued and taken over to Sweden when their Holocaust began.

The Maple Tree Behind the Barbed Wire

I am shaken by what is happening in Poland. It is no use trying to persuade yourself that these events might be random, that things will perhaps calm down. At the same time, I have no idea what I can do about not going back — where shall I go, who would I dare talk to about leaving the group? I have no passport, my only identification is my student card. I have to return to Poland, I think with relief, and finally decide there is nothing I can do — but Nina does not think so.

Nina must be aware of what is going on between Bodil and me. She is perhaps a trifle guarded, but does not bring up the way I have been living in Denmark, and I see no reason to take it up with Nina. Nina pretends that this affair with Bodil has nothing to do with her, and perhaps she is right. We see each other, but not as often as before. I am seldom at the student billet and have few opportunities of meeting her.

Nina ensures we have a chance to meet alone and she tells me openly what she is trying to do so as not to have to return. When I ask, Nina says hesitantly that she is doing all this although both her brother and Aniela are still in Poland and although she is not sure whether Rudolf is going to leave the country. Nina hopes that in the present situation, her brother will follow later if she manages to find a country to which he is allowed to come.

Nina has contacted her mother's large family in the USA - she knows them well from her yearlong stay in New York and Philadelphia shortly before the war. Nina has been to the American Consulate in Copenhagen, where they have told her she is well placed, but even for those with priority there is a queue and the consulate does not think she has time to acquire a visa to the USA during the short time she has left in Denmark. Nina tells me about her acquaintances in Sweden, among them Wiktor, another Mietek Tauman, whom I have never met, and she asks me if I am interested.

The purposefulness and inventiveness of this girl fascinates me, at the same time disturbs me in my present peaceful existence. I weigh up my dislike of what is happening in Poland, my curiosity, perhaps also my growing sympathy for Nina, then do as I usually do — try to keep all doors open and say to Nina that I am interested but have not decided.

So I am with her when on the student group's outing with Danish teachers, Nina manages to find a moment when we are alone with the rector himself, Professor Harald Bohr, brother of the Nobel Prize winner in physics. Nina tells him what is happening to the Jews in Poland and asks shyly but straight out whether he can give us any advice. Harald Bohr says we cannot stay in Denmark - which we knew, but he explains why. The Danish government has decided not to take any refugees until further notice, a decision directed at Germans fleeing their country, and it is feared some are trying to escape the current trials of war criminals, but the measure also affects others who ought not to be affected. We are on the shore in Skodsborg north of Copenhagen. Bohr looks across the Sound and says quietly: "Sweden is just over there, so near, and they do not have the same regulations there. Sweden accepts refugees." This is said in a friendly way, but is not much help. Bohr says nothing about how we can make our way across the Sweden.

Nina has already found out that Mrs. Bankir, whom she knows from Poland, is on a visit to Denmark. Shortly before the war the Bankir family emigrated from Poland to Sweden. I am with Nina when we meet Mrs. Bankir but nor did that meeting lead anywhere. Mrs. Bankir does not know how to set about getting to Sweden, and she also advises us against simply leaving without anything to live off. Sweden is a good country, Mrs. Bankir says well meaningly, but it is difficult to go there with no profession and no money to start a new life. We should finish our medical studies in Poland and then come. She thinks that in that case they would probably be able help if necessary.

I am also with her when Nina meets Wiktor, who has managed to get a transit visa and is living in Sweden - Nina has persuaded Wiktor to come to see us in Denmark. At first we think this meeting is not going to be any use either, except it is pleasant to talk about old times. But Wiktor gives us the address of the Emissary for the Jewish Agency in Copenhagen - Mr. Margolinski; he turns out to be the one to decide our future.

The Jewish Agency, formed in 1933 to help persecuted Jews in various countries, has already received international recognition for its efficiency. In some countries, there are permanent emissaries - Mr. Margolinski is one.

We are four Jewish students from Poland to visit him - Nina and I, Toska, who has found her own way to Margolinski and Helenka, who has changed her mind and also wants to come. Margolinski is an older man — anyhow, considerably older than we are — he reminds me of Professor Anisfeld, the rector of the Jewish gymnasium in Czestochowa. Margolinski looks fairly ordinary, not at all as I imagine an "emissary".

Nina, then Toska, do most of the talking. Margolinski listens with half-closed eyes and lets them talk on, then asks a few short questions on our circumstances in Denmark and previously in Poland, whether we have any relatives in Poland or in any other countries. His last question is about whether we are sure we want to leave Poland illegally — that is all he eventually has to offer. Then he looks straight at each of us in turn, his eyes alert as he listens to our answers. All four of us say we are sure we do, what else could I say now I have gone this far? I realise that here — faced with Margolinski - it is no use vacillating any longer, the time has come — has already passed — for the difficult decision.

The Maple Tree Behind the Barbed Wire

Margolinski seems satisfied with our answers and says we are not to reveal this to anyone, not to anyone, he repeats with emphasis as he looks at us. We are to come back to him the next day at the same time — is that all right?

The next day he again receives us in his small but simply furnished office, with no pictures on the walls. He is not so formal and guarded as on our first visit — on the contrary, he is almost cordial, and effective. The preparations take two days, and he describes briefly what will happen. We are told that we are to be there at exactly 13.00 the day after tomorrow.

We ought to leave our billet and the university "as usual". That means, says Margolinski, so that we don't attract any attention, we must leave our suitcases behind. At the appointed place there will be two young men waiting for us, Jews living in Palestine, and also a boat that will take us across to Sweden. We are given railway tickets to Stockholm and a little cash for unforeseen expenses. Unfortunately, it is not much, he says with genuine regret, as his organization has not much money. Any questions? If not, he again reminds us that under no circumstances are we to tell this to anyone here in Denmark - for what we are doing is illegal and he, like the two we are to meet on the shore, are taking part in an illegal action. As we are leaving he shakes hands with each of us. His handshake is warm, his look both encouraging and sad as he wishes us luck - I realise he really means it with all his heart, but also that he had wanted to say this was not going to be easy, though that is perhaps not part of his remit.

I feel some anxiety over what is to happen, but don't want to think about my whole future depending of having to meet Mr. Margolinki's associates the day after tomorrow to take that Danish boat — the decision has been made and trying to analyze it afterwards is too much for me.

That evening I find it difficult, very difficult, not to explain to Bodil and Margaretha. But this secret is not just my own, so I content myself by rather clumsily letting it be known that my visit to Denmark is shortly going to come to an end. Bodil says cheerfully that we have another two weeks, so we will not think about it that evening. I am the only one who knows, or rather think I know that this is our last evening together.

I have learnt to admire much more than just the beauty of this secretive, unusually lovely woman. As our farewell approaches, I realise I know very little about Bodil. She has never talked about herself; the little I know comes from the moments when I have been alone with Margaretha and she has said something at random about her friend.

Bodil and I have never talked to each other about our emotions or our relationship, perhaps because both know that it has no future. We belong in different worlds, meeting by chance one short summer. From

The Maple Tree Behind the Barbed Wire

the beginning it has been measured by destiny, like the life of a butterfly. Neither of us has tried to change this, and now it is too late. Perhaps it is just as well that to me Bodil will always remain a beautiful mystery and I to her a young Polish student on a brief visit to her country, to her life. If we had met under other circumstance I would probably never have dared approach her, and if I had, she would not have accepted my approaches.

In the morning, I say I will not be back that evening.

Helenka is the one to persuade Nina that we must say goodbye to Professor Beer. I think that is rash — he is the last person we should tell. He could be held responsible if he had known and not intervened to stop us. But once Helenka has decided, it is not possible to change her mind, no matter what argument I bring up — she seems not to listen. If the two of them are going, then it is just as well if all three of us go.

Professor Beer, relatively young but in Poland already recognized as a successful scientist and physician, is balding, rather thin, has a mustache - he receives us in his room at our billet and I am surprised that he makes no attempt to persuade us not to go - he quite candidly lets us understand that we are doing the right thing. Beer does not ask for any details, which we have agreed not to tell anyone, not even him, and wishes us luck, saying fairly unworriedly that several Polish students have already managed to make their way to England.

He is a brave man, Professor Beer, and in future is to show that he is even braver. His fearless behaviour and on his return to Poland his criticisms of the Soviet scientists and senior Polish officials made it impossible for him to stay there. Many years later, Nina and I go to see him at his home in Tel Aviv. For Beer was Jewish and several years after the visit to Denmark, settled in the free country of Israel. But when Nina and I meet him in Israel he is not the same happy forward-looking person, he is subdued and does not seem to be liking it, despite his professorship in experimental endocrinology at Tel Aviv University. Beer was probably too old to be pulled up by his Polish cultural roots and move to another country - even if that country was Israel.

Our departure from the faraway deserted quay outside Vedbæk, north of Copenhagen, our crossing and arrival at the deserted jetty near Landskrona are entirely undramatic; no one seems to notice that we have set off from Denmark and gone ashore in Sweden. The two Danish fishermen have said hardly a word to us on the crossing. They don't say goodbye to us until they point out on our arrival the road to Landskrona and the railway station. Then they are in a hurry to leave the Swedish coast. We have almost four hours to wait before the night train leaves so have time to look around our new country.   Denmark

The Maple Tree Behind the Barbed Wire

was unspoiled and orderly. But here in Sweden we are overwhelmed again by the abundance of such prosperity, the shop windows crammed with clothes in materials we have never seen before, articles we have forgotten about, or never even knew existed.

With a bit of the pocket money I had been given by the two Jewish boys on the shore outside Vedbæk, I buy a banana and an orange, to me exotic fruit I had last seen and tasted when I was fourteen, in a world long since disappeared — before the war. We go to the station in Landskrona in good time so as not to miss the night train to Stockholm.

I have crossed to Sweden, but have no long-term plans for my future except to take the night train to Stockholm and there report to the police.

I would never have believed it if someone had tried to tell me that Nina, many years later, would be chairing the Jewish Agency's Swedish organization - Karen Hayesod - the organization that made our crossing to Sweden possible.

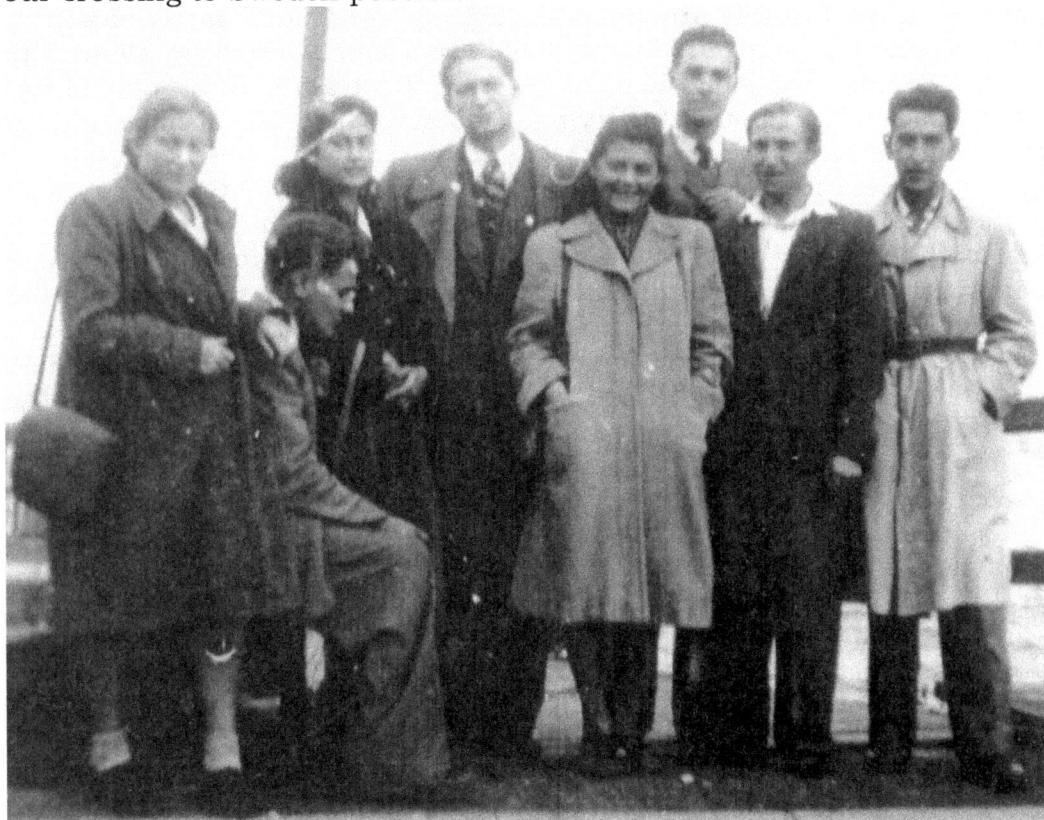

Margolinski's associates, Wiktor and the Danish fishermen who are to take us across the Sound to Sweden. When the four of us - Toska, Helenka, Nina and I - land in Landskrona, we are refugees

CHAPTER VII

REFUGEE IN SWEDEN

Gilel Storch

When we get off the night train from Malmö, two young men, Mietek Tauman and Natek Calel, are there to meet us. They tell us that before we go to the police we ought to meet their boss. They take us to the World Jewish Congress office at Grev Magnigatan 11 and for the first time I meet a legendary person — a hero or, if you like, a guardian angel. But Storch does not look like an angel.

We sit down on a sofa outside his big room and wait for him to see us, the door to his room open. Storch is an older, rather heavily built gentleman with a round face and rapidly balding head. Behind his desk is a comfortable armchair, though he apparently rarely sits in it. People come in and out of the room, speak or wait to be allowed to speak to him — it looks like the interior of a tram with an official but hopelessly scatty conductor trying to do several things at once, indeed it seems fairly chaotic.

Storch gets impatient if someone talks too much, but he may also interrupt someone expressing himself briefly. He himself can carry on an endlessly long tirade without there being any question of anyone interrupting him. In the middle of a conversation he may dismiss the person he is talking to with a wave and turn to another task, or take a telephone call. I have the impression of a domineering field commander, who likes his job and creates confidence, though at the same time he is fighting several battles simultaneously and so loses control of them all — but I am soon to find out that that is not at all true.

A little later, Mietek Tauman goes into the room and reminds him that we have come and are waiting. But Storch waves Mietek away — soon, he says without meaning it, instead sending Mietek off to arrange something else for him. After quite a wait, when Mietek again reminds him that we are there, he suddenly notices us on the sofa outside his room, although he could scarcely have helped looking at us before without seeing us.

Suddenly he softens and becomes another person — blind and deaf to the mess around him, he sweeps everything aside, comes out to us and tells us to come on in. On our way in he apologizes for keeping us waiting, excusing himself as he has so many things to do - though is apparently not very worried by this. He behaves as if we had been long expected, very welcome and important people. He calls out loudly to an older woman who is clearly his adviser and starts the conversation by entertaining us with matters that have nothing to do with our problems. He suddenly has all the time in the world for us and waves away anyone who comes without giving them a chance to interrupt. That seems good to us - we are no longer insignificant supplicants.

Storch gradually takes up our case. He says our situation is complicated. It is not good to come from Denmark as a refugee to Sweden - so I am suddenly a refugee? He tries to explain why our situation in particular is complicated - none of us understands his explanations but in the same breath he says he has arranged more difficult cases. Everything will be all right, says Gilel Storch, we need not worry. I am not in the slightest worried, but beginning to be aware that I am no longer a Polish student on a temporary visit to a foreign country.

Storch consults the older woman in a mixture of Swedish and German. She appears to be sensible and competent, he listens with obvious confidence in her, nods, turns to speak to us, then goes on taking time to do so.

Storch has not introduced himself, taking it for granted we know who he is, but he questions us on our families. Oh yes, Nina has a brother, and I have both a brother and parents in Poland. What do my parents and Nina's brother do? Oh yes, a lawyer is he? He asks us what our plans for the future are, which no one else has done before and he smiles particularly kindly when speaking to each of the three girls. He is genuinely interested. We are important people to him, which means we feel safe and are to carry that feeling with us for a long time after leaving his room.

Suddenly the phone rings — it is something important. "Ein Augenblick," he says to the person on the phone, waving us away after asking if we have had anything to eat and telling Mietek to take us out to lunch, then reverting to the phone call, but suddenly puts his hand over the mouthpiece and calls out as we are leaving the room that we must not worry, things will work out - then we leave this chaotic efficiency.

Despite all the disorder the man creates around him, he is efficient — very efficient. Our errand does indeed turn out to be very difficult, but he will arrange it, just as has arranged things for many Jewish refugees who happened to end up in Sweden, as well as for many others who have never been here, never seen him, never even heard of him. For this boisterous, apparently disorganized man has not only a network of contacts at the highest level in Sweden, but also in Nazi Germany, and when necessary he would be able to do so in other countries. He has an amazing ability to track down niches of communion with influential people who understood and appreciated his greatness and the importance of the matter for which he unselfishly fights for like a lioness defending her injured cubs, sacrificing everything he possesses for it, himself as well as his family life.

In Sweden it is mostly Tage Erlander, Olof Palme and Gösta Engzell, the cabinet secretary, who help Storch, but when necessary he reaches others — and all this for a cause — helping persecuted Jews and Jewish refugees.

Many years later I am present in the room when Storch, in the middle of a meeting of the board of the Swedish section of the World Jewish Congress, with no apology leaves and rings Tage Erlander and says to Erlander's secretary, who must know him well: "It's Storch, I need to talk to the Prime Minister." When the secretary asks if it is important, he irritably replies: "Of course it's important, otherwise I wouldn't be phoning." Tage Erlander interrupts whatever he was doing to hold a long conversation with his stateless friend Storch, and all of us sitting round the table have to wait, or go away and do whatever we want to - Gilel Storch is chairman, so the meeting cannot go on without him.

When Gilel Storch dies many years later only his nearest relatives and a few invited friends — among them Nina and I - are at the North Jewish cemetery chapel in Stockholm. After a brief funeral service the then prime minister, Olof Palme, comes in after waiting outside so as not to disturb the ceremony. He stands quite still for a moment by the lonely coffin to honor the man he knew was great, and equally quietly leaves the chapel after exchanging a few words with the widow, Mrs. Storch.

It is regrettable that this remarkable man's achievements during and after the Second World War have never been charted, analyzed and described, and that Gilel Storch has not been given the recognition he and his achievements deserve. In a historical perspective, it should be of less importance that he was boisterous, apparently disorganized, and with his impatience and speechifying could wreck any well-planned meeting to which many busy people had been summoned. For what eventually should be counted is the result, and the reason for his undiplomatic behavior was that he thought much more quickly, with more foresight than others did and he had no patience to listen to chatter he considered inessential.

Gilel was a fearless man. When help was required for persecuted Jews he could acquire channels to the dictator of Spain, Generalissimo Franco, or the SS General Kaltenbrunner or Heinrich Himmler - the much-feared head of Nazi Germany's Gestapo. His strength stemmed from a genuine passion, an almost clairvoyant ability to foresee historical events and the human reactions of rulers in combination with a calculating cunning, smoothly to pursue his aims, which were noble to him. It is likely that by exploiting his contacts with Heinrich Himmler's Dutch masseuse Kersten he laid the foundations for Folke Bernadotte's magnificent rescue expedition with the white buses and their brave drivers.

It is also likely that through the same contacts with Kaltenbrunner and Himmler, he contributed to preventing the blowing up of the great prison camp in Bergen-Belsen.

Professor Dov Dinar at Haifa University, the historian of the Nazis, has found in German war archives correspondence that shows how Gilel Storch saw through the belief in the myth of the power of the Jews all over the world in several Nazi potentates, among them Himmler, and how Storch heightened this belief with his superior tone in the exchange of letters with Himmler, who was convinced that Storch - a stateless refugee - must have great power as a member of the World Jewish Congress World Executive and as its representative in neutral Sweden. I was there when Storch foresaw Franco's need for rehabilitation at the end of the war and exploited it to create channels to Spain's neighboring Arab countries to help the Jews confined there.

Gilel Storch was an unusual man. I feel boundless humility when faced with his greatness and willingness to sacrifice himself and everything he possessed to help us and other persecuted people — and we were many, terrifyingly many during this period which was so tragic for the Jewish people. We needed people like Gilel Storch. I shall always be grateful for being allowed to meet him and for a short period towards the end of his life have the honor of working closely with him on important matters — for the man only wanted to work on important matters — everything else was uninteresting to him.

At lunch, which we have been longing for, Mietek Tauman explains what Storch had really said and also what he really means. We are to report to the police. He tells us which trams we are to take to get to Police Headquarters in Bergsgatan. We can do this whenever we like, but it must be that day. From then on we are in the hands of the police and they will question us. He says we are to be honest and tell them everything. But he also says that if Gilel Storch has said everything will work out, we can trust him. He asks us if we have any money to get through the day, gives us his telephone number, pays the restaurant bill and says he must get back to the office — good luck to you.

We stay in the restaurant, deciding we need not hurry to report to the police, the day is long and we have a little money left. I go to the cinema, then we take the two trams Mietek has described and report at the police reception in Bergsgatan.

It is quite late in the day. We are each taken in for a brief questioning; I tell them where I come from and why, give them personal information and show them my student card, which they

The Maple Tree Behind the Barbed Wire

keep. The friendly policeman informs me that I have entered the country illegally — which I know — and that I may speak to a special aliens policeman the next day.

My first night after my arrival in Sweden is spent in the police cells in Bergsgatan.

The police cells in Bergsgatan are like a better guesthouse with full board and lodging in Poland, a much higher standard than my student accommodation in Lodz. True, the room is small and locked, but nevertheless it is not as I had imagined a prison cell to be. Comfortable bed, good radio programs from several countries, a small shelf of books in Swedish I can't read and excellent food. As I had said on my arrival in answer to a question: "No, have not had any dinner today, and yes - I am hungry", I am given a late dinner — hamburger with filling dark brown gravy and onions, potatoes cooked just right, butter, bread and fruit juice. In addition, that evening I am given an open sandwich with sliced sausage and hot tea, coffee or cocoa, but may also have a glass of cold milk, which surprises me. I haven't drunk milk since Sarah stopped breast-feeding me; adults don't drink milk in Poland.

Having eaten my cheese sandwich, drunk a mug of hot tea with two lumps of sugar and switched off the radio, I fall asleep in my comfortable bed in the police cells in Bergsgatan in Stockholm.

I sleep well, as a young man should, exhausted from the multitude of impressions of a long day and after an uncomfortable night on the train from Malmö, but I wake early with a diffuse anxiety and a growing sense of insecurity. Breakfast is just as abundant and good as dinner the evening before and I feel slightly calmer after eating it.

Just after ten, I meet the man from the Aliens Department. During the long and exhausting interrogation I am made to realise that the step I have taken is irrevocable, that the door is closed on the life I have lived as a student in Lódz and all the plans for the future I had had. I realise this intellectually, but still find it difficult to accept emotionally, and the delay between intellectual insight and emotional acceptance — as usual in me — creates an ambivalence which unfortunately is going to mark everything that happens during the rest of the day.

The policeman in charge of aliens is a well-built gentleman in his early middle years — he looks like a policeman, although he is not in uniform. He is not unfriendly, but formal and seems quite devoid of emotions, perhaps just as an interrogator should be. He speaks German grammatically more correctly than I do, but not as fluently.

We already find it difficult to agree when he is to note down my personal details. Name and date of birth are all right, and which country I come from. But we get stuck on nationality - I reply Jewish.

The Maple Tree Behind the Barbed Wire

He does not accept that, saying there is no such nationality, and I am hurt. He does not understand that over all my years in Poland I have not been allowed to be Polish, and I do not realise that he is right, that I have come to another country and here in Sweden, I am a Pole and nothing else. I get the impression he considers me not only stupid but also obstinate, which makes me feel even more misunderstood. In the end, when he thinks this is all taking up too much time, he solves the problem in his way. Was I born in Poland? Yes, I was. Am I a Polish citizen? I suppose so. Are my parents Polish citizens? Yes, I suppose they are. He is no longer listening when I try to explain that he is simplifying it all, and suggest that the correct description could be - Polish Jew.

So the matter is settled by an alien official in the interrogation room in Bergsgatan. From now onwards I am a Pole. For all my fourteen years in free Poland I had wished for nothing better than to be a Pole, but was not allowed to be. And leaving Poland, going to another country, then I become a Pole - is this not this an irony of capricious fate?

My thoughtless obstinacy in the important early stages marks the rest of the interrogation. It is obvious we are finding it difficult to understand each other and I soon see that it is the policeman who has priority in interpretation, which annoys me even more. He is not inquisitorial, but suspicious. He skillfully returns to the same subject, perhaps putting it in a different way and against another background.

Was I member of a political party? That I have never been — he is not interested when I explain that my father has told me I should never get involved in politics. Instead, the policeman wants to know whether before, during or after the war I have written any documents or had any authorization carried out by any association or society. When I make an effort to remember and start listing the student corps in Lódz, the Jewish student club, the sports society friends of ISKRA society, he wants to know whether any of these had links with any political party. I wonder what he writes down when I reply that as far as I know they have not. Have I ever been to a meeting of a political party or had any contact with the youth section of a political party? Was I active during the war or had I any contacts with any underground resistance movement? We again find it difficult to agree whether ZOB - the Jewish resistance movement — was a resistance movement in the sense he thinks, if the couriers staying overnight at home, and that several of them were school friends of mine are the kind of active involvement or contacts he is considering with his question. No, I was not active myself in ZOB. He returns again and again to the same but differently worded question: Was ZOB part of the communist underground movement in Poland? I tell him over and over again about the Hanysh group in the forests round Koniecpol, who took over several of the ZOB cells when they managed to escape from the Small Ghetto; he will have to decide for himself whether ZOB was or was not associated with the communist underground movement. I don't know what he has decided as he taps out my answers on his big black typewriter.

The policeman has filled four sheets of paper, which he puts face down on the desk and inserts the fifth clean sheet.

Why had I left Poland? Because of the persecution of the Jews, the pogrom in Kiele and because Jewish students were being maltreated at Polish universities, two recently murdered at Lodz and others threatened. He says that is not clear and he makes me understand that is not considered a good reason for seeking asylum in Sweden, but I protest and try to maintain that it is reason enough to escape from a country.

Towards the end of this long interrogation he asks me to think about whether there were no other reasons. Certainly not, only the persecution of the Jews, but they are threatening our lives, I reply. In the end he tries to help me. Did I feel persecuted or perhaps threatened by the communist regime in Poland? But I put the nail in my coffin and he gives up when I maintain that Poland has an internationally accepted coalition government and is not a communist regime, and also that I am totally uninterested in politics, but he doesn't tap those answers on to his black typewriter.

He looks through his papers, says he has no more questions, and suddenly sounds really friendly when he asks me to think it over should I perhaps have anything more to add and would like to have entered in my record. But I don't know what he has written down and in addition want to put an end to this long interrogation — so I say I don't think so. He looks at my record again, thinks for a moment, then holds out his hand and lets me go. At last I get my late lunch.

I am feeling rather unhappy, dissatisfied with myself, considering I had no reason to be irritated with the policeman questioning me. No one has done me any harm, but again I feel like a person with no rights — this time not as a member of a large collective but as an individual, which is worse. A policeman I regard as irreproachably correct, not unfriendly nor particularly friendly, has a right to put personal questions to me and require that I answer them, while he then decides how my replies are to be interpreted. I feel vulnerable.

Presumably I shall never know whether it was my foolhardy behavior during this first and hitherto only police interrogation I have been through in my life, or whether it was other thoughtless actions I am shortly to commit, which were the reasons why I was the only one in our group to have problems with my residence permit in Sweden.

Later that day all four of us are taken in an open car to the refugee camp in Vikingshill outside Stockholm and after a few days we were moved to the camp in Kummelnäs. During my time in camp, all the

The Maple Tree Behind the Barbed Wire

consequences of my actions become clear.

It is no help that it is lovely August weather, that the refugee camp is surrounded by lush greenery, that we have a wonderful view over a beautiful bay and that I think we have been treated generously. I don't regret what I have done, but at the same time feel lonely and write every day to my parents, long letters that breath of longing and melancholy.

We go through a whole series of medical examinations. A suspicion of diphtheria is found in Nina and she has to leave the group and be alone in quarantine at the isolation clinic in Sundbyberg. She stays there during our stay in the refugee camp and during our return journey to Denmark.

On the second day of our stay at Kummelnäs, during lunch in the communal dining hall, I am handed a message from the camp office - I have visitors. A lady of my mother's age, her husband and their overweight son are sitting in the waiting room. The son is like his mother and seems less sympathetic than his father.

They speak Polish and have been living in Sweden for a year. The lady says she is Sarah's cousin — in reality she is a second cousin, her married name Gustava Seideman. Gustava tells me Sarah has informed her that I have come to Sweden. Her son Wladek has looked into it and found that I am in the refugee camp in Kummelnäs. Sarah has asked her "to take care of me", which she very much wants to do. As proof of this, she has with her sandwiches; newly made plum jam and homemade cakes of the kind we used to eat in Poland. It is nice of them to come and thoughtful to bring this food with them, though I don't know what to do with it, except perhaps the cakes.

The son very soon got bored. But the parents are sincerely kindly, tell me they have arranged leave for me and that Wladek can come the next day to fetch me to take dinner at home with them. The next day Wladek comes and he is really pleasant when we are alone.

The Seideman family has a cozy little apartment in Döbelnsgatan. Gustava serves up an eastern European-Jewish dinner with all the delicacies I know from home. We talk for a long time. They tell me what it is like to be in Sweden - a fantastic country, says the sympathetic Mr. Seideman. Gustava tells me that Sarah has made contact with her by a telephone she managed to borrow at the town hall in Czestochowa. It was a short call, but Sarah wanted me to live with them when I leave the refugee camp and they want me to. She shows me the sofa bed in the living room where we are sitting. Things seem better and that evening I don't write quite such a long letter home to Czestochowa.

The Maple Tree Behind the Barbed Wire

Two days later, Mietek Tauman and Natek Calel come to the Kummelnäs camp bringing with them a message and a greeting from Gilel Storch; he has solved our problem. "He is fantastic," they both say, and we nod dutifully, but the solution is complicated. Denmark is our first country of asylum, Mietek explains — starting out from that we understand what this first country of asylum means — but no one is persecuted in Denmark, so Sweden does not accept refugees from Denmark. Denmark does not accept refugees, but it is not considered to be the Swedish authority's problem what Denmark does with its refugees. So Storch has arranged for us to have a temporary visa to give him time to arrange something better. But we must first go back to Denmark, to have our visas stamped and then cross the Swedish border in a more legal way than we had with the Danish fishing boat; this is a temporary solution, but the only one that can be arranged. We will be sent to Denmark, they say, but we will come back to Stockholm and then there will be time to arrange something more permanent. This sounds rather complicated, but we trust Storch.

The next day, early in the morning, three policemen come to fetch us from the Kummelnäs camp — two male and one female — in civilian clothes.

We have plenty of time to pack the little we have with us and they do not hurry us. The older of the two men fills in various forms as we pass through the camp office. They are friendly, but the policewoman goes with Toska when she needs to go to the toilet. On the train they talk more freely to us, their German rather halting. They are watchful all the time, but none of us is even thinking of escaping. Where would we escape to?

On arrival in Denmark we are handed over to the Danish border police in Helsingör. They fill in three forms — a receipt for each of the three refugees they have received — the Swedish police bid us a fairly warm farewell, wishing us all the best, then turn back on the ferry to Sweden. That is the way three refugees are deported from Sweden.

Once the Danish border police have entered into their logbook what has happened they are fairly uninterested in what our future fates are; we have done nothing illegal in Denmark, and it is not illegal to leave the country in a fishing boat and they appear to be uninterested in how we left Denmark. They say we are to go to Copenhagen and report to the aliens police there — do we know where it is? They give us our railway tickets to Copenhagen Central Station.

The girl behind the counter at the aliens police in Copenhagen, two floors up in a large building, says we may sit down. After a while an older, uniformed policeman comes and tells one of the girls behind the counter how she is to register us. Then he turns to us and says in perfect English that we must report to the aliens police every day until our case has been dealt with. He asks us if we have understood what he has said and we are allowed to go.

The Maple Tree Behind the Barbed Wire

We phone our old friend, Mr. Margolinski. He suggests we stop overnight at a hotel — naming a cheap hotel nearby and asking if we have any money. Toska and Helenka take the tram to the hotel. I go to the railway station to buy a return ticket to Klampenborg.

Margaretha opens the door when I ring the bell, then calls for Bodil. It is already dusk and they are dressed to go out. Bodil's great eyes widen and her otherwise calm and controlled look is confused, but she quickly pulls herself together and seems more sorrowful than surprised. Margaretha starts off — couldn't I have said something before leaving, just disappearing like that, was that necessary? They were disappointed and Bodil is still miserable. I say nothing — what could I say?

Margaretha asks me into the living room I know so well. They talk to each other in rather agitated Danish - they have never done that before in my presence, Margaretha is not at all pleased, nor is she understanding when Bodil rather resignedly takes off her hat and her light summer coat, then and sits down in an armchair opposite me. Margaretha is to go on her own to the friends there were to meet, so I feel guilty, but can do nothing about it.

I have acted clumsily, but it had seemed natural to try to go to Bodil and I had very much wanted to. I know there is a telephone on the table beneath the mirror in their hall, but I have not their telephone number and have never needed to ring them before — a wretched excuse.

That evening is different from our previous evenings. Any luster I may have had as a student on a brief visit from an exotic country has faded, and with it my self-confidence. I am now a homeless refugee with no country of my own and with an uncertain future.

Bodil fusses round me, asking what I want to my tea. I sense that she quite justifiably cannot forgive me for simply disappearing, but she does not take the subject up. Margaretha has said what there was to be said, and I think there is no point in trying to explain — that would not make things any better. Between us, things are now serious. Bodil says little, I talk about myself in a more open way than ever before, and Bodil listens. We go to bed quite late that night and do not hear when Margaretha comes home.

The next day I report to the aliens police. Our visas have come. We can fetch our papers at the Swedish Consulate and can count on taking the night train back to Stockholm the next day. I go back to Klampenborg.

Bodil has pulled herself together and Margaretha has calmed down. They have made a simple dinner and are expecting me. Margaretha tells me that the Polish student group left several days ago. Some had defected — most to England. She tells me a little about Bodil, about Bodil's parents and I listen. Bodil is miserable, but so am I, and we don't try to hide it. I say that I shall probably get my visa the next morning and will be returning to Sweden. I am given a photograph of Bodil but have none to give her.

This last night we have together is also different. Bodil asks whether we cannot just hold each other, and we feel a calm, rather melancholy tenderness. We talk a little, but say nothing of importance; we both know that this is probably the last time we are to be together, but neither of us mentions it. With little conviction, Bodil says that I must let her know how things go for me in Sweden. After a while, she says things may be difficult for me, for the Swedes are not so open and kindly as people I have met in Denmark. We are silent for long spells. I can hear Bodil is awake, but the silence does not seem troublesome. We fall asleep or doze closer to each other than on any other occasion.

On several occasions I have thought of contacting Bodil. But at first I found it difficult, with nothing much to tell her. Later, I have not wanted to out of consideration for Nina, and after that out of consideration for Bodil - unwilling to trample into her life once again.

I can still think about how things have gone for Bodil, whether she is still alive, is still in Denmark? Presumably she is married, has children and I do sincerely hope she is happy, for she deserves that. I know so little about Bodil, and it would be difficult to track down wherever she may be. Also - is that appropriate? Is it not best to keep our memories of each other— as they are now? I still have a photograph — a half-length portrait of Bodil. It is in our photo album and I look at it when we leaf through the album.

Now, nearly fifty years later, as I write these lines, I still can't help wondering why this distinguished young lady wanted to be with me. Inviting a more or less strange young man back home was not her usual behavior - I know that. I think something had happened to Bodil just before we met and I happened to appear at the right moment. I had so little to offer, except genuine admiration, and perhaps I also turned out to be a warm person. Perhaps that was just what Bodil needed at that moment — unconcealed admiration and genuine human warmth, then it did not matter that I had no money — she had — or that I was not up to much as a lover, she could teach me that. We met at a point in time when we needed each other and were able to satisfy that need, and with it followed gratitude and warmth and those — gratitude and warmth — are not really all that little — in fact are quite a lot when I think about it.

At the Central Station in Stockholm, our faithful friend Mietek Tauman is there to meet us. He explains that we have a Swedish visa to stay for two months that we can apply for an extension, so we are now free to go wherever we want. I have a street map of Stockholm and walk from the station in Vasagatan to the Seidemans' home in Döbelnsgatan - though soon come to regret doing so.

The Maple Tree Behind the Barbed Wire

They are in mourning. The thoroughly nice Mr. Seideman has unexpectedly died only three days earlier and, as is the Jewish custom, had been buried the next day. Gustava Seideman and her son Wladek welcome me and for the rest of the day, they talk about their unhappiness, which is quite natural. Who else would they talk to otherwise? They have few acquaintances in Sweden.

All day, Mrs. Seideman again and again asks why has she survived the war, was it for her to be afflicted with this? I realize this is a rhetorical question I do not have to answer. She expects me to share her grief, which is profound and genuine. But I have met her husband only twice and am genuinely sorry about what has happened, nonetheless find it hard to grieve as she is. Both Mrs. Seideman and Wladek notice this and are critical. I try even harder, succeed a little and sink into a state that must resemble depression. That is not particularly difficult in my position, with thirty kronor in my pocket, no plans for the future and a residence visa for not quite two months, based on a travel arrangement in Denmark entitling me to only one single entry to Sweden with no re-entry if I leave the country.

The days go by and I don't take any initiative except to write even longer letters to my poor parents. I have sunk into an apathy that often afflicts people who have lost their future. The only glimmer of light is Nina's irregular but faithful visits. It had been a false alarm, and Nina did not have diphtheria. When she leaves the isolation hospital, she has to take her trip to Denmark, everything is better prepared and she is able to return to Sweden the same day.

Nina tries to talk me out of it, but not even she has any advice that I can take on myself — so instead I begin on the next letter to Czestochowa. After a few days I gradually begin to run small errands for Mrs. Seideman, who now expects me to address her as ciocia — aunt. Ciocia Gustava goes on sending me to the neighboring shop although she is seldom pleased with my purchases. I am also responsible for the washing up, laying the table and getting breakfast.

After yet another week — when the Jewish period of mourning, Shiva, is formally over but in reality goes on though in less ritualistic forms, Toska Roller comes to see me.

Toska is a stable person who does not allow herself to be disturbed by the atmosphere in the Seideman household; she behaves and talks as if she had no knowledge of the awful thing that has happened to the family. This is not particularly considerate to ciocia Gustava, but a blessing to me. Toska says, not in a whisper as most do in this apartment, but in a loud clear voice they can all hear that she has applied for an entrance test to the School of Chemistry at Stockholm University. She has spoken to the professor, I think she says Professor Silén, he has seen her student certificate and exam book from the equivalent in Lódz, and has said it is perfectly all right to apply. Toska asks if I want to do the same, adding that Silén has his reception time that same afternoon and the time for applying for the entrance test will soon have passed.

To me it is as if the sun had come out from behind thick black clouds. From the start I have found it difficult to choose between chemistry and medicine. Fate has decided I should come to Sweden, and that after all it was to be chemistry — not at all bad.

I say to ciocia Gustava that I shall go with Toska to Stockholm University and she says in a subdued voice: "If you want to." I fetch my student certificate, translated into Swedish in the refugee camp, my exam marks book which is still not translated, and go, not just to the nearby post office or to the corner shop, but with Toska as guide to Stockholm University School of Chemistry. Neither Toska nor I think for one moment about how we are to finance our studies.

Professor Silén is a slim, unexpectedly young, agreeable and helpful person. Of course I can apply but he adds that the test is difficult and wonders whether we know enough Swedish to understand the questions. "That will work out," says Toska brightly. "We can ask if there is anything we don't understand." "You do that," says Silén, then his voice changes. "But only the teacher supervising the entrance test and no one else."

I have just enough money for the entrance test fee. I am given a thin compendium, but Professor Silén says that all that is really necessary is gymnasium level in chemistry and mathematics and I have good marks, he adds encouragingly.

Back with the Seidemans, I read the compendium with the aid of the thin Polish-Swedish, Swedish-Polish paperback dictionary with a dark brown cover I have taken from the store in Vikingshills refugee camp; this my very first effort in the Swedish language. With the aid of the dictionary I am able to understand many Swedish words; other words are not in it, but most of them I recognize all the same, the Swedified international chemical and mathematical terms.

A few days later ciocia Gustava wishes to speak to me. Wladek is there and acts as prompter. She says she is my only relative here in Sweden. Sarah has asked her to look after me and she must take on the responsibility. "What you are doing is meaningless," says Gustava. Refugees, most of all those from non-Nordic countries, cannot get into a Swedish university — no one does, not even her Wladek. And if you succeed, how are you going to finance your studies? The best thing you can do is not to waste time on such childishness, get yourself a practical profession instead so that you can earn a living. Wladek prompts — in Sweden there are labour exchanges and he has found out that they arrange fee-free courses in fields where there is a shortage of labour. I can be given a loan for my keep during a course of that kind but not for long university courses — not even Swedes can get that.

The Maple Tree Behind the Barbed Wire

This is difficult. They pay for my keep and I live with them as a favor, but I am now on a newly aroused narrow path of hope and they do not succeed in knocking me down. I would fail anyhow, though not for economic reasons.

The written test consists of some easy, but many difficult and long questions; we have three and a half hours to answer them. My problems understanding the language contribute to that I am the last to hand in my answers just as the time runs out, and the teacher is looking impatiently over my shoulder as in a great hurry I am writing the last lines.

Neither Toska nor I pass the test. When we return to hear the results, Silén explains how close I had got to passing, but that is no help — either you pass and then you can read chemistry, or you don't. The next entrance test is in a year's time.

I go back to the apartment in Döbelngatan and the small services I do for Mrs. Seideman, for where else can I go? Again start writing long letters back home to Czestochowa, but this time I don't sink into my paralyzing lack of enterprise. There has been an opportunity, which I had indeed not managed, but if there have once been opportunities so more might arise — all roads are clearly not closed here in Sweden. I begin to go out to meet the few people I know here in Stockholm. As long as I am living with them, Mrs. Seideman requires that I am back at the latest by ten o'clock at night, otherwise she cannot sleep. I am just twenty-one and fall in with this.

Nina and Helenka have been given a six months' grant by the Jewish Congregation in order to be trained as laboratory assistants. In practice, they are already full-time assistants at the Wenner-Gren Institute in Nortullsgatan; it is just that their salaries come in the form of a grant from the Congregation, a grant that has to be repaid.

It is not easy to be a refugee in a foreign country and I don't think anyone chooses to be one voluntarily. You see yourself as without rights, even if in reality you are perhaps not, at least not entirely. You are torn up by your roots from your country, which you are beginning to remember in increasingly rosy colors, you miss environments you recognize and your previous plans for the future. You are alone, longing back to the country where people understand you and where you understand them. It is not just the language, but also a feeling for the customs of the country and for what people really mean when they say something.

I don't know the language, nor can I pronounce the words I have learnt. When I try to go to the main street of the city, the name of which Wladek has written down on a piece of paper, no one understands when I say it over and over again - Kungsgatan. "There is no such street. Anyhow, I don't know where it is, ask someone else", until an enterprising passer-by takes the piece of paper from me and reads out aloud, "Oh, you mean Kungsgatan"; then you do not feel happy. No, I don't think there are any "economic refugees" — no one chooses to become a refugee unless forced to, or is misled.

Mrs. Seideman goes on and on about that I should go to the labour exchange — as she keeps me, her words weigh heavily on me. In the end I go to the nearest labour exchange and am kindly received. "There's a shortage of galvanizers," says the young official, "so it's a safe occupation", he goes on — the course starts next week.

I very much wanted to be a tailor, but was not suited to that. My father had said that instead I would have to be a doctor or an engineer, and I tried to be that, but fate did not want it to be so, so instead I shall become a galvaniser. There is no shortage of tailors here in Sweden, the official replies to my question, and I know I would not be any good at that profession, but could I become a good galvaniser?

The Maple Tree Behind the Barbed Wire

Birkagården Folk High School

I don't really know who told me that there were adult education colleges called folk high schools in Sweden, one in Stockholm called Birkagården. Folk High School sounds good and I wonder what it might be. Two days before I am to start my training as a galvaniser, I go to Birkegården Folk High School at Karlbergsvägen 86B and have the good fortune to meet the rector, Gillis Hammar. Going there was a wise decision.

At critical stages in my life here in Sweden, I have been lucky enough to meet people with the ability to be generous with themselves, who have wanted to help me and have also had the prerequisites to do so. The first was Gilel Storch, to whom Nina and I return several times when no one else wanted to or was able to help us; the second was to be Gillis Hammar.

When I meet Gillis Hammar for the first time, he is already a well-known and appreciated personality in the important if not very glamorous sector of workers' education — the world of the folk high schools. Rector Gillis Hammar is a syndicalist; he has unrealistic expectations of society, but at the same time is a practical man of action. Rector Gillis Hammar and his wife Lisa - who supports him in everything he undertakes — seem content with their simple life, Gillis Hammar obsessed by his vocation to help ambitious young people who for some reason are finding life difficult. This presumably applies to several heads of folk high schools during this period, when the leveling out of social differences was only just beginning. Gillis Hammar considers I am one of the group of his potential protégés and contracts to take me in hand over several important months.

Birkagården Folk High School turns out to be the best possible introduction to a new country for a lost refugee with a thirst for knowledge, and Rector Hammar the best possible supervisor and teacher during the process. He takes me in hand at the just right moment - I have become sufficiently pushed around to have any realistic expectations, but have not yet got as far as giving up my ambitions.

Rector Hammar is a tall, slightly stooping man, his greying hair thin and usually untidy. He looks stern, but he isn't, though on the other hand he is demanding, while at the same time understanding the shortcomings of his students — a happy combination for the head of a folk high school. He speaks good German when he receives me in his simple, rather battered office, looks piercingly at me with his sharp pale grey eyes beneath bushy greying eyebrows, and he lets me talk for a long time, listening without comment as I tell him why I have come to see him.

The Maple Tree Behind the Barbed Wire

Gillis Hammar clearly finds it difficult to decide what to do with me. He has a habit of occasionally thinking aloud and I am not sure if he is talking to me or to himself as he sternly mumbles about the application date for his college has long since passed, that the student uptake is over and the autumn term already begun, I have a feeling there is hesitation in his voice, which contributes to me staying in his office and saying that I have had no chance of applying before — as if that gave me the right to be accepted. Rector Hammar looks at me for a while longer as I stand there, my arms hanging down, and he repeats — almost to himself — that naturally he has the right to take on extra students. I think he seems relieved to have decided, and he hands me a piece of paper to fill in with a few necessary personal details. Unfortunately, he has no room left if I want to live in, he adds, then he brightens and smiles his friendly but rare smile as he gives me dates and times when the course starts and says I am to bring with me the term's fees of ninety kronor. That includes the food we get in school over the whole of the autumn term, but not lodgings.

After I have filled up the form, thanked him and held out my hand to say goodbye, Rector Hammar looks searchingly at me and asks me if I have any money for the fees. "No, I haven't", I say cheekily. Uneasy in case this may make him change his mind, I add: "But it'll probably work out", although I have no idea how. Gillis Hammar is beginning to understand me and says resignedly that he can probably arrange a grant of ninety kronor from the Beskowska Foundation - no, there's no need to apply for that, all I have to do is sign a paper he hands to me. He then asks me where I am going to live and mumbles slightly irritably: "Why didn't you say so?" when I reply that I don't know. I can't bear the thought of staying on with the Seidemans, and anyhow I don't know if they would have me. Hammar seems to be indefatigable and also have unlimited sources of help for helpless young people. He makes a phone call and arranges for me to have a maid's room in a civil engineer's household in the large corner apartment house in Karlbergsvägen 46 in exchange for doing the dishes every evening when I get back from school.

That same day I meet pleasant Mrs. Lagerman and she thinks I will do, in spite of being a man and not knowing a word of Swedish. With the little I possess, I move in with them the very next day. I really have to move out of the Seidemans apartment as soon as possible and be free of ciocia Gustava's and Wladek's increasingly suffocating influence.

A new period of my life begins, a breathing space, when the fresh wounds of separation begin to heal and before new ones are inflicted.

The Maple Tree Behind the Barbed Wire

In the mid-1940s, the folk high schools of Sweden are gathering places and nurseries for ambitious young working class people wanting to acquire an education but cannot afford to. There are few grants for university studies, most vouchsafed for particularly gifted students, the state-funded student loans not yet invented. It is hard for young people who have grown up in financially poor families and for lone young people — like me — to find a wealthy person who will guarantee a loan from a bank. From an economic point of view, Sweden is still a divided society and the principle, long term most fundamental demand for equality — the same right and practical opportunity of an education — has still not been provided for.

That was to happen many years later, when the young Olof Palme was assigned by the Ecclesiastic Minister (in charge of education) Tage Erlander investigated and later as Prime Minister brought in Sweden's present grant/loan system for education, and when Ingvar Carlsson investigated and together with Olof Palme legislated for a coherent educational system. I share Ingvar Carlsson's view that this was the son of a rich man, Olof Palme's foremost and lasting contribution to the future of his country, for this was also the prerequisite to the mobilization of Sweden's slumbering reserve of talent. But in the autumn of 1946, these important reforms were not even planned and the folk high school was the only alternative for many ambitious working class young people.

Apart from lack of finance, a number of the students in our college are handicapped in other ways, among them myself, with fewer than ten Swedish words and that no one understands me when I try to pronounce them. In the same class is another Jewish refugee from Poland, the gentle Halina Zjaczkowska, who, however, seems more at home here than I am. She has her mother and older brothers and sisters in Sweden, and, most of all, she speaks better Swedish.

All students in our year are oddities in some way or other, perhaps why we accept each other. This is also the distinguishing mark of both the college and Gillis Hammar - accepting and being accepted — a wonderful milieu for someone with painful experiences of not being accepted.

For the majority of the students, Birkagården is their home during their period of education, those who are there all the time and have the luck to have a room at the college. Included in the term's fees are three good meals a day and snacks between, for four months — not bad for ninety kronor. But some of the male students already have wives and children and work in the evenings to support their families. They are older than most and it can be seen that they are tired.

Every evening, joint activities are arranged, sometimes organized, otherwise spontaneous, and if necessary, individual teaching for students finding it hard to keep up in some subject. I have a great need for both fellowship and individual teaching, especially in the

The Maple Tree Behind the Barbed Wire

language of the country, in Swedish. And I am given it, too, two hours three times a week from our Swedish teacher Signe Fagerholm. I have not found a single teacher in our college who does not work in the evenings whenever necessary, or heard any of them complain — they know what they have let themselves in for when they took on a badly paid job — no overtime exists, for the college cannot afford it.

My only formal teaching of the Swedish language consists of a term at Birkagården Folk High School. I am also given incomplete but anyhow fairly decent knowledge of the history of the country and I learn how a democracy and a society striving for equality functions. I also learn to oppose authority.

I have grown up in a hierarchical and authoritarian society, in a loving but authoritarian home, and gone to authoritarian schools. I would never have dreamt of questioning anything a teacher said, and certainly not openly. When I find out what it is like at Birkagården, I try out in my halting broken Swedish the ultimate limits — how far can one go? Maybe it is quite natural that I do so during Gillis Hammar's lessons — he is the highest authority in the college. To my amazement and astonished admiration, I find there are no limits. On the contrary, very skillfully, Gillis Hammar encourages the class to question things, and with his characteristic seriousness, he also takes part in the discussions. He can be impatient when an exchange of opinions between him and me becomes tedious and disturbing, but never does he make a fool of this troublesome student. He takes all my questions seriously. I recognize this — my father Pinkus also took all my questions seriously.

Being taken seriously is a prerequisite for self-confidence, for daring to think independently and reasonably unbiased. For - for good or bad — no human being can think wholly unprejudicedly.

My days an evenings at Birkagården Folk High School are filled with interesting and exciting activities. I meet people who accept me for what I am, and with whom I feel great fellowship. I learn Swedish folk dances, become quite good at the schottis, and in the sheltered world of Birkagården I grow into Swedish fellowship, learn and appreciate what I think is the innermost soul of my new country. My gratitude to the fellow-students of my year, my teachers and Gillis Hammar knows no bounds.

My letters to Czestochowa become shorter and shorter and intervals between them longer. I begin to take an interest in the girls of my year, which for a young man is a sign of recovery from the apathy of confusion, and I begin to meet, let us call her Ulrika.

Ulrika is slender, moves slightly indolently but lithely, and has short chestnut hair and green rather dreamy eyes. She is meticulously turned out, an ambitious and really clever student, taciturn but purposeful, and she has a strong will. Mrs. Lagerman no longer leaves

The Maple Tree Behind the Barbed Wire

the washing up to me in the evenings. I have become a member of the family and it hardly worries them that I don't always come back home to my maid's room at night.

Ulrika's mother often works at night. I am occasionally at their modest but soberly and tastefully furnished terrace house in its small well-kept plot of land. But I am given no opportunity to meet Ulrika's mother. Ulrika does not want me to. Sometimes we talk long into the evening, but I do most of the talking, about my plans or dreams for the future. After college, I am to try to get into university and - I am thinking aloud and speaking dreamily — reading chemistry or some other scientific subject. I read medicine before, but that's hardly likely now, but chemistry is also good.

Ulrika is a good listener, but refrains from commenting on my excursions into the future. She is more restrained, and has said nothing about herself until one day, she quickly tells me about her family circumstances — there is no father in Ulrika's life. But talking about it is painful for this otherwise so self-controlled girl, who is suddenly sitting resignedly close to me, and I sense an undercurrent of profound sorrow.

One evening Ulrika suddenly says, with a touch of aggressiveness in her voice: You'll never be allowed to go to university here in Sweden. Then she falls silent. I say nothing, miserable mostly because she doesn't believe me, because she has so brutally told me so, and because I've clearly talked too much. In future, I talk less about my dreams for the future, clearly tedious to Ulrika. Shortly after that our meetings come to an end when one evening, the course on a weekend outing, Ulrika rejects me for a sympathetic dark-haired leader who openly courts her. My male vanity is wounded.

Nina comes to see me once or twice at the beginning of my time at Birkagården, then, seeing things are all right for me, she stops coming. But one evening towards the end of November, Nina comes back, takes me aside and excitedly asks me if I want to read medicine at Uppsala University.

Nina likes being with people, but not the job of laboratory assistant at the Wenner-Gren Institute. Although she is a refugee in a foreign country, Nina finds it hard to accept that she may not become a doctor, what she has always wanted to be even when a small girl. Nina is stubborn and persevering, she ferrets things out and asks. Nina knows Kim Cramér, son of the professor of mathematics and rector of Stockholm University. Kim has read medicine at Uppsala, and on one occasion he has mentioned to Nina that there are some Norwegian students at Uppsala who, without the student exam, have been allowed to read medicine as extra-students. This gives us hope — if they can, perhaps we can.

The Maple Tree Behind the Barbed Wire

Nina, Helenka and Toska live with the same landlady in a villa in Häggvik. When it is not raining, Nina cycles to the Wenner-Gren Institute in Norrtullsgatan. She manages well on her grant, but she wants to save up and buy a bicycle. Older second-hand bicycles are cheap and you can save on train fares if you have the energy to cycle from Häggvik to Norrtullsgatan in the city centre every day.

Nina collects names and addresses of people she can turn to in Uppsala, takes out her bicycle, which she has already put away for the winter, and sets off early in the morning on the long way to Uppsala. There she meets Kim Cramér an older medical student at Uppsala - Harald Eliasch and Halinka Lis, her school friend from Lódz. Both Kim and Harald confirm that there are Norwegians who have been accepted to read medicine as "extra-students". They were refugees during the war and were allowed to go on with their studies. But they are not very encouraging, saying that not only was it in the middle of the war and they came from a neighboring Nordic country and could also speak Swedish. But Nina does not give up. In Stockholm, she has already heard about Hugo Valentin, lecturer in history at Uppsala University, who in various contexts has helped Jewish refugees, so she goes to see him at his home in Uppsala.

Hugo Valentin is a person who never in advance considers anything impossible. He has, as Nina has, a deeply ingrained conviction that all roads have to be tried first.

Valentin takes on our cause, speaks to Professor Gunnar Dahlberg, head of the Institute of Racial Biology at the School of Medicine at Uppsala. Dahlberg, in his turn, speaks to Professor David Holmdahl, head of the Department of Anatomy, in Sweden responsible for teaching the first term of medical studies. These two teachers at the School of Medicine in Uppsala discuss it together and come to the conclusion that there is nothing to prevent Holmdahl taking extra-students on to his course — at the time, professors had great power or thought they had, and acted accordingly.

When Hugo Valentin has accumulated these basic details, he meets Nina the next day and tells her she can bring her two friends from Poland - she has told him about Helenka and me — we are all to go together to Uppsala the following week to meet him first, then Dahlberg next, and finally Holmdahl. He thinks it should go well — under any circumstances, it is all he can do at the moment. "One course is not much," says Hugo Valentin. "But let's see what happens after the anatomy course."

We have lived a "day-to-day" existence during the war and have learnt not to think in the long term. So Nina is not all that worried about the time after the course in anatomy.

It has snowed during the night so Nina cannot cycle forty miles back in the snow. She leaves her bicycle in Uppsala, borrows money from Halinka for her train fare and comes to me to ask if I want to start

The Maple Tree Behind the Barbed Wire

reading medicine in Uppsala. Of course I do. Suddenly a possibility I had already rejected has arisen.

I go to Gillis Hammar. He says of course I can have the day off to go to Uppsala, but he adds that he thinks I ought to finish the second term at Birkagården, then I will have a better start in Sweden. Gillis Hammar is, as usual, quite right. I am not ready to leave college and my Swedish is still extremely bad. But the chance Nina has given me is something that is happening now and would perhaps never arise again. So Helenka, Nina and I club together to finance our railway fares to Uppsala.

Hugo Valentin is a modest yet impressive person, with friendly but obvious authority, sparse coarse wavy hair, greying and wild — he has the usual sorrowful eyes of a friendly old Jew and a soft melancholy smile — he has seen much Jewish suffering and radiates compassion and goodness. Our visit to him is short. He has spoken to Professor Dahlberg again, who has spoken to Holmdahl and everything appears to have been confirmed. Hugo Valentin wants us to come back after we have met the two professors, to tell him how things have gone.

We meet Professor Dahlberg in his office at the Institute of Racial Biology. Hugo Valentin has not told us he is confined to a wheelchair and has difficulty moving without help - battery operated wheelchairs not yet invented.

Professor Dahlberg is mostly a researcher, and for emotional reasons, but also from scientific conviction, is a combative anti-racist. He has become the head of this institute at the Faculty of Medicine in Uppsala in order to abolish it.

He seems tired but his gaze is strong and brave, not that of a weak and unhappy person. This meeting is also a brief one. Dahlberg tells us that Professor Holmdahl can receive us the same day at his Department of Anatomy. He has no teaching this week, so we can go whenever it suits us. Nina says it suits us to meet him now, at once. Dahlberg smiles his tired smile when he sees our eagerness and - while he is waiting for David Holmdahl to come to the phone - he asks us if we are aware that this is only one course, with no guarantee that we may continue training. Then he consoles us by saying that Holmdahl has promised to talk to the head of the Department of Histology, who is responsible for the teaching over the coming term. We need no consolation, but he has done his best to warn us.

His hand is cool and moist as he holds it out to say goodbye. This is the only time we meet this fine man with such a strong will in a weak body.

Professor David Holmdahl is the diametric opposite of Dahlberg - straight-backed, loud and bald, he appears to be constantly trying to convince - mostly himself — of his vigor. However, he seems rather stiff and clumsy, moving a lot, walking to and fro and gesticulating as he speaks. He does not bother to look at our Polish student marks translated into Swedish, but he wants to see our exam books that confirm that we had been at a university and had begun reading medicine in our home country. Holmdahl explains in his superior school German that it was on this basis that the Norwegians had been accepted as extra-students.

Our visit to Holmdahl lasts somewhat longer. Helenka and Nina do most of the talking about Lódz University, how the teaching was planned, which subjects we took, how the tests were organized. Holmdahl is interested, but surprised when he hears we were six hundred students in a course in Lódz. There are only twenty-five in his. He seems satisfied with our visit and finally says we are to be at roll call at ten o'clock on January 22nd. Meanwhile it would be good if we got hold of the three volumes of Rauber Kopsch's textbook in anatomy — there are only second-hand copies available — and preferably Corning's textbook in topographical anatomy as well, but that is difficult to find. All three of us confirm at the same time that we know that he can only prepare us for entrance on to his own course. We are downhearted when he fails to say anything about speaking later on to Professor Wrete, head of the Department of Histology.

It turns out that the warning we have been given from these three experienced older teachers is quite justified, and it is risky, really foolhardy to ignore their warnings. We are leaving everything we have begun to build up here in Sweden in order to go on to a single course at the Faculty of Medicine in Uppsala. But we take the risk, really without any further thought, and that is to turn out to be justified. Before then, however, a great deal is to happen and the final decision is up to other people, those seniors in the academic and bureaucratic hierarchy. But it was David Holmdahl and Gunnar Dahlberg, on Hugo Valentin's urging and Nina's initiative, who gave us the chance - without it, not one of us would have been allowed to read medicine in Sweden.

Both Hugo Valentin and his wife are genuinely interested in all that has happened to us during the day. Mrs. Valentin offers us tea and quantities of homemade cakes "so that we won't be hungry on the journey home". I now realise for the first time that I have not eaten anything since our early breakfast at Birkagården Folk High School.

After we had said goodbye, Hugo Valentin calls me back and hands me a postal order signed by him for 350 kronor — his fee for articles in Dagens Nyheter. Slightly nonchalantly and dismissively, he says it is an unexpected bonus. He gets all tangled up in an unnecessary explanation as he tries to say he doesn't need the money, and he doesn't know what to do with it. He makes it seem as if I am doing him

The Maple Tree Behind the Barbed Wire

a favor by relieving him of this burden, just so that we don't feel degraded by receiving this unexpected gift, a small fortune to us. We get the money out at the post office and share it between the three of us.

The autumn term at Birkagården is coming to an end. Gillis Hammar is disappointed when I tell him I am not coming back for the 1947 spring term. He is reserved, distant, but wishes me luck all the same when at the end of term I leave his school.

I am to keep contact with Birkagården Folk High School as well as Gillis and Lisa Hammar long after I left the college. Out of gratitude for what it has meant to me, as a qualified doctor I have lectured there for nothing, until the new rector, Lennart Seth, considered I had become too specialized to be any good as a teacher at his college. I am glad Halinka Zajaczkowska and I managed to go to see Lisa and Gillis Hammar shortly before Gillis died — they were pleased to see us and glad to know things had gone well for us. I am a member of the Friends of the College and still go to the gatherings, although I hardly recognize any of the old students. Recently I was honored to be asked to describe my memories of Birkagården in a pamphlet published for the college's seventieth anniversary.

At the point when I started at his school, the forceful but modest Gillis Hammar was at the height of his intellectual powers. He has at last been acknowledged for the contributions he made before, during and after the war as a fearless anti-Nazi and farsighted champion for human rights, during a period when those terms seemed to be empty phrases. Gillis Hammar also had his sixtieth birthday during my time at the school, and then, for purely formal reasons, he is irrevocably to be pensioned off — which is cruel and unjust. Gillis is to live on for another thirty years, his physique and intellectual strength unimpaired, but away from the foremost task of his life, before dying peacefully at ninety-five, physically though not intellectually impaired during the last years of his life.

The Maple Tree Behind the Barbed Wire

Student in Uppsala

There are a series of things to be done before I move to Uppsala - registering at the university, choice of which student "nation" — group I am to join, getting hold of textbooks, finding somewhere to live and — arranging for how to pay for my keep while studying.

At the end of the Birkagården term, through the labour exchange I manage to find a reliable source of income that suits me admirably — washing up at restaurants. My skills, evolved at the Seideman family and developed doing the dishes at the Lagermans, are to come in useful. This is temporary work. You are not allowed to wash up every night, but quite often. "My" restaurants in Stockholm are the Scandinavian in Fridhemsplan and the Bacchi Vapen in the Old City, near Järntorget.

A strictly hierarchical order prevails in a restaurant. At the top is the Head Waiter and with him, the head chef, then the waiters — they have to face the customers and are the aristocracy of restaurant staff — after that come the cold buffet and other kitchen staff, then right at the bottom come the washers-up. But I like the work, meet interesting people and earn good wages — by my standards, at first one krona twenty öre, then later one-fifty an hour, more at the Scandinavian, less at the Bacchi Vapen. My needs are small and I manage very well on washing-up three or four times a week.

Helenka and Nina tell me they have applied to the Jewish Congregation for a grant, or a loan for their medical studies. They meet the senior official of the Congregation, ombudsman David Köpnivsky, then later the Congregation's chairman - the bookseller Gunnar Josephson - but no loan was available. Both Köpnivsky and Josephson were friendly, obliging and wanting to help, but Köpnivsky explained that they could not give a loan of 20,000 kronor. I don't understand. Who needs a loan of 20,000 kronor? Nina tells me how Köpnivsky had calculated - 250 kronor a month, ten months of the year for eight years — that comes to exactly 20,000 kronor.

We refugees, whose standard of living has not risen since the war, do not require 250 kronor a month, nor do we think in such a long term as eight years. But Köpnivsky is right in principle. Medical studies do take eight years, and also the board of the Congregation cannot know who we are — whether we are serious about our studies, whether we will be allowed to go on after the preliminary anatomy year, or whether we are going to stay here in Sweden. So - no grant from the Jewish Congregation - not this time. However, I manage to acquire some starting capital. The time has come to sell that heavy silver cigarette case. I get 160 kronor for it in a jewelry store in Stockholm - I think that will do.

The Maple Tree Behind the Barbed Wire

By chance I get to know another Polish student who is to read medicine at Uppsala - Alexander Weinfeld. Alex comes from a religious but not orthodox Jewish family near the town of Kraków. He is older than I am and has an unusually wide higher education and experience. Alex has first tried theology - in a Yeshiva. Then he read practical philosophy, before deciding on medicine — an unusually widely read and intellectually inclined person, which I don't consider myself to be. We decide to go to Uppsala together to find somewhere to live — but that turns out to be rather less than easy.

There is a shortage of student lodgings. Largely lone older ladies find means to pay their own rents and make their own income go further by letting rooms to students. It is a landlady's market, especially when the new term is about to start, so it is natural that they make the most of the great demand and select, weeding out among the many applicants.

Not until our second visit to the student accommodation office do we manage to get three addresses, the most central Miss Björkman's at Järnbrogatan 10B — slap opposite the university. This is a vast apartment house with a large courtyard, called the "Scandal House" — not because the residents misbehave, but because the building is higher that the university building opposite.

Alex and I draw lots. I win and may choose first that day — if we manage to get a room. We put on our best clothes, clean our shoes and together go to see Miss Björkman. She is an elderly, quite authoritarian, taciturn lady with rather thin streaky grey hair. First we say I am looking for a room. I am thoroughly questioned and clearly succeed in gaining approval in Miss Björkman's eyes, so may have the large room Miss Björkman has to let, though there are a number of conditions. I may not use the bathroom or the kitchen, may not cook food in my room, may not use the telephone in one of Miss Björkman's own rooms, and I may not receive female acquaintances after eight o'clock in the evening. I may use the lavatory in the hall, and the rent is 85 kronor a month, to be paid in advance.

There is a large white washbasin in the room and two sterling towels hanging on hooks beside it. The room is not particularly nice, but is usefully furnished with drab dark furniture. Otherwise it is large and light and suits me perfectly. I pay 85 kronor in advance and ask whether I may move in on January 15th, which suits Miss Björkman.

Once this transaction is over, Alexander politely asks if Miss Björkman by any chance knows of anyone who might have another room to let, preferably in the same building. Miss Björkman refrains from answering, or perhaps doesn't hear the question. As we are to leave, Alexander Weinfeld bends over to kiss her hand — as gentlemen in Poland do when greeting a lady. Even several years after my arrival in Sweden, I constantly have to remember to control that innate reflex so as not to embarrass women acquaintances. But the stiff, formal,

The Maple Tree Behind the Barbed Wire

nearly sixty year-old Miss Björkman likes people to preserve the customs of their country. She is clearly delighted when Alex tries to kiss her hand and says slowly that she actually has another room, smaller and she doesn't know if it would suit, but she can show him it. There is a washbasin in that room, too, and the rent is lower, 65 kronor. This is a stroke of luck, bingo at the first address. We can live together and Alexander's room is only slightly smaller than mine. Somewhere to live has been arranged.

The next problem is choice of student nation. You have to belong to a nation to be registered at the university, pay the nation sub, receive an exam book and be allowed to read medicine. You are allowed to choose whichever nation you like. The only two provinces in Sweden to which I can consider myself to have any connection with are Skåne - where I landed from Denmark - and Stockholm, where I lived and went to the folk high school. At Uppsala there is no Skåne nation, students from Skåne have Lund University and would not even consider studying at Uppsala. So I register with the Stockholm nation, pay my subscription, and am given a receipt to show at the student office. It is not long before I find I have made the worst possible choice. In the spring term of 1947, the following circumstances prevail in Uppsala: if you want to dance, you go to the Småland nation — which farsighted Nina and Helenka have chosen. If you want to play bridge, you choose the Göteborg nation. If you want to be bored — which I don't — you go to Stockholm's nation. After a while, however, I realise that choice of nation is of no importance, as you can spend your time at any nation you like.

Finally I register at the university and am given my exam book, another fee to pay. All fees are small, but for me the sum is large and my start-up capital is fast dwindling. But that doesn't worry me, for now I am a medical student at Uppsala University in Sweden. That evening I write a happy and optimistic letter to my parents in Czestochowa.

I very much like being a student in Uppsala. The city is sufficiently large, you don't have to decide in the morning what you are going to do for the rest of the day, and it is great to improvise. If I feel like going to the cinema, I go down to Trädgårdsgatan, where nearly all the cinemas are — except the Fyris, which is in the Scandal House. If I want to play bridge, I go the Göteborg nation — where there is always a table and it is not long before there are three more who want to play. If I wish to bury myself in the history of Sweden, I go to the excellent university library, Carolina Rediviva. If I occasionally want to be left in peace and perhaps read a newspaper, I go to my always empty and desolate Stockholm nation. Everything is nearby, everything open and everywhere I am made welcome.

The Maple Tree Behind the Barbed Wire

It turns out that it is also possible to earn a living washing up in restaurants in Uppsala; three or four times a week is enough. "My" restaurants are the grand Flustret and the Gillet, but I myself eat at the cheapest place in town - Brunns Dining Rooms.

Like all other students, I receive a letter from the head office of Dagens Nyheter and find I can afford to subscribe to the newspaper — the cost of a student subscription is shamelessly low, but a wise investment to recruit grateful readers of whom many become faithful subscribers. For evening reading, I buy school textbooks on the history and geography of Sweden. These are also cheap, but I still need a Swedish-Polish and Polish-Swedish dictionary. With the aid of my dictionary and Dagens Nyheter, I continue to improve my knowledge of the Swedish language.

I go dutifully to every lecture and laboratory session, although there is no check on your attendance. Just as dutifully, I manage all compulsory oral tests, but I have no time for the demanding thorough mugging up for exams — that'll have wait until I am able to resist the temptations of student life.

Apart from the cinemas in Trädgårdsgatan, bridge at Göteborg's and dancing at Småland's nations, I have to do my stint of parties — student dances — arranged at the various nations. To my boundless delight, this happy student life explodes during the wild Walpurgis Eve, the following Walpurgis Night and the somewhat calmer spring parties at the beginning of June. I get to know a lot of new people.

I mostly mix with two of my friends on the course, Dag Hallberg and Josef Berglund, and quite often but not always, Nina is allowed to join us. We become a quartet, sometimes meeting almost every day. We go for walks, eat, go on little outings, play the fool and get up to mischief together, sometimes discussing serious subjects as we lie on the grass in the sun, or round a table late at night.

Towards the end of the spring term of 1947, Helenka and Nina are visited by a young newly qualified doctor - Herman Diamant. One of the foundations connected with the Jewish Congregation - the Israel Youth Association - has sent him to see how things are going for us. Herman Diamant takes his task very seriously and stays a whole day in Uppsala. He mostly talks to the girls, wanting a picture of their financial situation, their results, their outlooks for completing their studies, and he is curious about their plans for the future. But Alex and I are also allowed to meet Herman, a thoroughly nice man who, despite his assignment, behaves towards us like a nice somewhat older colleague, not as someone sent to investigate us.

Three weeks later, all four of us, Alex included, receive a letter with an offer of an interest-free loan of 150 kronor a month, beginning in the autumn of 1947. All we need do is to sign an undertaking to repay the loan after qualifying. Great deeds by the Israel Youth Association, the Jewish Congregation, Gunnar Josephson, David Köpnivsky and

The Maple Tree Behind the Barbed Wire

Herman Diamant.

This unexpected interest-free loan fundamentally changes my finances and makes my life easier. I go on washing up at the Flustret and the Gillet, but not so often and feel almost wealthy, so can allow myself various extravagances. One day I take lunch at the Gillet, wanting to see what it is like on the other side of the swing-doors to the kitchen. Eating a buffet lunch at the Gillet is over three times as expensive as at Brunns Dining Rooms. The food is better, the tables, chairs, cloths and service superior, but all the same, I think I probably prefer the simpler but homely Brunns Dining Rooms.

At Easter in 1947, Nina and I join one of the skiing camps on Marsfjället arranged by SFS, the Swedish Association of Student Corps, — a relatively cheap trip even we can afford.

From Wilhelmina, we are taken by bus to Saxnäs and — inexperienced as we are — put on our badly waxed skis for the almost eighteen mile trip to our cabin in the wilderness. We are tired after not sleeping all that well in sleeping bags on the train - Nina looks as she can't keep up any longer as we are to ski across Lake Kultsjö. It is covered with ice, on top of which is a thick layer of new snow that is hard going. The group moves quickly off while I stay behind to keep Nina company. Nina is later to tell me that it was then she "began liking me as a human being as well" - I still don't know what she meant by that.

I spend most of the coming summer of 1947 at one of the student camps arranged by SFS - the international student camp in Rottneros in west Värmland, close to the Norwegian border. It is hot. We spend our days semi-naked, harvesting on a large Swedish farm, hard but beneficial physical work in good company — in 1947, most agriculture work is still done by many people and few machines. We are nine cheerful youths from seven different countries and three continents, working by day on the land, in the evenings and weekends running riot at the popular outdoor dance floors of Värmland. Rumours spread and we are soon called the nine happy Ekeby Cavaliers. I read Selma Lagerlöf's wonderful Saga of Gösta Berling again, this time in Rottneros, Selma's own Ekeby. One Sunday we are invited to her lovely historical manor house. I don't think it looks as Selma Lagerlöf has so vividly described it.

The autumn term at the Department of Histology begins undramatically. No one seems to question whether we may continue our medical studies. I also begin to take this for granted, forgetting I am a refugee with temporary permission to stay in the country, and I do several things, which turn out to be thoughtless.

The Maple Tree Behind the Barbed Wire

For a period I meet a girl who takes me with her to concerts. I have never had any opportunity to go to concerts before. After each concert, we critically discuss what we have seen and heard, sometimes at some simple café with young people interested in music, or a student room, or at a nearby nation. I try to join in on the discussion and have some views — like all the others — but after a while realise that to me this is all just snobbery. Either I am unmusical or else am not attracted to sophisticated classical music, so the acquaintance comes to an end.

My next acquaintance - Maria - drags me off to museums. When we have done all the museums of interest in Uppsala, we go on to Stockholm. Maria has a thin body but a strong will and a flexible intellect, dark hair, dreamy eyes, is knowledgeable, is good at describing and explaining in a way that it arouses my interest. I have never been to museums before, except with my class in my schooldays in Poland. When else would I have done that? With Maria as my patient guide, I discover a new and interesting world — the Maritime Museum, the Natural History Museum, the Biological Museum, Skansen, and the National Museum. Afterwards we take a walk in some green area, sit in the sun at an outdoor café, eat a little and talk a lot.

Among my acquaintances is a slightly older woman student. She is a serious, thoughtful woman and one day she tells me about the discussion evenings the Clarté Society has in Uppsala. She takes me to one of these and later asks me if I would like to contribute with a lecture — perhaps on the situation in Poland. I am aware that the Clarté is on the far left of the political spectrum, but don't think this should prevent me from participating. I appreciate the intellectual debate carried out at the Clarté and go to a few more of their meetings before I grow tired of them.

In the autumn of 1947, the Polish parliament decides to offer an amnesty to anyone who has left the country illegally — they can now have a Polish passport and the right to return or visit the country without being punished. This is irresistible for Nina, Helenka and me, all three of us with relatives still in Poland. I go to the Polish Consulate in Stockholm to make my application, then later to fetch my consular passport. The Consul himself wishes to speak to me. He is patronizing, asks how things are going, whether I need any help, whether the Consulate can help me. Then he starts talking about how valuable it would be for Poland to receive information about Swedish industry. He makes no requests, and it sounds rather like a conversation about his problems, but I explain that I know nothing about Swedish industry anyhow, nor am interested. On the other hand, I do join one of the Polish-Swedish student club's cycling outings connected with and financed by the Embassy. With my consular passport and a Swedish return visa, I finally go back on a visit to Poland to see my parents.

We have a few wonderful weeks together, which means a great deal to them, perhaps even more to me. But I don't give a thought to what the Swedish authorities might think about this. A young man comes as a refugee and after eighteen months in Sweden, dares to return to his home country without being punished. He takes part in the Polish-Swedish club activities, has been to the Polish Consulate several times, has escaped from a communist country, but attended Clarté meetings and has himself lectured at them. Not only that, I am to contribute even more.

During my stay in Czestochowa, Sarah tells me that — not officially, but in practice — there is censorship of letters in Poland, and she asks me if I have an address to which she can write without the sender being identified. I give Sarah the address of the Stockholm nation in Uppsala and a cover name, so that the censor will not be able to identify the sender with the help of the addressee's name - Einhorn. Sarah sends lengthy letters to that address, on two occasions with banknotes in them, first one, and in the next letter two twenty-dollar bills. On this second occasion, there is a note on the mail board to the addressee with my cover name, and a request for that person to contact the chancellor's office. There I am given the letter, which someone has opened and seen the two dollar bills. This was also an incautious act by a refugee — receiving letters under a false name from his home country with, true not much, but nonetheless money in it.

Alex and I are now doing the chemistry course. One day we are summoned to Professor Blix. He is seriously worried and upset as he informs us of a communication he has received from the university Chancellor's office. From this it appears we are not to be allowed to continue our studies — he shows us a copy of the letter. It takes quite a while before I take in the content of this brief communication in bureaucratic language, but the contents become etched on my mind.

It has come to the knowledge of the national university Chancellor's office that four extra students have been taken on to courses at the Uppsala Faculty of Medicine. Owing to this, the office is compelled to inform Uppsala University that the concession previously made concerned special circumstances during a war. The office does not consider these circumstances any longer valid — and so on and so forth. Conclusion: the University of Uppsala has failed to consult the national university Chancellor's office, and it was wrong to allow us to begin our studies without any such proposal — we must leave. Signed Zacharias Topelius, Secretary to the Chancellor.

Professor Blix says he has been sent a copy, but as yet no request from the Rector's office. So for the time being we may continue on the course, but his advice is that we should go and see the Rector of the university, Professor Fredrik Berg, as soon as possible.

The Maple Tree Behind the Barbed Wire

Nina and Helenka receive the same message from their head of department. We meet in the afternoon, the girls bristling. We decide to ask our friendly, confidence-inspiring assistant lecturer, Bengt Nylén, for his advice.

Bengt tries to give us courage. He has heard about the communication from the Chancellor's office. Everyone knows about it — it is upsetting and must not be accepted. He also urges us to go and see the Rector. "Fredrik Berg is a good man," says Bengt Nylén.

But the result of going to see Rector Berg is not encouraging. He is friendly but formal when he says he is sorry. He will speak to Thore Engströmer, the Acting Chancellor of all universities in Sweden, but he does not hold out any hopes — the content of the Topelius letter is fairly unambiguous.

I see that others on my course are developing activities, which as far as I can judge concern this problem of ours. It is good that they are interested but what can they do? Dag Hallberg is the most active when it comes to collecting signatures from students on our and other courses. Sensitive as Dag is, he doesn't mention it to us that any such activity is going on. Friends on our course mobilize assistant lecturers, lab assistants and those in the university student office, go to see the professors whose courses they are taking or have taken, and are given support, perhaps not by all, but many. They go to see Rector Berg in full force — it is almost a demonstration.

I know nothing about this until the Rector summons us four, tells us about this widespread support for us, says that it also constitutes support for him, that he personally will go to the national university Chancellor's office in Stockholm. Rector Berg admits that our teachers, and with them the university, have committed a formal error. But they have done so in good faith, the regulations are unclear, and anyhow it is unreasonable that this should affect us — if we have been allowed to begin, we ought to be allowed to continue, anything else would be irresponsible. We are to continue our studies until we hear otherwise. That feels good.

Three more weeks later, a resolute Bengt Nylén comes to see Alexander and me — it has all been arranged, we may continue. The formal notification will also come in a few days. Sarah and Pinkus very much want to emigrate to Sweden so that we can be together. One condition for this is that someone will guarantee Pinkus or Sarah employment. I go round several large and less large gentlemen's tailoring establishments in Stockholm and tell them what a good tailor my father is, but that is no use. Most hopeful of all is my visit to Olympia Tailoring in Sveavägen, but the owner of Olympia finally also refuses. The repeated reason is that Pinkus is too old. Profoundly dejected, and also ashamed, I have to write to my parents: "I have not given up, but at the moment I cannot arrange anything here in Sweden."

The Maple Tree Behind the Barbed Wire

Instead, I make my second trip to Poland, to Czestochowa and my parents. Nina is on the same train, Helenka already gone. Packing is not my strong point. When I think I have everything ready, I remember at the last minute things I have forgotten. I get on the train with my big suitcase, which I think is bulging, but also with three loose paper carriers.

There are not many passengers — few people go to Poland in the summer of 1948. There are only three passengers in our compartment - Nina, Motek Birenbaum and I. The journey is long, we have plenty of time, and it is clear Nina and I enjoy each other's company. Nina looks critically at me as I rummage round in my paper carriers and she asks if she may re-pack my luggage. She puts the contents of my suitcase and the three carriers on the empty seats, methodically re-packs it and it all goes into my suitcase — which is not in the slightest difficult to close. That is the first time Nina takes me in hand so tangibly and I sometimes wonder whether this long journey and Nina's visit to Czestochowa was not the first time I thought how good it would be to live with her. But for the time being it is only a stray thought, for at the moment I am keeping company with the daughter of a rich shipping magnate.

I am tremendously pleased to be back in our old home in Czestochowa again with my parents and young brother - Roman. At the same time I realise that this is going to be my last visit, that it is going to be a long time before we meet again. Sarah is the first to tell me of their very advanced plans to leave Poland. She says, as if it were something encouraging, that things have been arranged with the help of Dr Zajdman, and they are going to Canada, not Sweden.

Sarah is aware it is going to be difficult, not least for Pinkus, who is established and has such a good reputation in Poland. On one occasion, Sarah says quietly - as if confiding in me a secret confession — that they themselves would probably have preferred to stay, for they are quite old and it will not be easy to leave and establish themselves in a new country. But with Roman in mind, they do not want to stay in Poland - he is sixteen. Sarah says they don't want Roman to grow up in this country. There is no future for us Jews in Poland, she says, and also Poland has become a communist country, like the Soviet Union. They hope I will follow them to Canada, that we shall be together again, she says, looking appealing at me.

The Maple Tree Behind the Barbed Wire

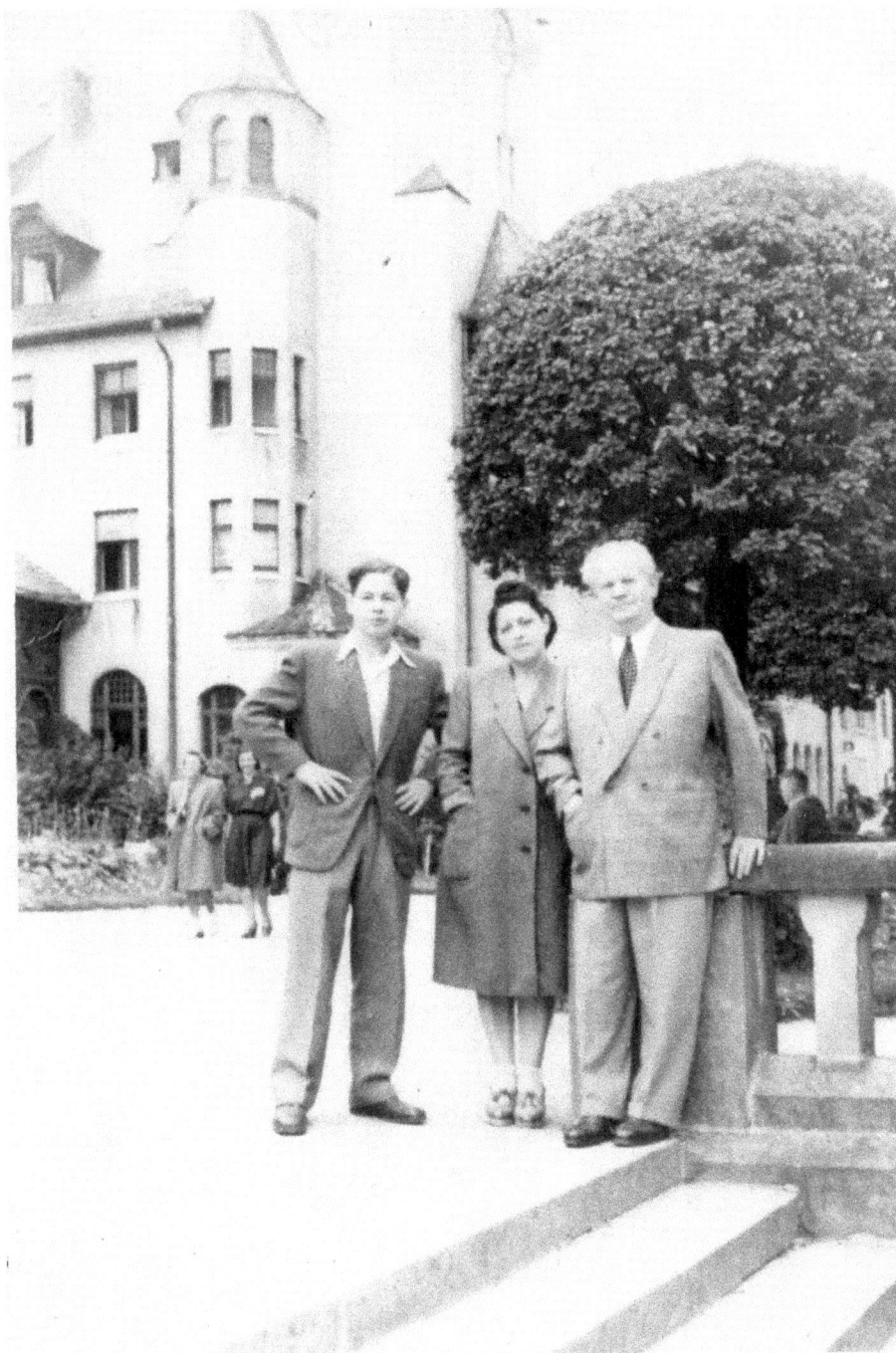

So that we can be together, Sarah, Pinkus and Roman want to emigrate to Sweden. In the autumn of 1947, I go round all the larger and smaller tailoring establishments in Stockholm telling them what a good tailor my father is, but it is no use. They keep saying that Pinkus is too old.

The Maple Tree Behind the Barbed Wire

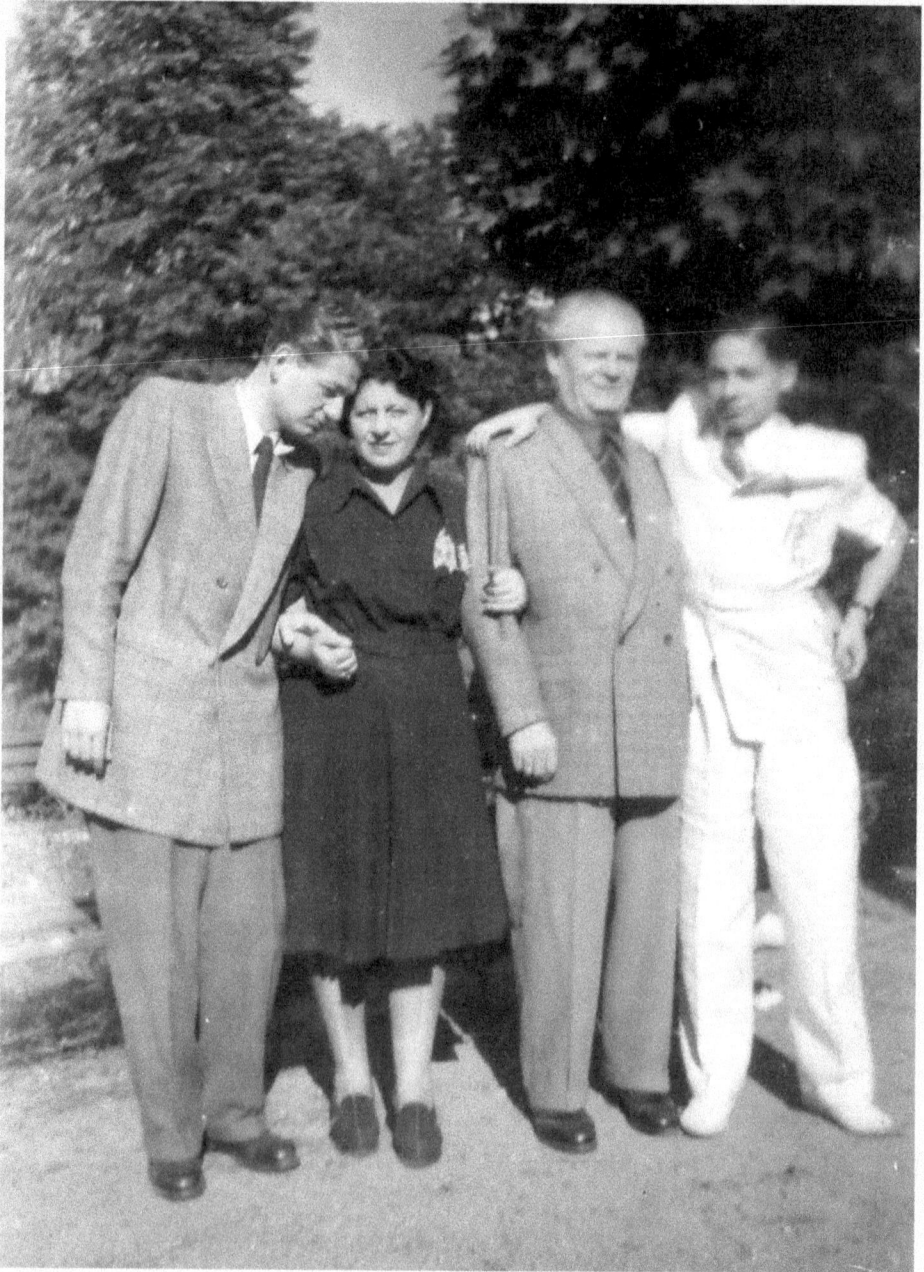

With my Polish passport from the Consulate in Stockholm, in the summer of 1948, I go to Poland to see my parents and brother. We have a few wonderful weeks together and I give no thought to what the Swedish authorities may think — that a man comes as a refugee and two years later dares to return to his home country without being punished.

The Maple Tree Behind the Barbed Wire

Dr Zajdman was born into a Jewish family in eastern Poland and his father had died early. He and his sister were brought up by their mother alone and they were very poor. At thirteen, he managed to leave the country on his own and ended up in Canada. He was badly undernourished and went to Scottish mission in Toronto, where they were distributing food parcels to the poor and where he fainted in the mission waiting room. They looked after him and let him finish his schooling, the mission then financing his theological studies at the University of Toronto. He graduated with high marks, was given a research scholarship and became a Doctor of Theology. Dr Zajdman converted to Christianity, then became like a child in the home of the head of the mission, whose daughter he married, and finally he was chosen to be his father-in-law's successor. "Actually, there is something strange about him," Sarah says. He is undoubtedly a profoundly devout Christian, but his wife calls him Mojsiele - a truly typical Jewish nickname — she has learnt to cook the most typical of east European Jewish dishes. They eat "gehackte leber" and "gefülte fisch", "knisches", "kreplach" and "kischke". Dr Zajman was made the Man of the Year last year in Canada. After the war, he went to Poland to look for his relatives. Pinkus is a distant relative of his, the only one he could find, probably the only one to survive the war. Zajdman is arranging for an entry visa for Pinkus, Sarah and Roman, and has promised to help them in every way when they come to Toronto.

Sarah has already closed down her dental laboratory. She still runs the home and the family in all practical matters, spoiling Pinkus and Roman, both of whom accept it. As if it were perfectly natural, I fall easily into the same role. Everything is just as it used to be, yet a watchful atmosphere prevails — the atmosphere of departure. One element in it is that my parents press on me a whole lot of things of varying value, which they want me to take back to Sweden.

Sarah buys a new suitcase, then during my stay there, fills it with handmade handkerchiefs, curtains made of thin material, an old bible someone had deceived them into thinking is valuable, some stamps we just think are valuable, but also a Leica camera. Before I sell that camera a year later, it is my most valuable asset. I pawn the camera when my money begins to run out towards the end of the month before the next month's loan comes from the Jewish Congregation.

In the summer of 1948, my last summer with my parents, my brother is sixteen. It is he who teaches me to swim in Czestochowa swimming baths during my stay in Poland - I am twenty-two and have had no opportunity hitherto to learn to swim. We go to football matches and theatre performances together. Not until now do we develop a mutual respect, a prerequisite for us becoming forever in future two brothers close to each other. It is a pity we have to live on separate continents.

The Maple Tree Behind the Barbed Wire

Pinkus will soon be sixty-four when he is shortly to be leaving his home country. He is marked by the war, but still physically and mentally a vigorous man. His hair is grey, almost white, though he still has his lion's mane, moves easily and purposefully, has kept his friendly but not ingratiating smile and his habit of looking the person he is talking to straight in the eye. He radiates self-confidence, wisdom and generosity. Working in his workshop is his life, his pride and his flight from reality. During my stay at home, we talk to each other more often than before and for the first time like two grown men.

During one of our evening walks I tell him about the shipping magnate's daughter. Later, I say I know it is scarcely appropriate to tie myself down until I have a profession, an established position, can be sure of supporting a family and give it security — perhaps at forty, as he had done. We continue up Aleja Wolnósci - we are both silent. Pinkus does not turn round, but walks on further than we usually do, realizing this is important. He is looking straight ahead as he slowly and gravely says: "That was in the 1920s. Now it is the end of the 1940s." What he had previously told me concerned him in the situation he found himself in. He turns to me, looks me in the eye and adds — with emphasis — "it was not meant to be advice to you. It does not apply to you today". We walk on for a moment before he admits: "It may be an advantage to marry young, to have children and see them grow up before you grow old."

That is all Pinkus says, but it is enough to free me from the false myth of a family that does not exist. That he married late was due to external circumstances, not his own free will. What he says is important — although it does not lead to me marrying the shipping magnate's daughter.

Nina and Helenka come for a few days to our home in Czestochowa. Nina gets to know my parents and my brother. Sarah, Pinkus and Roman get to know Nina. When I am to leave Poland a week later, my parents go with me to Warsaw and Pinkus meets Nina once again. All three of us take a horse-drawn cab - still the main means of communication in Warsaw. It is our last day in Poland and I am rather wrought up, aware that I will not be seeing my parents again for a long time and am therefore rather short with Nina - as young people can be.

First we drive Nina to her hotel. When she asks what time we are to meet at the station, my reply is rather unfriendly.

The Maple Tree Behind the Barbed Wire

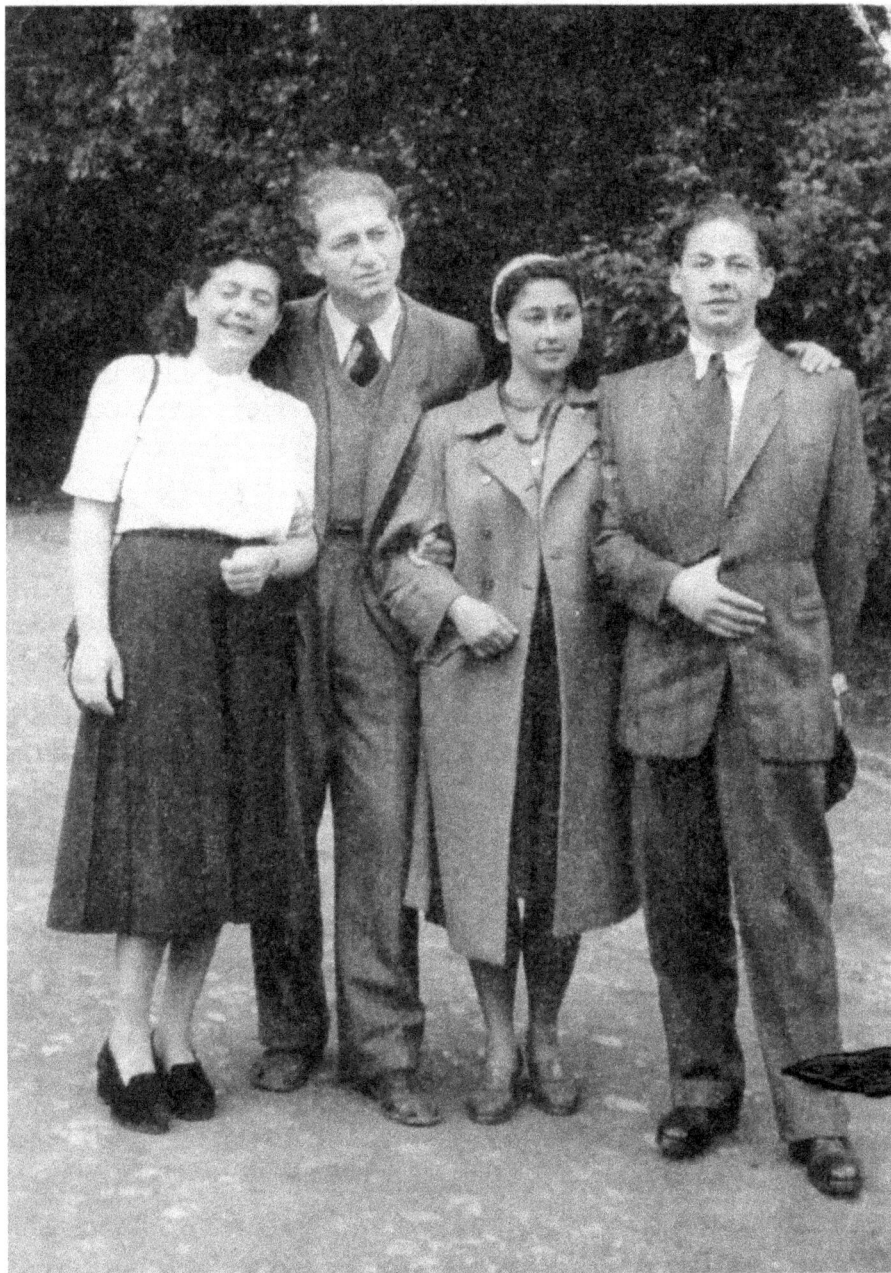

In the summer of 1948, Nina and Helenka spend a few days with us in Czestochowa. Nina gets to know my parents and my brother — and they get to know Nina. This was our last visit to Poland before my parents leave the country

The Maple Tree Behind the Barbed Wire

Pinkus is quiet after Nina has left the cab. All we can hear is the clatter of the chestnut horse's steel-clad hooves and the encouraging clucking of the driver on his high seat in front of us. Pinkus starts one of his rare admonishing speeches, this time containing criticism of my behavior towards Nina. There is no aggressiveness in it, only regret in his calm statement — he is speaking Yiddish, as always when he wants to be sure of choosing the right words. "How could you, Josele?" Silence. "Asaa lachtyk majdl" — such a nice fine girl asks you quite kindly — he repeats Nina's question in Polish, then goes straight on in Yiddish, "and how do you answer?" Pinkus is not looking at me, but without sounding unfriendly, he says: "I am ashamed of you." On our return journey to Sweden, I am unusually courteous to Nina.

This is the second and last time Pinkus and my future wife meet. But Pinkus has told me what he thinks of Nina - a lachtyk majdl, literally translated "a girl it glows round". He has already said previously what he thinks of my views on a suitable time to get married. He is to help Nina one more time, but then without meeting her himself, eleven years later, shortly before he died.

When Nina and I marry almost a year later and have our two children - Lena and Stefan - Nina, with her never failing generosity, is to urge me to go in for full-time research — "otherwise you will never be satisfied". At the time, there were no funds for research, so the prerequisite is that Nina can support all four of us. And Nina manages with her salary and our economical way of living to support the family on her own. On her intern's salary, she has to pay for the help she needs to be able to work full-time and take night duties, and from what remains of her salary find what is needed at home and supply me with pocket money until I finish my research training, defend my thesis and acquire the necessary academic start.

But I am ambivalent, wanting both, plagued by feelings of guilt because Nina has to work and is not at home with the children — as Sarah was when Roman and I were small. In our situation and with our ambitions, I have an unrealistic desire for our children to live a life that we had at home during my childhood. This discontent of mine creates tensions and affects us both.

When I have my PhD, and Pinkus in the spring of 1959, is seriously ill, dying of stomach cancer, through Dr Zajdman's intervention "at the highest level" - I am given a month's visitor's visa to Canada. Nina and I scrape the barrel of our funds to pay for the flight.

Tired and emaciated, but calm although he knows what awaits him, Pinkus lies in a bed Sarah has made up for him in his workshop. He wants to be there to help his only remaining employee. Pinkus has plenty of time to talk to me. We have not met for a long time and we know this is the last time we will be together.

When we are alone in the semi-darkness of the evening, full of regret and shame, I tell him that Nina is working full-time, although we have

The Maple Tree Behind the Barbed Wire

two small children. Lena is six and Stefan five. As always, Pinkus immediately realizes this is a serious problem for Nina and me. His eyes half-closed, he lies wearily back on his pillow, but then revives and says: "You have made your choice, Josele. You chose to marry a girl who with huge efforts has got herself a long training as a doctor. What do you want?" Zeby myla twoje garki? - that she is to spend her time washing your saucepans? We both say nothing, Pinkus because he is tired and has nothing more to say, I because I am thinking about what he has said.

The now constantly unhappy Sarah comes in to see to Pinkus; there is so little she can do for him. It is fortunate Sarah has not come in earlier, so I had time to take this important matter up with my father and Pinkus was able to reply.

Neither Pinkus nor I say anything more about Nina working, nor is there any need to. He has said the only right thing, all I needed to hear from him in particular, and it is enough. Many years later, Nina says that her life became happier after my visit to Toronto and that is probably also true of me.

But I have no idea about all this when eleven years earlier, in August 1948, I return from my last visit to Pinkus and Sarah in Czestochowa.

Shortly after my return to Sweden, late in the summer of 1948, my residence visa runs out. Nina, Helenka and Alex all receive an extension, but I do not. After weeks have gone by without hearing anything from the police, I go to the police station and the woman official tells me that they have heard nothing from the Aliens Department. She adds consolingly — occasional delays of this kind are not unusual. I content myself with that — am not aware that this is the prelude to increasing uncertainty and a gnawing unease which is the result of this continuous state of uncertainty.

The spring term of 1949 is the fifth and last term of our medical studies before my Bachelor degree. I have dutifully followed all the courses and passed all the orals, but have only done one exam for my degree. At the approach of the end of the fourth term, the 1948 Christmas vacation, I pull myself together. I have to make up for four terms' neglect by — apart from the current course — doing all the exams in medicine, and it actually seems to be going well.

Nina, much further on with her studies, fails anatomy. Anatomy is the major subject that is the most demanding but also the dullest subject of the Bachelor degree, like learning by heart the two fat volumes of the Stockholm telephone directory. Sensible Nina hates it and thinks it an unnecessary demand for a doctor-to-be to be able to rattle off the smallest little bone, the smallest muscle — with its origin and attachment — every blood vessel, fissure, anastomose, nerve, and nucleus of the brain and spinal cord. Nina has interviewed several doctors who say they have forgotten most of it a month after the

The Maple Tree Behind the Barbed Wire

anatomy exam and assure her that despite this they manage well as doctors. Also, who bothers about every single muscle round the ring finger of the left hand? Possibly a hand surgeon — her torrent of words is unstoppable - Nina goes on complaining, although she has realized long ago that she has to learn all the bones, muscles, blood vessels, fissures, anatomoses and nucleus to qualify as a physician. She tries to mitigate her misery by asking me if we can't work on this awful subject together — "I can't do it on my own", she says. I say yes, why not, it would be nice — having no idea I am thus sentencing myself to a happy lifelong relationship with this unusual women.

The demands for a good pass in anatomy are high. It takes a lot of time to learn everything in Rauber Kopsch's three fat volumes and complementing it all with Corning's excellent but even fatter topographical anatomy. The time before the exam day turns out to be limited, so we have to work for longer and longer days and nights to catch up. It is not long before the inevitable occurs.

Nina shares a room with Helenka. I have a room of my own. So we have to work in my room. Miss Björkman knows that Nina is with me all day, but does not protest. She seems to like Nina; everyone does. I actually find a certain pleasure in learning anatomy, but most of all being with Nina - experiencing a calm pleasure in having her to myself all day. Nina has accepted her fate and complains less and less — that does not help anyhow — and works dutifully at all the unnecessary details of human anatomy.

It is late in the evening, Nina is bored stiff, adding to her exhaustion, so she lies down to rest on the thick dark green bedspread on my bed. I go on working at the big desk, trying to make out a timetable that may help our maltreated brains to force in a whole mass of not very stimulating Latin terms. I am also rather tired and try resting my head on my arms lying on all the books on the desk, but feel I must lie down too and rest to be able to go on. The problem is there is only one bed in my room and on it is Nina, her face to the wall, and, as I think, asleep. So I lie down on the same bed with my back to her for only a tiny moment — and fall asleep.

I don't know how it happens, but when I wake, Nina is lying facing my back. She is warm and soft. I lie still so as not to wake her.

It is not out of desire, but from an overwhelming tenderness, an insight into how fond I am of Nina, how much we have in common, that I slowly turn over and see that she is not asleep.

I am unable, nor have I any desire to resist my imperative need to put my left arm round Nina in the semi-darkness — its wonderful to hold her — at close quarters. I look into her grey-blue eyes and my happy fate is sealed.

The Maple Tree Behind the Barbed Wire

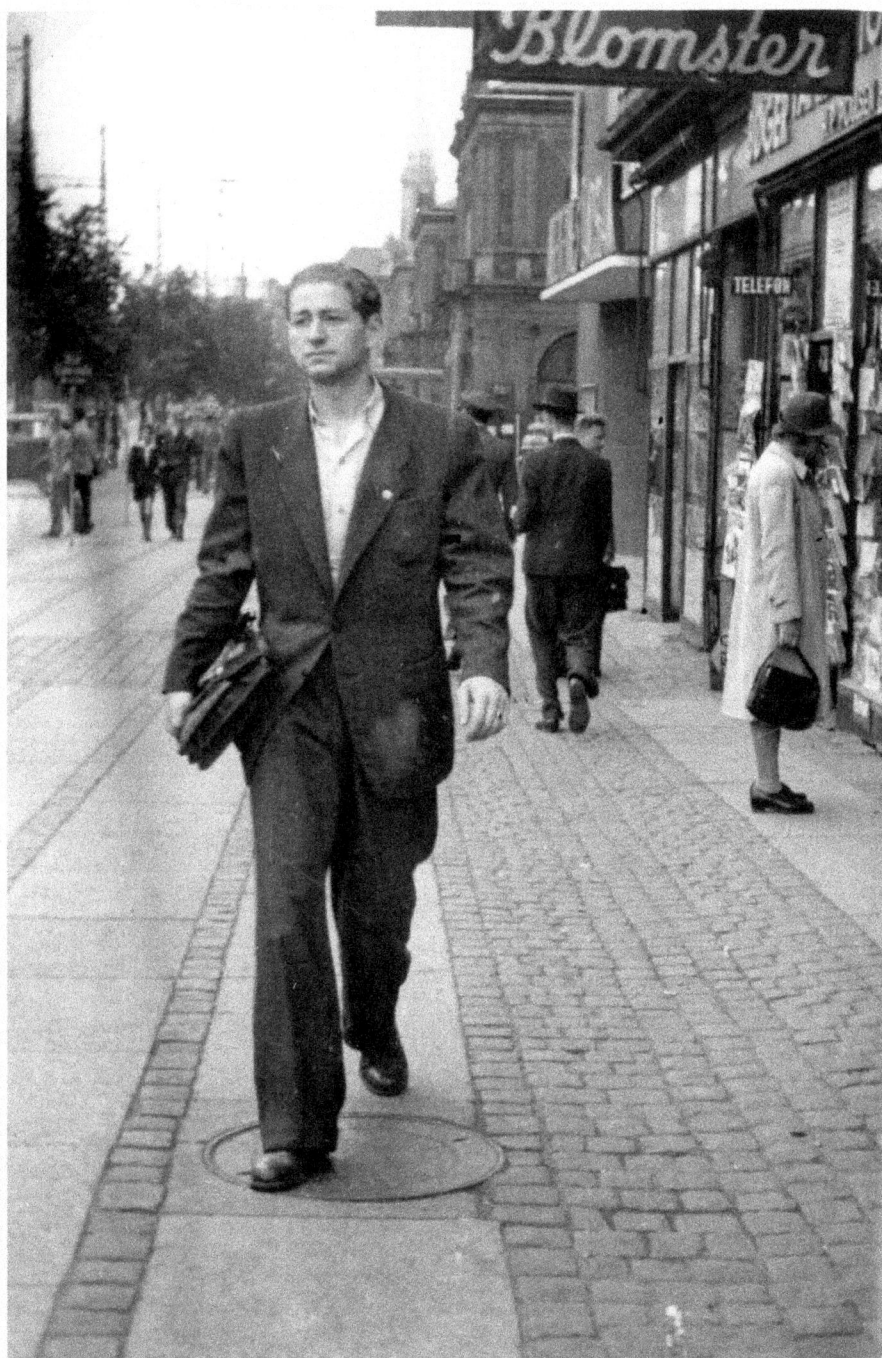

Perhaps what was decisive was that Nina saw through me, realizing that beneath my boastful exterior, I was uncertain, that I needed someone to look after me. And that task attracted her when I proposed on October 1st, 1948, in Uppsala.

The Maple Tree Behind the Barbed Wire

I have long known that if I take up with Nina, then it will be serious — if I do so without meaning it, I shall hurt this fine girl, whom I like, whom no one is to hurt. So perhaps I am nonetheless probably aware of what I am doing, even if I am being guided by my emotions, not my reason. Nina does not retreat. Her eyes are wide open and she moves easily against me. I hold hard and tenderly on to her. She smells good.

The room is quiet for a while, perhaps several minutes. To my astonishment, but not unexpectedly, I whisper into the warm ear close to my mouth — "will you marry me?" Instinctively wise, Nina does not answer, just lies still against my chest and the room is quiet again. I am beginning to worry now. Is she hesitating or had she not heard? I ask slightly more loudly — "will you, or perhaps you don't want to?" She still says nothing, then a little while later she mumbles: "Jurek, it's too soon."

I am panic-stricken now. Things haven't turned out as I thought they ought to. She doesn't throw her arms round my neck, weeping with joy. It is no simple matter of course that I can have her whenever I want to. I don't know what to do or say. But Nina adds, slightly louder, she too: "You must qualify first." It is at least five and half years until then, and a lot can happen in that time — what do you mean, Nina? But Nina stays lying there, softly pressed against me as I mumble — in five, six years, we will be twenty-eight, no, twenty-nine. Nina hears and says quietly, gently and consolingly: "I mean the Bachelor degree". It is only six months until then.

Nina usually lets herself be guided by her wise instincts. With their help, she has put me exactly where I ought to be. I am not the one to grant Nina a favor by proposing. It is Nina who grants me a magnificent favor by accepting my proposal. I am relieved — we are in practice engaged, although no one has mentioned the word. There is no need to.

We talk quietly about her brother Rudolf, about Roman, about my parents, about Nina's parents, who are no longer alive but whom she remembers so well and mourns, about ourselves, our dreams, our plans for the future. It all feels so right that from now on we are to share our plans and our future. Not until late that night do I pull off the thick bedspread and we creep in under the bedclothes. I can't help noticing that she is shy and inexperienced, but lovely. This is genuine unreserved and eternal love. Actually, for a very long time, perhaps already in Lodz, I have loved this girl and been vaguely aware that she has long been prepared to love me for what I am.

The Maple Tree Behind the Barbed Wire

We both fall asleep in my bed despite Miss Björkman saying I may not receive ladies after eight o'clock. But Nina gets up early, dresses, kisses me lightly on the forehead and silently leaves my room and the apartment before anyone has woken.

It is getting lighter. I am happy about what has happened, but unhappy that she has left, fall asleep again and sleep for a long time. My first thought the next morning, with satisfaction and no loss — is that on my part this is the end of student parties and temporary girlfriends. I am pleased — as long as Nina wants to be with me.

Periods of many difficulties, divergent opinions, even quarrels await Nina and me, particularly after the children are born and all the strains that entails. Periods of that kind await many young couples trying to build up an everyday relationship. Much patience and thoughtfulness, preferably love, too, are needed before two people learn to make the great sacrifices demanded, to accept the considerable limitations to their freedom necessary to learn to live together, sharing everything — even their defects and imperfections. But from that evening when consciously or unconsciously, Nina moved softly against my back and I turned to face her — from that moment neither of us needed to face any adversity, nor any success, alone and — most of all — neither of us need live in a loveless state. For we had genuine love from the start, still have a surplus of it and over the years it just becomes more and more.

I like it when we are together and become deeply unhappy every evening when Nina leaves me to go back to her room in Banérgatan. Nina seems surprised but not troubled by the passion I have suddenly developed and agrees with some hesitation that we should move in together. But this means we must find somewhere else to live. We manage quite quickly to get hold of another room with its own entrance with a young married couple in St Persgatan 45, smaller than my room at Miss Björkman's, but with its own toilet and the young landlady has no objections to us living there although she doubts there is room for us both. We buy a second-hand double sofa bed at an auction. There's plenty of space in our room in the daytime but when we pull out the lower bed and make the bed up for the night, there is no room to stand in the room — anyone who does not go to bed has to be in the toilet.

In this room in St Persgatan, we marry.

In the last days of February 1949, Pinkus, Sarah and Roman leave Poland and on March 7th, 1949, they arrive in Canada.

The Maple Tree Behind the Barbed Wire

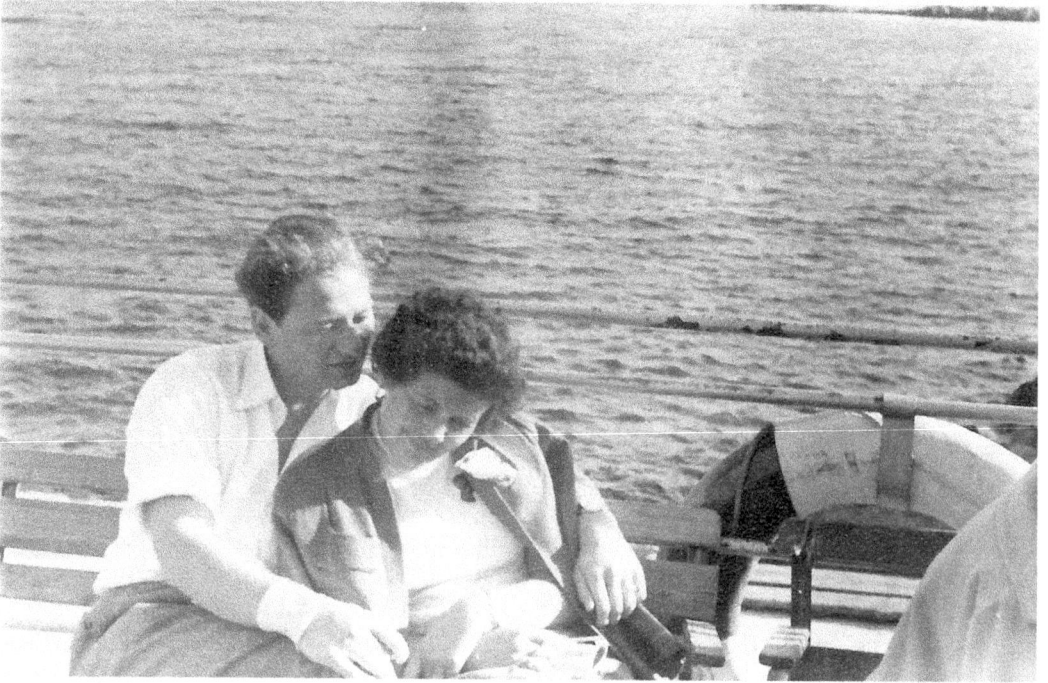

I see myself as a violin, which with her gentle hands Nina first tunes, then plays on — and in all our life together tempts out the best sound the violin can produce.

During the stormy crossing, the worst period of a sea voyage on board the old-fashioned Polish passenger ship M/S Batory, Pinkus is very seasick — he is in a bad way when they arrive. After their arrival, Roman, now seventeen, has to help support the family by working at cleaning out steam locomotives at the great Canadian railways marshaling yards in Toronto. In her letters to us, Sarah mentions this as something positive and does not mention any financial difficulties. Despite this, Nina and I collect up everything I had brought with me from Poland and anything else we can find to sell. We put an advertisement in a daily paper and try to sell everything by phone, blocking the telephone for a whole day from kind Mietek Tauman and his wife Marysia - both live in Stockholm. An elderly man, Mr. Byk, reads the advertisement, rings us up and comes to the Taumann's. Nina and I show him what we have and he buys the lot. I hurry to send every cent to my parents in Canada.

We have little left now, not even the Leica camera which I pawn whenever necessary. But that does not worry us. We can go on washing up more often, and we do not feel poor. You don't if you have faith in the future — and we have.

The Maple Tree Behind the Barbed Wire

The professor of internal medicine at Uppsala University, Erik Asp-Uppmark, is responsible for the first course after the Bachelor of Medicine, the preparation course for clinical studies. Ask-Uppmark says officially he is not prepared to provide places on his courses for the four Polish extra-students, and he is unwavering. Helenka Zymler asks to meet the professor and he explains mathematically why we have no practical chance of getting on to his courses.

If there are to be any places over for extra-students on his course, he takes them in the following order: first students from Germany, then students from other west European countries, then students from East Europe who are not of Jewish origin and last of all students from East Europe who are of Jewish origin. So it pointless for us to wait, for we are in the last category. The professor finds it rather difficult to explain just why German students come first, but he complements his queuing order by putting male students before female. At a concert at the Östgöta nation, Helenka meets a sympathetic older medical student called Gunnar Svantesson. They fall in love and are to marry. Helenka will be called Svantesson, will be Nordic so from then on will be able to continue her studies wherever she likes — she moves away from Uppsala. The three remaining foreign students in Professor Ask-Uppmark's last group with great sorrow, will have to break off their studies at Uppsala University. Alexander Weinfeld is given a place at the newly created medical faculty at Göteborg University - he is to defend his thesis there and build up Göteborg's first and still only Department of Hematology. Alexander becomes an internationally appreciated researcher in this difficult field and is to train and take to PhD level several of the most outstanding physicians and hematologists in the country. Nina and I apply and are given a place to continue our studies at the Karolinska Institutet in Stockholm.

We are not aware of the wide body of opinion that Martin H:son Holmdahl, the pugnacious and fearless member of the board of the Medical Society and of the student corps in Uppsala and the equally pugnacious editor of the student newspaper Expo, Per I. Gedin, manage to arouse, first in Uppsala, then with various authorities in Stockholm. The parliamentary ombudsman, Uppsala Student Association, several faculties and finally the Chief of Police in Uppsala and the Uppsala Society of Physicians are activated. Long after we had left Uppsala, the stubborn human rights champion Martin Holmdahl and the clever young writer Per I. Gedin continue their campaign against a professor's autocratic ways and the tendencies they give expression to. But we do not find out about all this until many decades later when I happen to met Martin Holmdahl on Frankfurt airport. By then Martin Holmdahl is himself Professor of Anesthesiology at Uppsala University, and Per I. Gedin is chairman of the Swedish Book Publishers' Association.

The Maple Tree Behind the Barbed Wire

I managed to pass all my exams for my first Bachelor degree during my last term. When I proudly and expectantly arrive at the student office, it turns out that I ca not have my marks written into my exam book. Another communication has come to the registrar's office from the university Chancellor's office in Stockholm. In it, it says I may not be awarded the Swedish Bachelor degree, as this would bind me to Sweden and it is not certain whether I may stay here. No such communication has come to the other three medical students from Poland. So Nina and Alex and Helenka, the latter soon to be known as Svantesson, receive their degrees — but I do not. No, the friendly assistant at the student office does not think that prevents me from continuing my studies here in Sweden. "If you want to do so without receiving your degree," she adds. No, she does not know why this has happened.

In connection with my next visit to Stockholm, I gather up my courage, make an appointment and for the first time personally meet the Secretary of the Chancellor at the national university Chancellor's office, Zacharias Topelius. He is the man to have signed this latest communication. Topelius does not seem in the slightest troubled; all he has to say is that he made his decision after consulting the Aliens Department. He admits that this is an unusual decision — then the conversation is over.

The Aliens Department gives Alex permission to live in Göteborg and Nina to live in Stockholm. But I am given no permission to move and am forced to stay on in Uppsala, but may not continue my studies there.

The Maple Tree Behind the Barbed Wire

Locum

Nina and I are no longer surplus extra-students and are included in the quota of fifty students accepted on the preparatory course in the autumn of 1949 at the Karolinska Institutet. The course is held at St Erik's Hospital in Fleminggatan, led by Henrik Lagerlöf, future Professor of Internal Medicine at the Karolinska Institutet.

In Uppsala, we were twenty-five students on the course. Here in Stockholm, the acceptance regulations with additional high points for military service, mean that Nina is the only woman among forty-nine male students. As in Uppsala, we are at once accepted by all the others and as the only girl, Nina is also the course favorite. Luckily she has already been laid claim to — by me.

Student life in Stockholm is not as in Uppsala; students rarely meet after lectures as the long distances are an obstacle. Nina and I also have the problem of our daily train journeys. We still live in St Persgatan in Uppsala and every day as well as some weekends we have to make our way to Stockholm - it is tiring and also makes severe inroads into our already frail economy.

Professor Kristensson, head of the Department of Medicine at Serafimer Hospital, makes an unconditional demand that no one without a valid reason may be absent from his morning lectures. These begin at eight o'clock. Our compulsory attendance is probably necessary - Professor Kristensson's lectures are so dull that otherwise not many would attend. The arrival times of trains from Uppsala are not adapted to our lectures. We have no valid reason for being late, so have to take the first morning train from Uppsala at 5.40, and we get back late in the evening. There is no time for washing up at a restaurant, except sometimes at weekends.

Although I have not yet received my first degree, I have done all the exams and Nina and I are married on October 1st, 1949.

Nina buys a piece of medium-blue nylon cloth, blue thread of the same color, though slightly darker, then makes her own wedding blouse with lovely wide frills. I buy nine dark red rosebuds and am allowed to marry my beautiful Nina. We still have the nine roses and every single leaf of the green sprays that go with them. Nina ruins three fat textbooks drying and pressing every rose and spray, but I don't think we still have Nina's blue wedding blouse.

We were married by the mayor in Uppsala Town Hall. We are to be married properly before a rabbi beneath the traditional canopy and with the bridegroom's customary breaking a glass wrapped in cloth when — we hope soon — we are to visit my parents in Canada. Helenka Zymler and Dag Hallberg are witnesses, and with Halinka Lis, Josef Berglund and Alex Weinfeld, we are seven people at our simple wedding lunch at the Glunten. I have managed to get the only window table in the little restaurant.

The Maple Tree Behind the Barbed Wire

Some time goes by before Nina and I can afford to go to Canada, so we still have only a civil marriage. Nina laughs with some satisfaction, but says I am crazy when I go on and on about wanting to be married to her by a rabbi. Nina says we are too old for that now we have grown children and grandchildren. In the end, Nina agrees to be married by a rabbi, but not until our fiftieth wedding anniversary — our golden wedding on October 1st, 1999.

But now it is the snowy winter of 1949-1950. The streets of Uppsala have not yet been plowed when, weeping in the semi-darkness, Nina plods through the snow to the railway station in Uppsala. Once or twice, I am on the point of hailing a passing taxi so that Nina doesn't have to get her feet wet, but we can't afford taxi fares.

Despite this, we don't envy the others on the course. Some of them have bought or been given a car by their parents, others have acquired motorcycles. Car, motorcycle, an apartment of one's own are all pleasant to have, but are not essentials for life. If your standard of living is low early on and you don't keep looking sidelong at what other people have, if you can hope that one day you will be able to afford them, too, you can manage on very little for a long time, and be quite content.

Our usual dinner in the evening is spaghetti or rice, which we always have at home, and soup cubes - that's good if you are hungry. If the weather is fine, Nina and I go for a walk in the evening and people stare at us as we walk with our arms round each other. Things are good as long as it does not snow in the night and Nina doesn't have to trudge through the deep snow early the next morning.

Sometimes I have to explain why I have not received my degree, though actually I don't really know why myself. But I constantly dwell on it, wondering why just me.

One day Nina says she is going to the Aliens Department and asks me whether I have any objections. Nina wants to "explain that I have done nothing wrong". I have forgotten all about it when a few weeks later, Nina tells me she has met Wiman, the deputy head of the department and they had had a long talk, at least half an hour. Wiman had listened in a friendly and interested way and promised to look into the matter himself, but he was not able to promise anything. I just hope Nina has not wept when with Wiman. Neither he nor the young assistant present during their meeting has said a word about why the extension of my residence permit has constantly been delayed, why I may not live in Stockholm and am not allowed to receive my medical degree.

Towards the end of November, Dag asks whether we would like to spend Christmas at his home in Hudiksvall. This is the first time Nina and I have been invited into a Swedish home. For us it becomes two wonderful weeks, just what we needed to rehabilitate our souls.

The Maple Tree Behind the Barbed Wire

We are welcomed as warmly appreciated guests, filled with good food and are comfortable in a way we have almost forgotten existed. But most important is that we can recover in the warm atmosphere of this lovely family and again see the world in a brighter light.

Nina spends most of her time with the motherly Mrs. Hallberg, who showers us with her care — she is always worried whether there will be enough food. Dag's younger sister is there, too and the three women seem to have a lot to talk about. I spend my days with Dag, often with his father, Dr Hallberg, an elderly, commanding and assured gentleman with unusually large ears.

I am troubled when one evening after dinner we are all sitting around in the comfortable leather armchairs in the big living room and Nina brings up the subject of my residence permit. But when the Hallbergs show some interest, I start. I tell them I cannot receive my degree — which seems unjust — and am not allowed to live in Stockholm, but I say nothing about Nina crying on her way to the station or the financial consequences of all this. I tell them about my uneasy wait for my permit, that no one tells me why. I give them a long list of my "sins". It is a relief to me to say all this in the Hallbergs' safe home without it arousing the slightest hint of suspicion or them disassociating themselves from it. Instead, the Hallbergs are upset, thinking there must be some mistake — which is a great relief. In our presence, Mrs. Hallberg asks her husband if they can do anything.

Dr Hallberg is head of the Surgical Department in Hudiksvall so, as in other medium-sized Swedish towns during the 1940s, is thus a highly placed person with much say — in his own town. The Hallbergs invite Mr. Lehman, the managing director of the largest industry in the district. They know each other well.

Mrs. Hallberg offers freshly baked, still warm buns, small open sandwiches, fresh coffee and tea. They must have told Mr. Lehman beforehand, for he at once asks us about the Aliens Department's dealings with my residence permit, and also whether I have been told "why" — which I have not. He shows a genuine interest but makes no comment on what we tell him. It is Dag who later says that Lehman and his father have both agreed to intervene. He is pleased and encouraging — this good Dag Hallberg, our friend.

After our stay in Hudiksvall, somehow our troubles seem to be easier to bear. Nina stops crying on her way to the station — perhaps because there is less snow or because we have been helped by friends who believe in us and have influence, at least in Hudiksvall. We no longer feel totally vulnerable.

Almost two months later, at the beginning of March, two letters arrive almost at the same time, in brown envelopes - I have permission to live in Stockholm and a residence permit in Sweden for three months — longer than on previous occasions.

The Maple Tree Behind the Barbed Wire

I don't know whether this is due to the intervention of Director Lehman and Dr Hallberg, or to Nina's long talk with Wiman behind it all. Perhaps all those together, or something quite different. Under any circumstances, we can now move to Stockholm.

Today, fifty years later and several years after the collapse of the Soviet Union, it may be difficult to understand the Aliens Department's dealings with my case. But the second half of the 1940s was the beginning of the Cold War, a period of espionage trials and a paralyzing fear of communism. This fear spread like wildfire all over the democratic world, unjustly and badly affecting many innocent people. In the United States, it was the beginning of the McCarthy era, which the President, the wartime General Eisenhower, put a stop to when Senator McCarthy and his associates in their arrogance approached the president's own co-workers and friends. In Sweden, no such devastating national hysteria arose, but some people were nonetheless affected, among them me and with me, poor Nina.

Worst of all was that I did not know — and still do not know — why. I felt as if my wings had been clipped and five years were to go by before I recovered and in the early autumn of 1955, one sunny morning in the middle of Kungsträdgårdsgatan in Stockholm, I realized my wings had healed and I could fly again.

Through a friend of a friend, Nina has an opportunity to find a little apartment of our own, one room and kitchenette — but we have to make a quick decision.

The very next day we go to the quite nearby Mälarhöjden to look at the apartment — it is small, but pleasant; this could be our little paradise here on earth. The rent is no higher than for a room at second-hand, but we have to pay 1,500 kronor "key money" — that sum is for us insuperable — if we do not get a loan. Nina and I have got quite far with our studies by now, so we hope that someone will stand guarantee for a bank loan of 1,700 kronor — we need the 200 kronor to buy furniture.

I again start the round of various wealthy people, but fail with them all. We need two signatures and I fail to get a single one. In the end, Nina says we must go to Gilel Storch.

I am not keen on the idea. Gilel Storch helped us stay in Sweden - are we also to ask him to take a personal financial risk to help us? Supposing everyone he had helped came to him with the same request, I say to Nina. But both of us very much want that apartment — so we try. We meet Storch at his office adjoining a carpet store in Kungsgatan - his own firm and the family source of income, which he neglects for his work for the Congress.

Gilel Storch receives us in his boisterous way. He immediately takes over the conversation, wanting to know how things are going for us.

The Maple Tree Behind the Barbed Wire

He has heard that we live in Uppsala, are reading medicine — "is that so, that's right, good, then we have two doctors to go to", he says in his benevolent way, so that we don't feel like poverty-stricken supplicants. Finally, Storch asks us why we have come to see him. He interrupts me when in my lengthy explanation I mention the guarantee. "Have you the personal guarantee paper from the bank? Give it to me". He signs it without any further questions — "Good," says Storch, "a young couple should have a place of their own. Good luck to you." The conversation is over.

On our way out of his room, Storch asks: "Whose is the other signature?" I start off on another long explanation — we don't know yet, but it will be easier now we have one signature ... Storch interrupts me again — he is quite annoyed now: "Why didn't you say so? Nina - come back, sit down!" Slightly confused, we sit down opposite him at his desk again — and he makes a phone call.

"Calle - I have two great young people here. Two students from Poland who need a guarantor to get a bank loan. It's about an apartment in Klubbacken in Mälarhöjden. I have already signed," says Storch, "but you know, the banks want two guarantors — what about it?" "Which bank? Skandinaviska Enskilda." "Good, when can they come? Great, thanks, how long will you be there? Thanks, goodbye" — he doesn't even mention the sum we are thinking of borrowing. What a difference from all the questioning we have had in our previous searches for guarantors.

Gilel Storch scribbles down the address on to a piece of paper he tears out of his diary. We are to go there at once to get the other signature — he's busy now.

Calle Berman starts by signing, after which he hands back the bank guarantee and chats to us for a brief spell. Then he ends the conversation: "Anything else I can do for you?" And he means it.

That is how Nina and I get to know this great person - Calle Berman. We are to meet on many occasions in the future.

It is an amazing feeling, equipping your first ever apartment - and for me, to do so together with Nina. In one respect, it can be an advantage not to take for granted that most things come to you as a gift. There is a certain pleasure in slowly collecting what you need and to know you are doing so by your own efforts. Our first table, the four chairs, two beds of our own, our first frying pan, two saucepans, four place sets of plates and cutlery for when we have guests, the first two tablecloths — a kitchen cloth and a Sunday best, every new acquisition is like a step forward. It doesn't matter that most things are second-hand, as they are all in good condition. Things are good for Nina and me.

The Maple Tree Behind the Barbed Wire

During the 1950s, the health service is given high priority in Sweden and is being rapidly expanded. There is a shortage of doctors, for there has not been time to train the medical personnel required. Medical students with sufficient training may be permitted to work temporarily as physicians and in the summer of 1951 my medical training has reached that stage. From the stenciled list brought out every week by the Association of Young Doctors containing vacant posts, I choose a smaller hospital - Domnarvet Hospital in Borlänge. I send in my miserably short CV, and after a brief telephone call am appointed by the senior consultant as the summer locum for seven weeks — he does not mention a salary and I have a feeling it would be bad manners to ask. Instead I go to see the lawyer of the Swedish Medical Association at Villagatan 5. He says my post is as an extra doctor for which the salary is usually about 500 kronor a month, though it is possible to negotiate for more.

For the first time since that evening in Järnbrogatan 10B twenty months ago, Nina and I will not be together for a longer period, and that weighs heavily. On the last day before I leave, we go for a walk in the woods near our apartment. Nina usually picks wild mushrooms there.

It is a lovely late afternoon, cool, the sun occasionally emerging from between the high, almost white banks of clouds. Nina has helped me pack, everything is ready for my journey tomorrow. We hold hands, our everyday problems forgotten, and we are thinking only about each other. It is melancholy to be parted, but lovely to feel like that. We feel how strong our emotions have become, how dependent we are on each other and that this dependence feels good — it is mutual and unconditional. I do most of the talking, about how fond I am of her, how I will miss her. Nina finds it difficult to talk about her emotions, but she holds even harder on to my hand when I say all this. She herself says "look after yourself, we will soon be seeing each other again, phone — if you can". Nina never makes demands that may make things difficult for me — "... if you can". I have forgotten my anxieties on our walk — how am I going to manage my first locum?

I get to Borlänge and Domnarvet Hospital in the middle of the day, so that I can take a look round before beginning my duties the next morning, and I am overwhelmed by how much responsibility is to be put on me — a young, still not fully qualified physician. The housekeeper shows me my room on the top floor of the hospital, large and light - I sleep uneasily that night.

But things go well once I have started. My uncertainty and anxieties slip away and I like being a doctor in a small hospital in which everyone knows each other. This is where I first experience the confidence patients have in their doctor, the great delight and satisfaction entailed in discovering that you are able to help. I have chosen the right profession, I think — how fortunate that I failed the entrance exam for the chemistry course at Stockholm University.

We are two physicians, one a consultant, the other an intern, and there is a great deal to do. The intern is on duty six days a week and is woken several times in the night — weekdays and weekends. The Domnarvet Iron Works runs a three-shift system and is working well beyond full capacity. Swedish products are in demand all over Europe. The other European countries have not yet built up their industries destroyed by the war, and it is a matter of Sweden making the most of this flourishing market. At the same time, in the 1950s the safety and industrial health services are not what they ought to be - every night injured or acutely ill workers are brought to the hospital. Many of Borlänge's patients prefer the hospital to the provincial doctor, and also it is the only the hospital open at night.

Only thanks to the experienced nurses can the absurdly heavy workload be managed by one single doctor. They see when I am simply incapable of doing any more — often at two or three in the morning — and take on most of the responsibility without waking me. The next day, patients come to show me the injuries the nurses have stitched up or plastered.

I am on duty the next day after night duty. The day begins with my morning round, admissions and discharges of patients in the hospital's open ward. That actually goes well though there is no time for anything except work. I soon realise that I learn a lot from taking independent responsibility. I am pleased I can cope and am beginning to acquire the self-confidence a physician needs — without becoming arrogant.

Every Wednesday, my clinic is shorter than usual, and when the consultant takes over duty at two o'clock, I fall into bed and sleep the dreamless sleep of the exhausted but contented, until the alarm clock goes off at seven o'clock the next morning and the morning round of our ward starts at eight. My room is comfortable and airy, the food in the hospital dining room is good and plentiful, and the staff open and pleasant — but an intern has not much time for that.

Working hours are not regulated — whether for doctors or nurses. But the physicians receive performance bonuses for the patients they take into the open ward — a modest sum per patient per day, slightly more but still small at night. However, it does come to quite a lot because of the unending stream of patients all round the clock and the huge workload. My salary from the hospital is, as told me by the lawyer, 500 kronor a month, but that is only a smaller part of my income. In my first week in Borlänge, I earn more on the open ward and duty cases — and ask Nina to come to see me. We agree on a suitable Thursday, which I can take as my day off after eleven o'clock — and Nina comes to Borlänge with Halinka Lis.

The Maple Tree Behind the Barbed Wire

Suddenly I feel like a wealthy man. I stand Nina and Halinka lunch at the best restaurant in Borlänge - Nina is uneasy and asks if we can afford it. When we get back to the hospital, I unlock the desk drawer in my reception room and show her all the banknotes. Nina calms down and is full of genuine admiration.

We go to a jeweler's - I have chosen it beforehand — and exchange the copper rings with which the mayor of Uppsala has married us for proper wedding rings — of twenty-four carat gold. But Nina keeps our copper rings — after all, they are the ones we were married with.

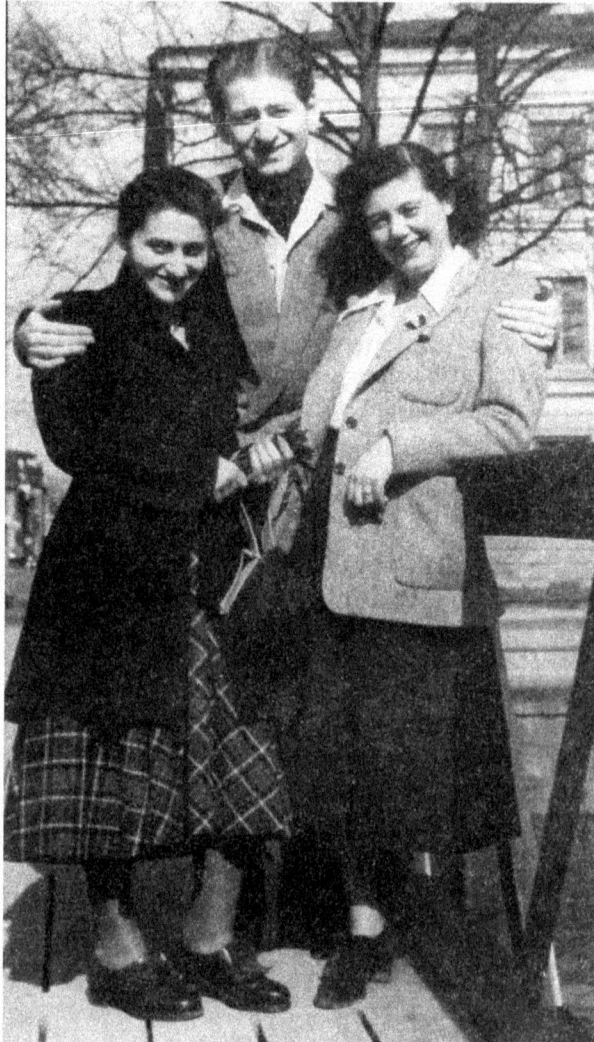

In 1951 I have my first locum, at Domnarvet Hospital in Borlänge. Suddenly I feel like a wealthy man. Nina and Halinka come to see me. We go to a jeweler's and exchange the copper rings with which the mayor of Uppsala had married us in 1949 for proper twenty-four carat gold wedding rings

The Maple Tree Behind the Barbed Wire

Little Lena

Our way of life, even after my post in Borlänge, would by most people be regarded as extremely economical, while I think we can afford anything and start giving Nina small presents. Sometimes it's a flower — always red — or a pastry. But I mostly stop at the EPA department store by the bus stop on my way home and spend a few kronor on something Nina doesn't really need and probably doesn't want.

During vacations and other free time from our studies, we do locums as physicians. I like working in small hospitals where you quickly learn the practical elements of the many-facetted art of being a doctor. These hospitals usually have two doctors, a consultant and an intern who is on night duty six days a week. I spend some time at the now closed Maria Albert Hospital in Trollhättan, then take a temporary appointment at the hospital in Vetlanda, where I am able to learn a great deal from Dr Jacobsson, a calm clever man who is generous with his wide medical knowledge. On each occasion, I earn in a few weeks what covers our needs for several months.

The next summer I take a temporary appointment as a general practitioner in Stenstorp, roughly halfway between Falköping and Skövde. Being a provincial doctor turns out to give me great satisfaction, perhaps even greater than working as a junior in a smaller hospital. As a provincial doctor, I cover a catchment area of about five thousand inhabitants — almost three times as many as the state-appointed general practitioner of the 1990s — with no secretary or nurse, no health centre, only two reception rooms and a small, very simple laboratory. But we have continuous medical cover. A provincial doctor at the beginning of the 1950s is on duty seven days a week, except the weekends he exchanges with the neighboring district doctor. Then the next weekend you have double the number in the catchment area, about 10,000 inhabitants, and none of us would even dream of not making a home visit, anywhere in the district, when a patient or a relative rings.

A provincial doctor soon gets to know the whole of his or her own district and after a few weeks everyone in the district — sick or well — knows his or her provincial doctor. I have never before or since had so many gifts as during my summer as provincial doctor in Stenstorp and I appreciate them all — a basket of fresh eggs from someone's own hens, fruit from a patient's trees, fresh home-grown vegetables, fresh home-made bread made from the farmer's own wheat. On leaving Stenstorp, I am given knitted gloves for the winter and a hand-made Christmas crib I am proud of, and still have in the attic.

The Maple Tree Behind the Barbed Wire

Before I decide on my future as a physician, I want to see what it is like working in a specialized hospital clinic, so take a three-month autumn appointment at the newly opened women's clinic in Kalmar. The consultant, Dr Ahltorp, has recently moved to Kalmar from Lund. Ahltorp wants help, most of all in the operating theatre, in which he is clearing up cases of uterine prolapse in older women living in the county. We have two interns there, I am on duty for only three nights a week and haven't nearly so much to do on those nights as in the small general hospitals. Working hours are not regulated and there are no bonuses for working duty hours.

In my fourth month, in December 1952, I go to Karlstad, where Nina has already been working for three months at the much larger women's clinic. In Karlstad, they have problems with two Dr Einhorns at the same clinic. The senior nurse in the operation department solves if by calling me "Dr Einhorn's husband". On the women's clinic board for planning the future day's operations, it says either "Dr Einhorn" or else "Dr Einhorn(husband)".

Medical training is long, in the 1950s on an average eight years - and then remains a four or five year period of specialist training. The reason why I started working as a physician so early was that we had to earn a living. During my first years, I was influenced in my choice of post by my desire to acquire broad clinical experience, but also by curiosity and a search for my own identity within the enormous field of medicine. After a few years, I had managed to work in Sundsvall, Gävle, Borlänge, Vetlanda, Trollhättan, Kalmar, Karlstad, Stenstorp and at the South Hospital in Stockholm.

When one works in so many places, particularly as a physician perhaps, meeting so many cultures in different parts of the country, one gets to know the customs and the people. People I meet during my locums in various parts of the country have minimal schooling, are often taciturn, but trustworthy, basically honest people with a deeply anchored sense of personal integrity, but also with great respect for each other — a prerequisite for mutual consideration. I realise that democracy is not only, not even first and foremost, a form of constitution. Democracy is first and foremost the attitudes people have towards each other. So democracy cannot be forced upon a country or a people, which we Europeans, in our well-meaning naivety, all too often try to do, and do great harm by wrecking social structures that were not ideal, but which functioned.

Perhaps better than those born and grown up here in Sweden, I am able to compare, and am grateful that chance took me here. I was so generously received - I was not used to that. I am grateful for having been given my entire medical training here without having to pay a cent and without my parents paying the country's taxes. With all my defects, I feel accepted by people I meet in Sweden and hope that even the Aliens Department will eventually accept me.

The Maple Tree Behind the Barbed Wire

I have done all the revision for my exam in surgery and Professor J. P. Strömbeck is satisfied. After writing the result in my exam book, Strömbeck asks me if I want to be a surgeon. If I do, after I have qualified he would find me a post at his department at the Serafimer Hospital.

I have no ambitions to have an academic career, but I am flattered by this offer of specialized training at a teaching hospital. Surgery suits me as a basis for continued specialization and I need no time to think it over. I say to Professor Strömbeck that I would be grateful if I may work with him at the Serafirmer Hospital - it is best to decided at once when made such an offer. Strömbeck leafs through my exam book and asks me whether I am reckoning on finishing my studies during next spring, which I confirm, and he says I may begin at his department at the beginning of the summer of 1954.

My future as a physician has been staked out, or so I thought.

Towards the end of July 1953, Nina and I work out from a review of our assets that they need reinforcing before the autumn term. In the latest list I see a locum is required at the Radiumhemmet, the department of ontology of the Karolinska Hospital and Institute in Stockholm. I go to see Dr Lars-Gunnar Larsson that very afternoon. He is responsible for the medical appointments in the general department of the Radiumhemmet. I can start immediately, to fill a vacancy that has unexpectedly arisen.

The Radiumhemmet is different from everything else I have tried hitherto, a rigid, markedly hierarchical order prevailing there. A junior physician takes responsibility for only simple matters the head of the department is quite certain he can manage. Lars-Gunnar explains why this is so. Every cancer patient has only one chance. It is a question of doing the very best to make the most of it. Almost all the patients are seriously ill, often anguished, as are their frightened relatives. It seems particularly important to look after these severely afflicted people. The demands are great and I have a sense of working at the front line of medical science and the art of healing.

A secret that has made our marriage easier is a joint promise that we are never to go to sleep on a disagreement. A symbol for this is a large pillow I brought with me from Poland - the only thing I have left from my home in Czestochowa. It has served us well in our long marriage — we have never fallen out for twenty-four hours. Instead we share our thoughts every night as we lie on that big pillow.

At the beginning of October 1953, before we go to sleep that night, Nina says slightly diffidently: "My period hasn't come." The next morning Nina leaves a urine sample for a pregnancy test at the nearest chemist, and the result comes the very next day — we are to

The Maple Tree Behind the Barbed Wire

have a child. When we lie down on our big pillow that night in our apartment in Klubbacken in Mälarhöjden, we talk about the child we hope is to come. Nina adds — if all goes well.

Nina works it out that she will have time to complete her courses and exams before the birth, and will be able to work at home and rest. That night we talk for a long time after going to bed, and we fall asleep late.

When an immigrant has been in Sweden for at least seven years, the time has come to apply for citizenship. In exceptional cases, when there are special circumstances, Swedish citizenship can be granted after five years, but that applies only to immigrants considered particularly valuable to the country, well-known scientists and teachers, experts, world class athletes — not us. Nina and I plan to hand in our applications for Swedish citizenship in the autumn of 1953, almost seven years after that Danish fishing boat put us ashore on an abandoned jetty outside Landskrona. We know it usually takes at least a year before any decision is made.

It is important to us to be Swedish subjects. After all these years in Sweden, Poland is no longer our country. We have no country we can call our own. I have no flag, no government, no parliament and no embassy to which if need be I can turn should anything happen to me when I am abroad. All these are symbols, to the majority so ordinary that they are considered trivial, but if need be they can become common security mechanisms. A refugee is more aware of the significance of them if he is a twenty-eight year-old father-to-be and has experienced the disadvantages of being without this security since the age of fourteen. I see myself as a person with no homeland and am not sufficiently strong to ignore this — as today's world looks and national states are organized.

Nina is in her seventh month and doing her last course before her degree — in dermatology — diseases of the skin — at Karolinska Hospital, where on the morning of March 21st 1954, I take my last exam for my license as a physician.

That evening, we celebrate in our new apartment in Holbergsgatan 98 in Blackeberg. This also has only one room — but a larger one — and it also has a proper bathroom in which there is enough room to see to the baby, and a proper kitchen. Nina has cooked a good dinner, bought a little gateau with a candle, which she lights and I blow out. I know Nina is worried about our finances and also because I may have to leave Stockholm. There is a shortage of vacancies, particularly in the university towns and not many doctors want to take their holidays in March. Despite this, Nina says we must do as we had previously decided. I shall take a week off, read books and listen to the radio. I have earned it.

The Maple Tree Behind the Barbed Wire

It rains that night. Nina gets up early. I wake when she kisses me lightly on the mouth. She is already in her outdoor clothes and on her way out. I don't have time to embrace her before she leaves — "Don't fuss now, go to sleep", she whispers. I fall asleep and am woken by our newly acquired telephone.

It must be late in the day. It has stopped raining and the spring sun is shining in through the pink-and-green patterned thin white curtains. Have I slept that long? The insistent telephone goes on ringing. I lift the receiver and mumble a yes. It is Sixten Franzén, an older colleague from my appointment at the Radiumhemmet.

Sixten is known for his persistent attempts to diagnose cancer with the aid of a thin needle and an empty syringe to suck out cells from lumps suspected to be tumors. On a microscopic slide, he smoothes out and colors the content of the needle, insisting that on a smear he can recognize cancer cells through the microscope. The pathologists rage — this is quackery. You can't make a diagnosis from single cells. For that, a piece taken with a surgical knife is required — an operation and not a prick with a thin needle. But some of the older doctors at the Radiumhemmet, Lars-Gunnar Larsson and the head of the department, Sven Hultberg, let him go on, perhaps because Sixten is so enthusiastic, or because they are hoping for a breakthrough, a possibility of diagnosing without having to cut into a cancer tumor. It turns out that Sixten is right, and not the authors of all the textbooks or the professors of pathology.

The always cheerful, unworried Sixten Franzén finds it difficult to put things into words in conventional scientific terms. He cannot write an article any self-respecting scientific journal would publish, or write an application for a grant any sensible research committee would approve. Sixten Franzén, who pays no attention to formal academic norms, is a long way from the generally cherished prototype of a scientist. Sixten is to be responsible for the greatest discovery in the long history of the Radiumhemmet. His aspiration biopsy and Franzén's syringe are to be responsible for a breakthrough on the research front. With his work, Sixten is fundamentally to change the future diagnostics of cancer, and with that, the treatment of cancer all over the world. He is to take away work from a great many surgeons, and also prevent much unnecessary suffering for a great many patients, making possible earlier treatment of tumors with no unnecessary waiting for the operation wound to heal, opening up new opportunities for routine follow-ups and early evaluation of the results of cancer treatment.

Sixten is to be the author of classic scientific publications and new textbooks in pathology for which others are to regard it as an honor to be allowed to write for him. But two decades are to go by before he receives international appreciation and before the Swedish government

The Maple Tree Behind the Barbed Wire

award him the title of professor. Meanwhile, Sixten Franzén has to work his way up a steep hill only few would be able to manage — but despite this he is content and happy.

I am surprised at Sixten telephoning. He asks me cheerfully how things are going. I tell him proudly about my last exam, about how Nina and I have celebrated it. "I have a week off — and need it" "Oh yes," Sixten interrupts me. "That's good, but it will have to be next week. Gun Persson is ill and we have a vacancy. Can you come, at once?" Disappointed that my time off is disappearing into an uncertain future, but also flattered - I must have done well during my appointment in August - I answer without thinking that I will come as soon as I can. When? says Sixten, it's urgent. In two hours at the most, I say hesitantly. I have only just woken up and have to get dressed, have a cup of coffee and it takes time to get from Blackeberg to Karolinska Hospital. But Sixten is adamant. "You may get dressed," he says. "Then take a taxi. We have a waiting room full of patients and are short of staff in the clinic. Get yourself here in half an hour, please. I will phone and book a taxi to pick you up in thirty minutes. I will tell Sister Vera so you get some coffee and a snack when you arrive. OK?"

No one can refuse whenever kind Sixten, always helpful to everyone, asks for something. So I scramble out of bed, do as he has said, take the taxi he has booked, arrive at the Radiumhemmet, note all the waiting patients, swallow some coffee and start work without the cheese sandwich Sister Vera has left in the little writing room next to the doctor's reception.

It is a hectic day, with unexpectedly many patients coming, several with major problems. During a brief snack lunch in the staff room at the patient reception of the Radiumhemmet, I again meet the man responsible for medical appointments at the clinic, Dr Lars-Gunnar Larsson. "It will be two weeks," says Lars-Gunnar. "Gun has got tonsillitis in her old age and she won't be coming next week, either." He doesn't wait for a reply, taking it for granted I will come — and I do.

The greatest surprise of the day comes when after the patient reception, I go to see Nina at the skin clinic and tell her about the post at the Radiumhemmet. Nina squeezes my left arm hard and starts crying, with relief and delight. I had not realised until then how insecure she had been feeling with her great belly and a husband, indeed recently qualified, but who has no job. Though all the same, to be so happy over a two-week appointment?

It was to turn out that Nina knew better, perhaps even had some idea about the future. For it was not to be two weeks, nor two months, nor two years. March 22nd, 1954, is the first day of almost thirty-eight years working at the Radiumhemmet. Three months later, at the end

The Maple Tree Behind the Barbed Wire

of June, I am rung up by the medical appointments doctor at the surgical clinic at Serafirmer Hospital, who says I can start as assistant doctor in two weeks. He is surprised when I ask for time to think it over. Nina says — "You must decide this yourself". Lars-Gunnar says — "You are to stay here". I don't ask anyone else. I stay at the Radiumhemmet, although at the Serafirmer Hospital I have the head of the department's promise to have my specialist training in surgery at his clinic, and at the Radiumhemmet only a promise of a temporary post over the summer.

It is hard to say why I chose to stay at the Radiumhemmet, a decision which is to govern my whole future and life. Perhaps it is because I want to take care of the seriously ill — it sounds noble, though is perhaps because the Radiumhemmet has a reputation of being one of the leading cancer clinics in the world, and I would be given a good training. Perhaps it is quite simply that I like it there and I have learnt to appreciate Lars-Gunnar Larsson - he is stringent, but as reliable as a rock. Or perhaps I stay because Nina wept when she heard that I had a locum at the Radiumhemmet. Nina said: "You have to decide this yourself" — but I know my Nina nowadays. She has a way of saying more than what her words mean — presumably unconsciously — with the nuances in her voice. Nina can say Yes or No or Perhaps in a great many different ways, and nowadays I know what she means.

We are three young doctors starting at the Radiumhemmet at the same time. When we have been junior registrars for a year, we are all summoned to the head of the department. Professor Hultberg receives us in his big office. He is friendly — but formal and serious. Once we are seated on the visitor's sofa to the left of the door, Sven Hultberg starts by saying that he would very much like us to stay in his department. That sounds good. But then he goes on. At the same time he feels it his duty to point out before we choose which direction we are to take in our training how poor the future outlook is in this specialty. "We have recently had a generation change," Sven Hultberg goes on. He does not reckon on any new appointments in the foreseeable future being made in Sweden. So there will be a long time before any post falls vacant and the competition for it will be great — he names all older colleagues at the Radiumhemmet and other departments of oncology in Sweden. Sven Hultberg ends the conversation by saying: "I am taking this matter up with you only on this occasion. I will not bring it up again." He repeats that we are welcome to stay at the Radiumhemmet, if we want to.

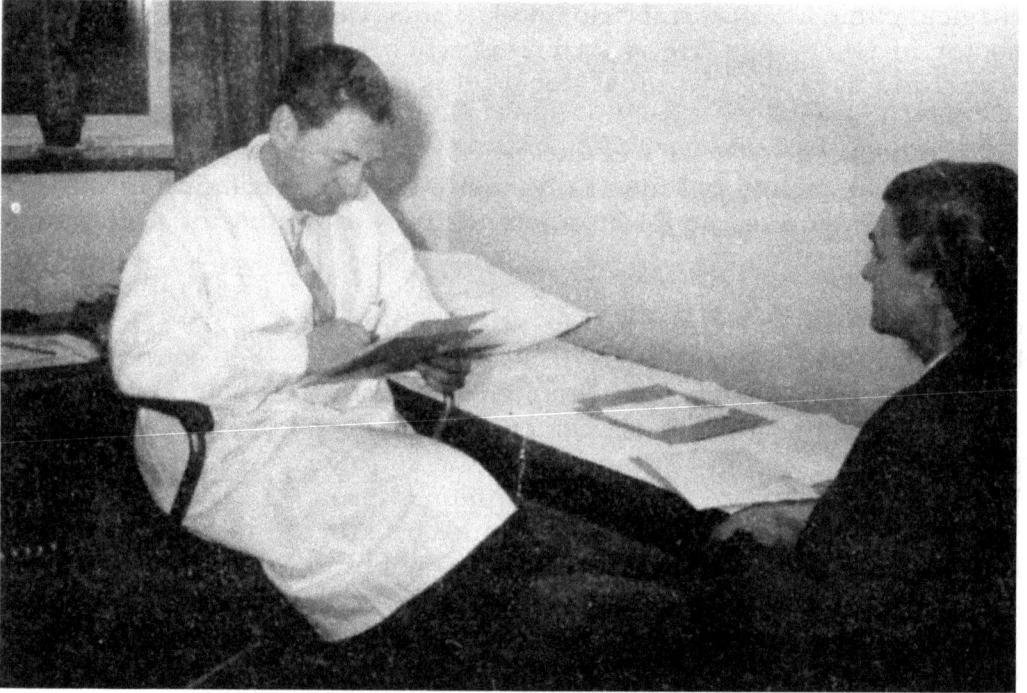

I am an intern at the Radiumhemmet and enjoy working in the big department to which doctors from many parts of the country remit their patients.

Herman Hjort, recently married to a pretty nurse in Ward.5, who is expecting a child, leaves and becomes a diagnostic radiologist. Both Herman and his wife leave the Radiumhemmet. Folke Edsmyr and I stay. I have decided now, and so has Folke. In time, we become close friends and running-mates at the Radiumhemmet, and in a few years, I am to refuse offers from other countries as well, in order to stay at there.

Eight years later, I have been in the United States for four months on a grant from the Medical Association and Nina and our two children are on their way by air to New York. The first night, we all sleep in the same room at Nina's Aunt Mary's in Brooklyn. After the children have fallen asleep. I tell Nina quietly in the dark — so as not to wake the children — about all the unexpected offers I have had — four professorships at various universities in the USA. Two of these are the universities considered leading ones in the country - Harvard in Boston and the University of California in Los Angeles - two are at smaller, newly formed universities — in Minnesota and Florida. After a while, Nina whispers that she will come with me to the USA if I like —

then she falls silent, lying against my left shoulder, and I can feel she is tense. I ask, and Nina replies, reluctantly. She says: "The children are small — so it would be all right to move." Nina understands the possibilities these offers mean to us, and she also has a large family in New York and Philadelphia, but she would prefer not to move - Nina adds even more quietly, then goes on: "We have changed countries once. It was difficult. Are we to move again?" The big family is good, but she does not want to be dependent on them.

Nor do I really want to move, despite the fact that in 1963, there is an acute shortage of specialists within the rapidly expanding field of oncology, so excellent opportunities for a young trained oncologist. At the time I had only two years left of a three-year appointment as junior registrar at the Radiumhemmet, and no one would be more surprised than I if someone had tried to tell me that one day I was to be Sven Hultberg's successor.

But I have not the slightest idea about all that when in March 1954 Nina is squeezing my left arm and crying with relief and delight because I have got a two-week locum at the Radiumhemmet.

Nina almost, but not quite, succeeds in finishing her medical studies before the birth. I have to phone Professor Bosaeus at the Department of Legal and Forensic Medicine to ask him to postpone Nina's exam for a week, her last before her degree. I tell him Nina has been admitted a few days earlier than expected to the maternity department of Karolinska Hospital. Bosaeus answers the phone himself and questions whether a week is long enough, and I say that is what Nina has said. Nina wants to do her last exam before she has to leave the hospital — and she manages just that, too, both the delivery and the exam. Nina receives her degree on May 30th, less than two months after me. She is purposeful and clever without making too much fuss about it, my Nina.

I am there when Lena is born in the evening of May 14th, 1954, and find it difficult to control my explosion of happiness when I see that little red bundle with raven-black hair. This is the first newborn baby I think is quite different from all other children and the prettiest newborn baby I have ever seen.

When Lena Fanny was born, my life was given new content, a new dimension and I have another responsibility and another future. I am so infinitely grateful to little Lena for being born, yelling loudly, as Nina's and my daughter — though she really had no choice in the matter. But Nina can be pleased with our child first when we are alone and I count to five. "Yes, she has five fingers," on her small hands and there are also five toes on each of Lena's fat little feet - Nina breathes out with relief.

The Maple Tree Behind the Barbed Wire

Later that evening, our friends come. It is after visiting hours, but they can look at the little miracle through the window. Sonja and Jacob Igra come, the people we helped at weekends to start up their umbrella factory in a garage — it is to develop into the largest umbrella factory in Sweden - also Hanka and Jakob Ringart, who often invited us back to their home and let us eat our fill during our student days.

Not until that night when I fall asleep alone on our big pillow does the thought strike me. That little child is stateless, for she was born of stateless parents. It is to be hoped that all goes well for little Lena - Nina's and my daughter.

The Maple Tree Behind the Barbed Wire

Swedish Citizen

Apart from Ward 4, Lars-Gunnar Larsson is responsible for the Radiumhemmet's isotope unit, which includes a junior post he now gives to me.

Only recently have we learnt to produce radioactive isotopes from different basic elements, which give off ionizing radiation which we try to use to make diagnoses and treat diseases. A new field has opened for medical research and a new unit at the Radiumhemmet - the isotope unit.

In the second week of May 1954, an elderly man arrives with a tumor on the base of his tongue — an unusual malformation entailing the thyroid gland, normally at the lower part of the throat, having moved up to his tongue. To us, this patient is of interest to see if with the aid of a radioactive isotope, it is possible to diagnose a goiter on the tongue - Lars-Gunnar delegates to task to me.

The laborious examination takes a whole day and turns out that all the radioactive iodine and thus the thyroid gland is on the tongue, and nothing in his throat. Lars-Gunnar is enthusiastic — a case of this kind has never before been diagnosed using radioactive isotopes and we are to be the first.

Lars-Gunnar allows me to write the first draft of the article on the patient with a lingual goiter. When I hand over my effort, he mumbles "it's good", then turns the whole article upside-down, shows me what he has done and sends it in for publication.

It is unremarkable, with the aid of a commercially available radioactive isotope, that it is possible to establish that an elderly man happens to have his entire thyroid gland tissue on his tongue. With the naked eye, it is quite possible to see a purplish swelling in the middle of the patient's tongue, and it is not difficult to guess it is a lingual goiter — there are good pictures of it in every textbook. But Acta Radiologica accepts the article for publication. I am proud to be first in the field when I tell Nina, and she makes an effort to be impressed. Then comes the disaster.

Lars-Gunnar says I am to submit the paper on the lingual goiter diagnosed by a radioactive isotope to the Swedish Radiological Society's spring meeting in the main auditorium of the Karolinska Hospital. I do as he says, our paper is accepted for presentation, allotted ten minutes, with five minutes reserved for questions.

At first I do my three slides. One is a photograph of the large purplish swelling on the base of the tongue. The second shows the result of the survey from the front, and the third the survey in profile. When this is done, I write out the paper — word for word, changing words and the word order, rehearsing my lecture at first silently to myself, then aloud, deleting and adding so that it is exactly nine and half minutes if I speak slowly — the remaining thirty seconds are necessary to get to the platform and back again.

On the day I am to give my first paper, I know every single word by heart, every emphasis, pause and question mark practiced. Despite this, I get up before five o'clock — cannot sleep anyhow — and go to the hospital. In the early spring sunlight, I walk along the out-of-the-way hospital street between the Radiumhemmet and Department of Tumour Pathology, all the time practicing my lecture. In the end, I don't even have to look at the manuscript to check whether in every individual sentence I use the exact correct word order, emphasis and pauses. In good time, I head for the large auditorium of the Karolinska Hospital.

The chairman of the Swedish Radiological Society, Folke Knutsson, Professor of Diagnostic Radiology at Uppsala University, is to chair the spring meeting scientific proceedings. He takes the three steps up to the platform, sits down alone at the long table in front of the white screen, tries out the microphone — it works — and summons the first lecturer.

Everything goes well, questions and answers, everyone keeps to their allotted times and Professor Knutsson keeps everyone in order. When the time for me to give my paper approaches, I calm down — people usually do, but I also become reckless. When my name is called I leave my manuscript on the lowered, light-wood lectern in front of my seat, then with deliberately measured steps I go up to the platform, walk to the lectern, take a firm grasp on it, turn to the chairman and start quietly: Mr. Chairman - he is quite close — then with well-rehearsed calm and in a slightly louder voice as I turn to the great auditorium - Honored colleagues, ladies and gentlemen. That's it — it is deathly quiet. I look down on to all those expectant faces turned towards me — most of them unfamiliar. How did the actual lecture begin?

I sweat, but pull myself together, grasp the lectern even more firmly, almost convulsively, hoping the rest will come if I start from the beginning. In a slightly less sure voice I repeat my Mr. Chairman, Ladies and Gentlemen. But nothing more comes. My poor head whirls and I can feel the sweat running down my spine, although it is not hot. I would like to run away, but may not.

The great hall, almost full, is totally silent as, with my head down and my eyes fixed on the floor, I leave the platform, go back to my place, pick up my manuscript and return again. I am painfully aware that no previous speaker has succeeded so completely in capturing the interest of the audience, and I feel like a little rabbit surrounded by a pack of inquisitive hyenas. Tormented and as rapidly as I possibly can, I reel off the text of almost four typed pages and manage to do so

The Maple Tree Behind the Barbed Wire

without once looking up towards the audience. No commas, no full stops, no pauses for effect, no practiced changes of tone. The showing of my three poor slides is not particularly well integrated with my hyper-swift gabbling, but I don't care as long as the torment and shame is over.

Despite my two failed introductions and two walks between platform and my seat, my lecture takes less time that my allotted ten minutes, and not a single question comes from the auditorium. To fill in the time before the next lecture, Professor Knutsson speaks to the audience. He asks those present for indulgence, explaining that the program committee of the Swedish Radiological Society is not able to question every lecturer in advance before the lecture is accepted for presentation at the Society's scientific proceedings.

I hardly hear what he is saying, but take in the content, and I must be as scarlet as the roses I had given Nina when we married, wishing I could sink through the floor or escape. But I have to stay in my seat and suffer all the way through the remaining lectures. A thought has flashed through my poor head, but has been discarded — for it would be even worse to try to slip out of the hall, bearing my shame — so I stay where I am, as if nailed to my chair, although I don't take in a word of what is being said for the rest of the scientific deliberations of the Swedish Radiological Society in the spring of 1954.

My first publication is something of the most banal an international scientific journal could be thought to publish. My first public lecture is a disaster. But one thing I have learnt — and advice I would give to the reader — never rehearse a lecture to death. In future, I am never to have manuscripts at my lectures.

But Lars-Gunnar Larsson knows how to handle a complete misfit. Three days later, he says to me that I am to give another lecture. I am to do so at the end of year of the Sophiahemmet's college of nursing. This time it goes better, despite its idiotic title - Bloodhounds of Medicine.

Over a year has passed since my application for Swedish citizenship was made to the king and handed in to the Ministry of Justice. We have heard nothing. Our friends the Igras help us acquire a four-roomed apartment nearby, in Duvedsvägen 20 in Vällingby, for a rent, which does not ruin us.

The summer of 1955 is the first I do not have to apply for a locum. I am already junior registrar at the Radiumhemmet. Peter Reizenstein - a young doctor like us — asks us whether we would like to share a villa with them and Jan and Git Pontén they are to rent for the summer in Värmdö. The villa is large and there is plenty of space for us all — we are three young couples with a small child each.

The Maple Tree Behind the Barbed Wire

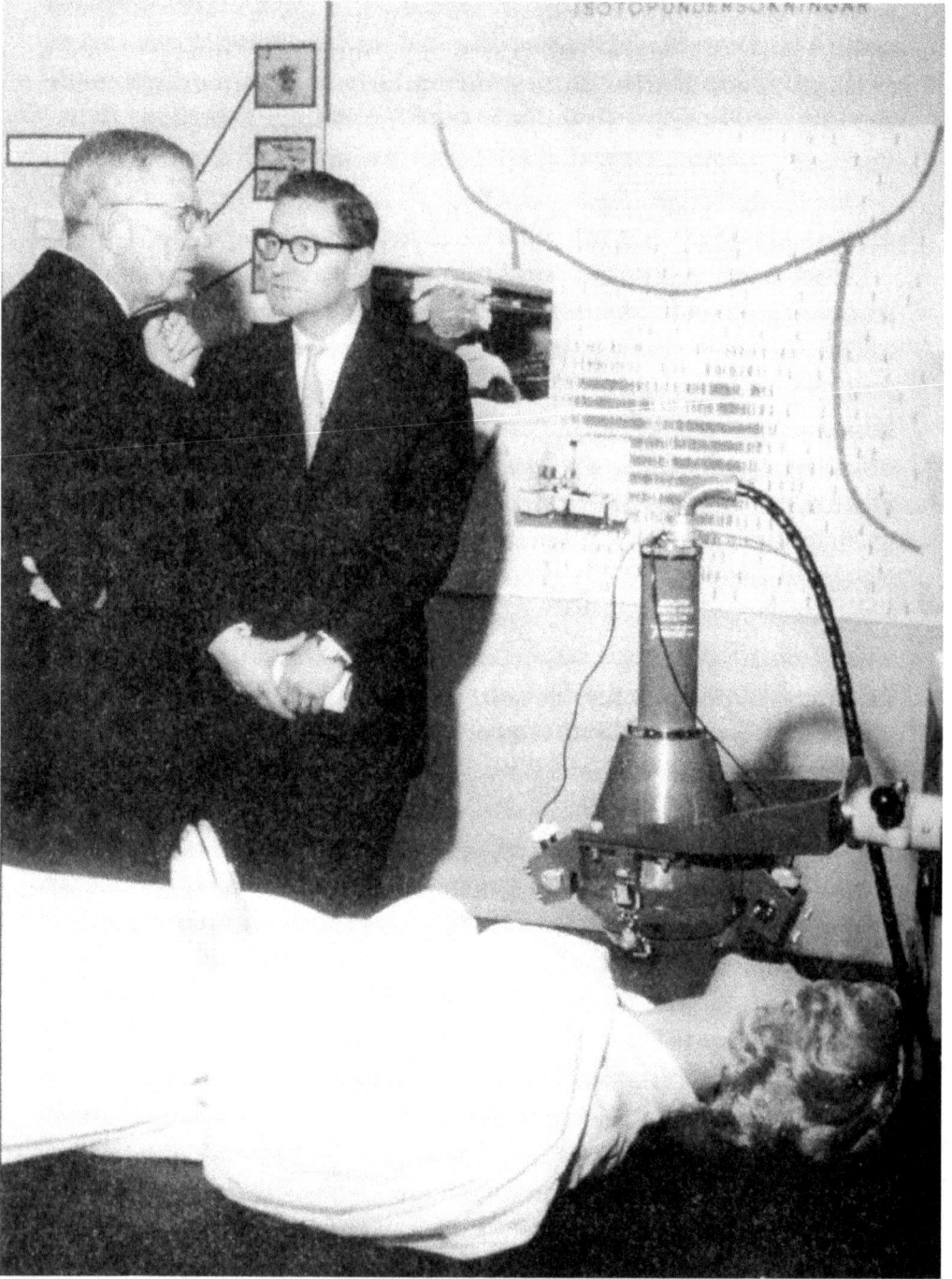

When the atoms of radioactive isotopes fall apart, they give off rays used to make diagnoses and treat diseases. King Gustaf VI Adolf is interested when early in the summer of 1955 he visits the isotope unit of the Radiumhemmet.

The Maple Tree Behind the Barbed Wire

It is a long way from Värmdö to the Karolinska Hospital in Solna. Three young breadwinners have plenty of time to exchange experiences, plans and hopes. Jan Pontén is to be a pathologist and tells us about his already begun research project, Peter talks about his plans and ambitions as a researcher. In this company, I cannot help thinking about the possibility of starting in research myself — if they can, perhaps I can, too. But I realise that to make a meaningful contribution and acquire a decent research training, full-time research is required over a sufficiently long coherent period — and we cannot manage without my salary. I am the breadwinner.

One evening, on our large pillow, I share my thoughts with Nina. Nina listens, understands, but says nothing. What is she to say with a small child to look after and another growing in her rapidly swelling body — we are to have our second child in October - we have no savings, no family, no friends who could help?

At the beginning of August, a letter comes from Sarah - my mother asks whether she might come and stay with us, preferably towards the end of the summer. It is demanding to have a small child, look after it and then have another so soon after - Sarah writes, so Grandmother wants to be here to help.

Sarah comes in mid-August. We move and welcome my mother at our new apartment in Vällingby. She has aged, is more worn, but calmer, having lost some of her previous exuberant joy and the infectious vigor of her comments, and she is more thoughtful, but still holds her head high, her stately posture and proud charm still there. She is a beautiful, attractive elderly lady.

It is over seven years since I have seen my parents and my brother. Once Sarah has settled in, made herself at home and starts talking to us, a picture slowly emerges what it is like them as immigrants in Canada. One evening, when Sarah, Nina and I are alone after dinner, my mother tells us about their difficult early years.

With the help of means they had managed to take with them from Poland, Pinkus has acquired the bare necessities required to open a tailoring business in Toronto. They put up a notice:

P. Einhorn & Son's
Taylor Studio

and began to wait for customers who did not come.

Doctor Zajdman ordered two suits — one for himself and one for his eldest son. When they were finished, Pinkus made suits for himself, for Roman, and a dark-blue suit to send to me at the earliest opportunity — all from cloth he had brought with him from Poland - Sarah brings that suit with her when she comes to Sweden. After that, Pinkus has nothing to do. They put advertisements in the local paper, then tried sending out personal letters to selected groups. But they soon realized that this was using up the little capital they had left and was producing no results. Sarah tells us about another immigrant who cheated Pinkus. He had several suits made for him, borrowed sixty dollars, then disappeared without paying a cent. "But he did not give up" — says Sarah proudly, with some melancholy.

A long time goes by — almost two years — before the first "real" customer appears. Sarah does not know how it happens that this distinguished, well dressed, grey-haired and slightly lame middle-aged gentleman finds Pinkus' workshop. Both Roman and Sarah are out when he arrives, but this customer does not allow himself to be put off by having to wait to be able to talk to the tailor through his wife, a still fairly diffident interpreter. He is pleased with his first discreet dark-grey pin-stripe suit, tells his friends and acquaintances about this new master-tailor from Poland. Then another comes, and another, several "real" customers. The business has taken off and Pinkus employs an assistant — and although he speaks Yiddish and a little Polish, Pinkus gets on well with him. Pinkus is not good at languages and is also too old to learn another language. He doesn't know a word of English and is dependent on Roman or Sarah when he is to receive customers. But they can now live off Pinkus' tailoring workshop, simply, but putting a little aside every month. With the help of these savings and a bank loan, they have bought a small, not particularly well-maintained old house in Avenue Road. In it, Pinkus has his workshop, the fitting room and upstairs the kitchen and two rooms. They take in a lodger to eke out their finances.

Roman has graduated from school in Toronto. As I have not become a tailor, nor does he want to. He follows in his brother's footsteps and like me wants to read medicine. Roman has excellent marks from school and gets into the university in Toronto. They all like it there and are all right, says Sarah, but with no joy in her voice. Pinkus is unhappy because Nina and I are not with them in Toronto. He hopes we will come and that we are planning to do so.

Sarah tells us how Pinkus used to say that when Roman has qualified, Nina, me and our children, his grandchildren, are to come to Canada. He will retire then and close his workshop; Pinkus is already seventy - and the two Einhorn brothers and Nina, three doctors, are to set up a practice in their house at 52 Avenue Road. They are to hand over their house to us and our joint practice as soon as we want it. In the expectation of this, Pinkus has registered his firm in the name of "Einhorn and son's, Taylor Studio", although he now knows neither of us is to be a tailor. Sarah has tears in her big brown eyes when she shows Nina and me the letter-headings and visiting cards they had printed with this nostalgic firm's name, "P. Einhorn and son's".

Sarah and Pinkus make long telephone calls they probably cannot afford. They are a fine old couple, my mother and father, and it is a pity we cannot all be together. For both I, and Sarah, too, know that Pinkus' dreams of Roman's, Nina's and my joint practice in the house in 52 Avenue Road can never be realized — and I suspect that even wise old Pinkus also knows it. But he wants to keep his hopes of reuniting his little family and to keep the dream of his life about the firm "Einhorn and son's". If it cannot be a tailoring business, then at least an Einhorn and son's medical practice — as it says on the heaps of notepaper and visiting cards my mother leaves as a souvenir for Nina and me when she goes back to her Pinkus.

Sarah enjoys being with us very much, though she does weep a little with longing and joy after every telephone call with Pinkus. For the rest of the days, she goes around with Lena in her pram, or Lena in her arms, spoiling our little daughter as grandmothers should, hardly letting anyone else look after her first grandchild, and Lena loves being with her grandmother. Nina relies on Grandmother Sarah and for the first time for a long spell is able to relax a little and truly rest.

Mid-September has gone by and we have still heard nothing from the Ministry of Justice. Nina is getting bigger and bigger — is our second child also to be born stateless?

On October 1st, 1955, when Nina, Lena and I come home, in the post are two brown official envelopes from the Ministry of Justice. In each envelope is a white paper -we can fetch the evidence of our Swedish citizenship. We must take forty kronor with us for stamp duty. The office hours are given at the bottom.

Just like that, a printed standard letter — we can come and fetch it as long as we pay forty kronor each.

It is too late to do it that same day, for the office is already closed and does not open until nine the next morning. But I have time to phone the Radiumhemmet and warn Lars-Gunnar. I am sorry but I shall be late at the clinic in the isotope unit - I don't say why and Lars-Gunnar doesn't ask. He takes the reception of patients after his round of Ward 4 until I come. I promise to hurry.

The next morning I put on my best suit — the dark blue one Sarah had brought with her from Toronto - white shirt and a dark-red, discreetly patterned tie. On October 2nd, 1955, I am the first to arrive at the Ministry of Justice office dealing with these matters, only a minute past nine o'clock. I go into a drab little office. There are two comfortable upholstered chairs by the wall to the left of the door and a small two-seater sofa. But I prefer to stand at the highly polished counter and wait with the paper I had received the day before in my hand, until the young woman has finished her preparations. She moves expertly and quite quickly, unlocks and opens a cupboard, then the cashbox, takes out an inkpad and several rubber stamps, some stamps in various colors and values.

The Maple Tree Behind the Barbed Wire

When everything is ready she stands there behind the counter and looks questioningly at me — she is thin, smiles a brief smile and looks to me sympathetic. She glances with some recognition at the paper I have handed to her and says: Forty kronor. Those are the first words that have been spoken since, still the only visitor, I have come through the door. She seems only moderately interested in what is happening — to her this is routine. I hand over my forty kronor I have had ready in my hand and the woman on the other side of the counter says thank you. Now everything goes quickly. She takes out two twenty kronor stamps, moistens them on the dirty-brown pad, sticks them on to the given places on the white paper, franks the two stamps, then puts everything into the big brown Ministry of Justice envelope and hands it back — here you are — then she loses all interest in me. Forty kronor, thank you, here you are — that's all that has been said.

I stand at the counter, totally at a loss. Is that all? She looks at me — surprised now — then she smiles her quick smile, which for a moment lights up her face. I am troubled. What shall I say? I realise she does not understand, or understands and does not know what to do. I turn round slowly and head for the door, then walk the short stretch to Kungsträdgården, where I stop to think. Why am I disappointed? I have been given my Swedish citizenship and no longer have to wait for answers to my application for a residence visa. I am to be an authorized physician, is that not enough? What had I expected? A long emotional statement from the mayor of the city, warm handshakes, kisses on cheeks and fanfares?

A swiftly approaching airplane making a great deal of noise makes me and the others in the street look up. It is a cool but sunny morning; in the almost crystal clear pale blue sky, four air force planes are flying in perfect formation unusually low over the streets of Stockholm. I watch and think: they are my planes, the pilots up there on a training flight are flying them to protect Nina, little Lena and me. And I can feel my eyes filling with tears, tears of relief and joy from a forgotten but long yearned for feeling of security. I look over at the front façade of the nearby Royal Palace and think: I have a king, and the flag indolently flying above the Palace is my flag. And I look at the pompous Parliament building and think: that is my parliament - I may vote at the next election. I cannot help the tears pouring down my cheeks.

At shortly after nine in the morning, a great many people are walking along Kungsträdgårdsgatan. Many of them pass quite close to me and no one stops, but some stare in surprise. I must look foolish, a mature man in an unbuttoned pale grey trench coat, elegant dark blue suit and dark-red tie standing in the middle of Kungsträdgårdsgatan, weeping without being miserable. I am not ashamed but look gratefully at the passers-by and think — now I am one of you, like everyone else. I am no longer a refugee, no longer stateless. I have a country and a people to whom I belong — the Swedish people.

I cannot resist the impulse. In the middle of the street I open the brown envelope and through a mist of tears, I read:

HIS MAJESTY through the resolution of this day has admitted the licensed physician

Jerzy Einhorn, born July 26th, 1925 in Czestochowa, Poland and resident in Stockholm as Swedish citizen.

Similarly His Majesty has resolved that this naturalization decision shall also include the daughter of the applicant, Lena Fanny, born May 19th, 1954.

Herein and hereafter the above resolution is thus declared confirmed.
Stockholm, September 30th, 1955.

At my desk, in our house in Stockholm, 3.30 p.m., August 26th, 1999, 44 years later.

AFTERWORD

Who Are We Jews?

Persecution influences an individual's view of himself, our identity. It may damage us for life or make us stronger. Persecution on the grounds of race or religion may lead to shame and denial, or to adherence to a group, the identity thus strengthened. In me, my Jewish identity has been reinforced. A natural consequence is that I try to read into what exists in writing an image of what we really are, we Jews, whom Hitler decided to exterminate. The image I try to portray is personal to me. I cannot exclude that it is subjective and it would be surprising if it were not.

There are better and not so well founded explanations for anti-Semitism, as well as attempts to divide it according to original sources. Hitler's anti-Semitism has its origin in the pseudo-scientific anti-Semitism originating in France, and later developed by H. C. Chamberlain in England into a similarly unscientific racial biological science. In Hitler's interpretation, that science was extended to extreme consequences into large-scale systematic extermination by the authorities of Jews, gypsies, Germans handicapped in various ways, and, in the long term, certain non-"Aryan" people.

Who then are we Jews?

In the obscurity of pre-history there is a story about a fairly small tribe — seventy families — which emigrates to Egypt and in slavery reproduces its numbers into a people who return to the country that Abraham's family left owing to famine. The Jewish people have acquired their identity, their God and their religion during this deliberately long forty-year wandering back to what their strong leader, Moses, called the Promised Land. There are not many facts that speak for this country ever being flowing with milk and honey, as the scouts sent out by Moses told the people during their wanderings in the desert. But in the history of our people, in our daily prayers, it was to remain the promised land that we could constantly look forward to.

The Maple Tree Behind the Barbed Wire

During our almost four thousand year-old history, our people have experienced periods of independence and a short period of what some people persist in calling "days of glory", for about seventy years, two kings - David and Solomon - and two generations, and we were allowed — with brief interruptions — to live for two thousand years in an area of land that was ours.

The first to drive the Jews out of their country were the Assyrians. They expelled ten of the twelve tribes and these "the lost tribes" have as far as can be seen never returned. The Babylonians drove the two remaining tribes into exile, but they were not dispersed and were already able to return after a generation or two.

The original Jewish people must have been fairly refractory. The Romans, otherwise tolerant of people they ruled, found it necessary — after the last Jewish rebellions were crushed in 70 AD and again in 135 AD, one thousand eight hundred and sixty years ago — first to kill or sell as slaves, according to several researchers, up to 500,000 Jews and then exile the rest, as well as to change the name of the depopulated country.

The Jewish people were split into small groups which settled in many different places in the vast Roman Empire, from what was to become Cologne in the north to the ancient city of Memphis in the south, from Cordoba in what was to become Spain in the west to Babylon near the Persian Gulf in the east. And this continued, often parallel with the spread of Greco-Roman culture as far as what became Great Britain in the north, and India and China in the east. Many people abandoned their Jewish identity, this occurring en masse in some places. But other groups kept together and retained their Jewish identity. In China in the 1200s, there were twenty-one known Jewish congregations, several of them having been there for over five hundred years, and some had their own synagogues.

Certain periods in the history of our Diaspora are sometimes called Golden Eras. A period of that kind was experienced by the Jews under Moorish rule in Spain. Jews there were able to partake in the development of their own and other cultures, as well as to contribute with renowned philosophers, doctors, cartographers, leading politicians, administrators, diplomats and poets. But every Golden Era was followed by ferocious persecution — in Spain and Portugal by the Inquisition.

The oppression of the Inquisition forced the mass conversion of a great many Jews. Others fled, primarily to the Arab countries in North Africa, and to the Caribbean Islands. This occurred almost immediately after Columbus discovered America. Of the crew on his ship, five were recently converted Jews and their interpreter was also Jewish. But the Inquisition followed, and they were only able to survive in the Dutch possessions in the Caribbean and in South America, then later in the British possessions in North America.

The Maple Tree Behind the Barbed Wire

The mass-immigration of Jews to what became the Polish-Lithuanian Empire began in the 1200s and 1300s. Under the pressure of mock-trials, expulsion, discrimination, economic blackmail, pogroms, forced isolation in ghettos and forced conversions under the threat of death over nearly all western Europe, large groups of Jews fled to the country which offered them protection and freedom to exercise their religion, the country at the end of the 1300s a federated united Poland-Lithuania.

Poland-Lithuania extended from the Baltic Sea to the Black Sea, including the Ukraine and White Russia in the east. Almost all the people, including the nobility and many princes, were illiterate, and on the other hand many Jews could calculate, read and write. The new great power needed its Jewish population to develop the country's trade, later on also its culture, and the nobility began to use Jews as scribes and sometimes as managers of their estates, primarily in the eastern parts of the country.

At the end of the 1800s, over 800,000 Jews were living in Poland, amounting to almost three quarters of all the Jews in the world. That was also where the cultural centre of world Jewry lay. The end of this Jewish sanctuary in Poland-Lithuania began in 1648 with the mass-murder of over 100,000 Jews during the Consul Bohdan Chmielnicki's Cossack uprising. It ended with the division of Poland, which entailed the areas where most Jews lived belonging to the rapidly growing Russian Empire.

The secret police of the Russian Czars fomented and exploited the hatred of Jews as an instrument to divert the large peasant population's discontent with serfdom under the Boyars nobility, the peasants in practice ruthlessly exploited slaves of the landowning noblemen. That was when the secret police produced the myth of the Manifesto of the Wise, the myth of the Jews striving for domination of the world, and revived mediaeval myths that Jews killed Christian children to have blood for the Jewish Passover bread. Restrictions, prohibitions and taxes were imposed on the Jews, which very soon reduced the Jewish population to destitution. One of the Czars, Nicholas I, alone established over six hundred anti-Jewish laws, the Jews were isolated in defenseless ghettos, and twelve year-old Jewish boys were taken for twenty-five years of military service in the Czarist Army. Discriminated against and persecuted also in military service, some of these lonely children did not survive the pressure and converted. Even more astonishing is that many endured the brutal treatment and, as forty year-old men old before their time, returned to continued poverty and persecution, but also to the traditional, warm Jewish fellowship of the ghettos.

The Maple Tree Behind the Barbed Wire

Nearly all Jews in the ghettos of Eastern Europe lived in poverty. Many were craftsmen such as tailors or shoemakers, others supported their families with temporary unskilled work. During this difficult period, a network of aid-activities developed — those who had a little helped those who had nothing. The oppressed, isolated, impoverished and constantly threatened Jewish populations sought hope in their religion. It was under these circumstances that several false Messiah figures appeared and gained adherents.

Respect for learning, however, lived on within the east European Jewry. A scholar was a suitable husband for the daughter of a better-off man, even if the scholar were poor. People kept to the tradition that all boys were to start school at five, in crowded cheder in the teacher's home — often a single room where the teacher both lived and taught his pupils — younger and older children in the same room from eight o'clock in the morning until six in the evening. But the children learnt to read, write and calculate, were taught the history of the Jews, and much time was spent on studying religious scripts. Girls had shorter schooldays, but most could read and write. However great the poverty, education was not to be neglected and was the most important occupation in Jewish life.

The Talmud attitude that "every view must be taken into consideration" contributed to small Jewish communities in closed ghettos being relatively democratic, each Jew considering that his or her ideas were of the same value and had to be heard.

With the period of revolution and enlightenment in the 1800s in Europe, among more forward-looking and progressive people, this oppression began to be questioned. Jewish revolutionaries took part in the hopeless Polish rebellions against Russian predominance, or became involved in the Russian people's revolutionary movements. In other rapidly growing groups arose the dream of a Jewish country of their own in Israel, open to Jews from all over the world, and where no one would be able to persecute us.

After the First World War, the collapse of the Russian Empire and the division of Germany and Austria, many Jews again ended up in Poland, which in 1918 acquired her independence.

In 1800, we were a nomadic defenseless people dependent on the goodwill of others. Our tradition says that we are Jews if our mother is a Jewess, but we have not always desired and periodically not always been able to adhere to that. Also, a hundred paternal generations separate us from the original Jewish people. Although our religion is not evangelical, over the years many people, on several occasions an entire people, have gone over to Judaism and been accepted as Jews, an example of which is the Khazars living in a large area north of the Black Sea and the Caspian Sea.

The Maple Tree Behind the Barbed Wire

Today there are white Jews in Europe, black Jews in Africa and oriental Jews in East Asia. Many of the young people who go to Israel today from Russia, White Russia and the Ukraine are fair-haired, blue-eyed and have Slavic features. The small boys who during the war in Poland reported us to the Germans would never recognize them as Jews, but they are Jews in that Judaism is their religion and culture.

It is unreasonable to maintain that we belong to a race, should anyone persist in maintaining that in today's world there are people belonging to limited races. We have deserved to be called a people — the Jewish people.

For long periods of our dispersal, it was easy to change religion and escape persecution, to be allowed to own land, exercise our professions, go to school or hold office. And yet sufficiently many succeeded in holding on to their Jewish traditions and their Jewish identity — to survive as Jews for a hundred generations — until the phenomenon of Hitler decided to deal with us.

Who was he, this Adolf Hitler, and what circumstances contributed to him acquiring the confidence of the German people?

We were over three million, a third of all the Jews in the world, living in Poland on September 1st, 1939, when the Second World War began with Germany's invasion of our country.

The Maple Tree Behind the Barbed Wire

Germany's Elected Chancellor Adolf Hitler

Forty years after the end of the war, now that the anguish that keeps emerging with memories has become more manageable, I begin to take an interest in the explanation for the German people's actions, as I had been able to observe it in the micro-world of Czechoslovakia. I try to understand how this could happen to the leading cultured people of Europe. Who and what could bring this educated people in the mid-1900s to plan and then systematically carry out genocide of Jews and gypsies and, with fundamentally the same motivation, murder its own handicapped people? This is my picture of the historical background and my attempt at an explanation. Others may choose other facts from the same sources and draw different conclusions.

The formation in 962 AD of the Germanic-Roman Empire with King Otto the Great of Germany, crowned by the Pope as a Roman emperor, confirmed the position of the German people as the major power in Central Europe. In the 1600s, the Thirty Years War led to the fall of this powerful nation. Large areas of land populated by Germans had to be surrendered to neighboring countries and what was left was periodically divided up into four hundred minor states. For two hundred years, constant fighting tore apart this already divided and weakened country. The collapse was formalized when the powerless emperor was force to relinquish his imperial crown in 1806.

By creating the Federal Republic of North Germany in 1867, Bismarck succeeded in laying the foundations of German reunification. France, who had annexed large areas of land with German-speaking populations, felt threatened, tried to stop the current reunification, and the result was war. For the first time for several hundred years, what was to become Germany appeared to be more or less united — and was victorious. The Franco-German war of 1870-71 restored the slumbering German sense of nationality, but many years were to go by before the loosely joined federation of twenty-five German states could be welded together into one single nation, with its own colonies — all in a peaceful way.

Reunited Germany was striving for acknowledgement as one of the world powers and for a fair share of the international market. Wilhelm II, Emperor of Germany and King of Prussia, was moderately talented but, at least in his statements, a belligerent person and the German military were arrogant. But the new German military men were not alone in being arrogant, and many other factors in conflict-filled Europe contributed to humanity being afflicted with the First World War in 1914. The factor that directly gave rise to it was not Germany, but the desperate Austrian Emperor Franz Josef's ultimatum to Serbia caused by the insane assassination of the heir to the throne, Arch-

The Maple Tree Behind the Barbed Wire

Duke Franz Ferdinand. Together with the Austro-Hungarian Empire, Germany lost the war.

The Treaty of Versailles was an astonishingly naive product of the victorious allied powers. The peace treaty was a profoundly unjust result of negotiations behind closed doors with all the participating gentlemen — for there were only gentlemen partaking — making their own claims, all of which were approved without consideration that the whole might bring with it tremendous consequences.

The German naval fleet was handed over to the victorious powers, the army was limited to 100,000 men and the German defenses of the Rhine were removed. Germany had to hand over all her colonies. But on top of that, the victorious powers chose to humiliate the German people by forcing their leaders to sign an agreement stating that Germany was entirely to blame for the war — which was not true — and so was condemned to reparations, not just for damage caused by Germany, but also those her allies and the Allied powers had caused in their own and other countries. More than anything else, reparations were to contribute to what became the inescapable development. Germany was quite incapable of paying for them.

The German people were humiliated and burdened with debt, their national self-respect crumbled to dust, and the country sentenced to economic misery. This unjust peace created a store of gunpowder, which sooner or later was bound to explode.

The Treaty of Versailles was based on a series of principles, but Germany was also discriminated against in the application of them. The most important was the principle of nationality. According to that, language was to be the leading national bond and decide the boundaries between the different countries, with one exception - Germany. Large German minorities were cut off from their mother country. This happened to the German minorities in Czechoslovakia, Poland, Romania, France and some other countries. The Emperor went into exile, the remaining princes abdicated, the republic was brought in and an attempt was made to set up a democratic form of government on command.

With the lack of traditions anchored in parliamentary democracy, the German people were torn apart, now by rivalry between the ten "major" an—d innumerable smaller political parties, all with a seat in parliament. Governments were formed in constantly changing coalitions and resigned.

When payment of the impossible reparations was not forthcoming, the German people were again humiliated by French troops marching into and occupying Germany's leading industrial area — the Ruhr. France confiscated everything of any value, this ruthless exploitation in practice making it impossible for Germany to go on paying reparations. The German people produced the only defense they had left, passive resistance. The Ruhr was paralyzed.

The Maple Tree Behind the Barbed Wire

Germany's main remaining source of income became the mint presses, which printed banknotes of increasingly higher values. People had to pay 1,247 thousand million marks for what three years earlier had cost ten marks, a postage stamp was twenty billion. Savings became worthless and many pensioners became destitute, the middle classes — which after the abolition of the nobility had stood for stability in German society — were impoverished. Inflation brought with it rapidly rising unemployment, the wages of those still in work often at a corresponding existence level — the economy collapsed.

When the victorious powers came to realize the effects of their actions, they brought in reliefs to their demands for reparations and the French troops left the Ruhr in 1929. Then the beginning of stabilization of the German currency and the financial infrastructure was wrecked by the world economic crisis.

The severe social distress afflicting the already previously impoverished country became a natural seedbed for extremist parties and motivation for political coups. The state of emergency was not able to alleviate unrest in the population. Governments appointed by President Hindenburg could not acquire a majority in parliament, the country had to be governed by emergency decrees against which parliaments protested, and had to be dissolved.

The Germans were rightly disappointed with all the alternatives offered hitherto. Democracy did not work. It was quite natural in this situation that a longing for uniform strong leadership arose in the population. Unfortunately, that strong leader was to be Adolf Hitler.

Adolf Hitler was born and brought up in Austria. He was Austrian until the age of thirty when he was given German citizenship.

The young Hitler's relations to his father, a customs official, were poor, his relations with his mother good. He had several brothers and sisters, of whom only he and a sister survived. He failed at school, according to his teachers owing to a lack of self-discipline, and he changed schools. But in his new school he passed only a few subjects and had to leave without any leaving certificate.

Hitler dreamt of becoming an artist. In 1907 he applied to the Academy of Art in Vienna, but was not accepted. After a while, he applied to the School of Architecture in Vienna and was again turned down. He was profoundly disappointed and considered he had been unjustly treated, but he did not abandon his dreams of being an artist - painter, architect or composer. He made great plans for his future studies that never materialized. He did comprehensive and detailed drawings for the rebuilding of the whole of the nearest town - Linz. He went on painting although no one wanted to buy his paintings. Among other things, he composed a pompous musical drama, but no one wanted to publish or play his compositions. He never acquired any proper employment. Apart from contributions from his mother, he earned a living from temporary work - painting postcards and leaving his paintings in second-hand shops.

After the death of his mother, Adolf Hitler lost his foothold in life as well as his financial support from home. He lost his home, slept on park benches, and was finally taken into an institution for the homeless in Vienna, where his clothing had to be fumigated. On several occasions he was to be found in the records of the Vienna police, and an Austrian enlistment commission declared him unsuitable for military service. Together with a friend from home, he moved to Munich in 1913, where he lived a somewhat more orderly life, but still maintained his unrealistic dreams of becoming an artist.

The fate of the world would have been different and many more people would have lived if the young Adolf had succeeded in something of all that he so ardently desired. That would probably not have helped him himself - owing to his personality, he was condemned always to have greater ambitions that his abilities allowed - but he might nevertheless have been a happier person if he had had his first successes earlier than at the age of forty; but that we shall never know.

Hitler himself wrote that he fell to his knees and prayed to God when the war broke out in 1914. He volunteered for the German army and was overwhelmed by happiness when he was accepted. He served as a courier, was wounded, received two honors, one of them the Iron Cross, and was promoted to corporal. Although judging by these honors he was a brave soldier, he was not particularly liked by his comrades. As a result of being gassed at Ypres, he was in hospital when the war ended, and he afterwards wrote that it had been the happiest time of his life. As was his habit, Hitler maintained that the war was lost owing to the treachery of socialists, Jews, politicians, and the cowardice of the leaders back at home. He wholeheartedly adopted the stab-in-the-back theory — again it was other people's fault.

Hitler delayed his demobilization as long as possible, and finally became one of the badly paid informers of the National Defense, his task was to attend political meetings and report back to their intelligence service.

The event that was to change his life and shape the destiny of the world occurred on September 12th, 1919. Adolf Hitler had been assigned to attend a meeting arranged by the German Party. The meeting was taking place in a smoky beer cellar. Although he was supposed to be there as an observer, he was provoked by a speaker agitating for the independence of Bavaria. He stood up and made his first political speech, a passionate appeal for German unity. Among the twenty guests in the beer cellar happened to be Anton Drexter, the first person to notice Hitler's talent as an agitator. Drexter invited him to an internal meeting of the party. Hitler became member number seven, was put in charge of the party's propaganda, transforming the hundred or so registered small parties in Bavaria at the time into a mass movement. He changed the party's name to the National Socialist Workers Party, was elected chairman in 1921, demanded unlimited powers as the party Fuehrer and within the course of two years turned it into a factor of political power in Bavaria. Then, in 1923, he made his first major mistake as a politician.

As usual with Hitler, the mistake was due to an over-estimation of both his own and his party's abilities. The attempt with the aid of a party with 15,000 members to take over power via a coup was doomed to failure, despite the fact that he had succeeded in persuading the hero of the nation, General Ludendorff, to head the march. Hitler was profoundly shaken when the police let through a small group round Ludendorff, but barred the way to the rest of the instigators of the coup, and when they refused to stop, shot down several. That was when he decided to change, not the aim, but the tactics for achieving power in Germany.

He was brought to trial and skillfully exploited a courtroom with the free press as a forum for his political statement — he became a known personality all over the country. Hitler was given a five-year sentence, but spent only a year in prison. As a well-known person, he was given good conditions by the prison authorities and also received the help of a secretary and the faithful Rudolf Hess towards writing his book, Mein Kampf. My copy of the book is 637 printed pages full of his ideas — with several real but not particularly profound observations, a great many subjective interpretations, half-truths, pure nonsense and simple clever nationalistic propaganda. In it Hitler describes quite openly, as he does in his public statements, what he is striving for, which means he will use and what he will achieve. He is to come into power the democratic way in order to abolish democracy, he is to establish a "thousand year reign of terror" and right all the wrongs that have afflicted Germany.

Hitler was a clever demagogue. Many politicians are, but he was cleverer than most. He had a gifted fanatic's ability to capture the masses, and he possessed an unerring sense of what they wanted to hear and how he ought to say it. And the masses were jubilant, my goodness how jubilant they were. But he also possessed the ability to attract and convince individuals, perhaps not intellectuals, but several leaders in society of the worlds of banking, business and industry. Alfred Hugenberg was not the only one of a whole series of bankers and industrialists who with their financial support made possible the financing of expensive mass meetings with bands, innumerable flags on tall flagstaffs, and the most modern and most expensive loudspeakers available.

The Maple Tree Behind the Barbed Wire

When necessary, Hitler was a skillful, calculating bluffer and a grandiose actor, who on critical occasions exploited these talents in order to frighten or convince, and he could also be astoundingly honest.

His actions were marked by preconceived opinions. He read a great deal, but interpreted fairly freely what he read in order to adapt it to what he himself thought and wished for. He liked to build his views on pseudo-scientific publications, which he took very seriously when the conclusions suited his way of thinking.

Before he had taken power, many people were to regard him as a ridiculous figure in boots and leather breeches, a phenomenon soon to disappear into the margins of the confused history of the interwar period. But that was a gross underestimation. Once he learnt to use his abilities, he was never again a ridiculous person. He was masterly at exploiting his limited talents and predicting the reactions of individuals and of the masses. From the day Adolf Hitler took his place in the arena of Germany's politics, both he and his ideas should have been seen as profoundly frightening as he purposefully — in his hoarse guttural voice and well-rehearsed gestures — seduced and carried with him the irresolute masses.

He said to the German people what they wanted, and in their degradation what they needed to hear:

You are not worse — you are better than all others. You have an historical task, to lead the world to new times and I, Adolf Hitler, shall lead you.

Poor German people. Under the prevailing circumstances, to many he must have appeared as a saviour in their need.

Adolf Hitler came into power via democratic election. When at two consecutive elections his party had become the largest in parliament, he was appointed as Chancellor by the president of Germany. The rest was easy to foresee. He had simply done what he had promised, abolished democracy and brought in "the Third Reich of Terror". The free press was silenced, concentration camps set up for opponents who were not murdered. And also, unemployment was abolished. Germany was covered with a network of autobahns and heavy industry was inundated with orders. He gave the unemployed occupation that seemed meaningful, wages which were not high, but nor were they at existence level. He turned recession into a forced boom. He offered the German people a grandiose spectacle, giving them back their self-respect and providing scapegoats for them to hate. And he was lucky. Economies were beginning to turn all over the world, the surrounding countries had incompetent, almost foolish leaders, and he himself was clever at exploiting that.

The Maple Tree Behind the Barbed Wire

But he adhered to a characteristic, which was forever to dominate his personality and guide his actions. His unlimited ambitions were constantly greater than his abilities. That, together with a lack of objectivity and an inability to listen to other people, meant that Adolf Hitler was fundamentally destructive. That was why he failed in everything he had previously undertaken in life, and that was also why he was to fail to manage the great confidence the German people had placed in him.

For undeniably, the people had supported him, in great numbers and in important circles in the commercial world. The rest were swept along with his spectacular initial successes and gave him their perhaps not entirely unreserved, but nevertheless wholehearted and periodically enthusiastic support.

When he came into power, great singing crowds poured out on to the streets in a spontaneous triumphant procession. In this victorious procession were many intellectuals, many military men, among them the young officer von Stauffenberg, who today symbolizes that there was nevertheless some opposition. For when eleven years later, the same von Staffenberg and his co-conspirators were to attempt to organise an assassination of Hitler, the war was already lost, and they knew it.

When times were relatively good - in 1929 - only about 800,000, scarcely 3% of the electors voted for him. But as times grew worse, the number was nearer fourteen million, 37%, giving him a 210 mandate in a democratically elected parliament. A few months later, in November 1932, some pulled themselves together, but almost twelve million gave him a mandate of 196 and that was enough for the president of the country to appoint him Chancellor. Then there was no return. Once he had power, he would never hand it over voluntarily - only over millions of dead German soldiers and their newly acquired wives. He did not relinquish power until the whole of Germany lay in ruins and foreign troops were at the entrance of his own bunker.

He was like a gambler at a casino who however much he wins goes on playing until he has lost his last cent — then commits suicide. This restless, lonely man was also doomed to fail in this the greatest task of his life by taking this incomprehensible chance the great German people had given him.

Did they not realize this on one single day - July 27th, 1932 - 60,000 people listening to him in Brandenburg, 60,000 in Potsdam and 220,000 in Berlin, as they raised their arms and screamed Sieg Heil, Heil Hitler? Did they not realize how humiliating the situation was, or his megalomania when they were to greet one another by raising their right arms and saying Heil Hitler?

The Maple Tree Behind the Barbed Wire

The proud, great well-educated German people were treated badly by the outside world for several hundred years, primarily by the neighboring western countries ruthlessly exploiting their weakness after the Thirty Years War. When they managed to restore their national unity and lost a war, Germany was hugely humiliated and exploited economically. The country had an unworkable constitution forced on to it. Naturally, the German people desired an effective government, but it is impossible to ignore that the alternative they chose in free elections was Nazi storm troopers ravaging the streets all over the country. They chose a party which in the three weeks before the last election fought 461 street battles registered by the police, leaving about a hundred dead and thousands injured, and that because of the progress of the Nazis, leaders of other parties had to request police protection. Was this a better alternative?

Hitler was a captivating speaker, a gifted propagandist who surrounded himself with other clever propagandists and administrators, skillfully exploiting people's preference for flags, uniforms, marching and glossy jackboots. He was the first in the world to use film for political purposes, and one of the first to use recordings bellowing out his message from vehicles through mobile loudspeakers.

But did the German people listen to what he was saying? Did they think it was their task to be the world's Herrenvolk that their vocation was to rule the world? Did they really want to have their people, "their race", freed from weak elements, from the less gifted and the handicapped? Did they want to take on the responsibility under Hitler's leadership of bringing in a thousand year reign of terror? Did they not realize that what he was yelling in his provocative voice from hundreds of loudspeakers was a hotchpotch of truths, half-truths and propaganda — essentially astonishingly naive propaganda? Did they not realize that they were gross simplifications when he screamed that the will is more important than wisdom, and action better than thought, and that these messages were bound to lead to spontaneous violence? And if they believed in all that ingratiating stuff about himself, which he so cleverly marketed, did they also believe that the world would be a better place if we — the Jews - were exterminated? Did they believe that a whole people can consist of evil parasites?

Why did not more statesmen read his declaration of intent — the book he published — why did they not listen to his speeches? Why did those who did listen not believe what he was saying? After all, the man was a fanatic and fanatics usually ruthlessly realize what they are promising.

The Maple Tree Behind the Barbed Wire

Whenever has it happened before that a democratically elected head of state has killed his recently acquired wife, he himself committed suicide at the age of fifty-six, several of his closest men have taken their own lives, and one of them killed all nine of his own beloved children? Those who ruled the German people over this period must have been aware that what they were doing were serious crimes.

Adolf Hitler was a lonely, often discontented man, who constantly had grandiose but unrealistic plans and finally failed in everything he undertook. He was a man who needed war to still his restlessness. If it is possible for one single moment to ignore his deeds, he appears to have been a pitiful person.

INDEX

The Maple Tree Behind the Barbed Wire

www.ingramcontent.com/pod-product-compliance
Lightning Source LLC
Chambersburg PA
CBHW050400110426
42812CB00006BA/1751